Immune Infertility

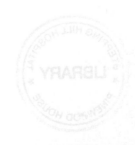

Walter K. H. Krause • Rajesh K. Naz

Immune Infertility

The Impact of Immune Reactions on Human Infertility

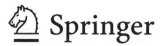 Springer

Prof. Dr. Walter K. H. Krause
Universitätsklinikum Marburg
Klinik für Andrologie und
Venerologie
Zentrum für Hautkrankheiten
Deutschhausstr. 9
35033 Marburg
Germany
krause@med.uni-marburg.de

Prof. Rajesh K. Naz
West Virginia University
School of Medicine
Reproductive Biology
Morgantown WV 26506
USA
Rnaz@hsc.wvu.edu

ISBN: 978-3-642-01378-2   e-ISBN: 978-3-642-01379-9

DOI: 10.1007/978-3-642-01379-9

Springer Dordrecht Heidelberg London New York

Library of Congress Control Number: 2009934299

Cover design: eStudioCalamar, Figueres/Berlin

Printed on acid-free paper

Springer is part of Springer Science+Business Media (www.springer.com)

Preface

Infertility is defined as the inability to conceive after having unprotected intercourse for a year. Infertility is increasing worldwide and has various causes both in the male and the female partner. Immune reactions to sperm can contribute up to 2–30% of infertility. The sperm has both autoantigenic as well as isoantigenic potential, and is thus capable of producing antisperm antibodies (ASAs) and sperm-reactive T cells in both infertile men and women. Also, over 75% vasectomized men produce autoantibodies to sperm that can cause a problem in regaining fertility even after successful re-anastomosis in vasovasostomy. Early claims regarding the incidence and involvement of ASAs in involuntary human infertility were probably overemphasized because of unreliable techniques and naivety concerning the complexity of the immune response and antigenic nature of the sperm cell. These factors, the lack of well-designed and controlled experimental studies, and the dearth of effective therapeutic modalities resulted in the confusion of the occurrence and importance of ASAs in human infertility. Consequently, evaluation of infertile couples for ASAs and their possible role in infertility was not considered a significant proposition. The development of more accurate assays and the discovery of mucosal immunity capable of responses independent of systemic immunity have caused inclusion of sperm cells and genital tract secretions in the analysis of ASAs. Furthermore, with progress in assisted reproductive and hybridoma technologies, recent developments in proteomics and genomics have tremendously increased our understanding regarding the induction and role of ASAs in infertility. It is becoming clearer now that any immunoglobulin that binds to sperm cannot be called an "antisperm antibody" unless it is directed against an antigen that is relevant to fertilization and fertility.

Although there are numerous reports on ASAs and their role in immunoinfertility, there is no book comprising various aspects of immunoinfertility under a single comprehensive treatise. This book is unique and the first of its kind in bringing together our current knowledge on immune mechanisms, proteomics, and genomics of sperm structure and function, and diagnosis and treatment of ASA-mediated infertility. Also included are chapters on the application of these immune reactions in the development of novel nonsteroidal immunocontraceptives.

This book has 18 chapters, arranged into four sections, written by well-renowned experts in the field of immune infertility from all over the world. In Part I, various sperm antigens involved in immunoinfertility are enumerated. Chapter 1 describes the protein structure of spermatozoa, the proteome, followed by a chapter dealing with the methods of analysis. In Chap. 2, the proteins inducing immune reactions that cause an impairment of sperm function are summarized. Section II is dedicated to the different aspects of the nature of ASAs. First, the status of immune privilege of the testis is discussed. The following chapters describe the immune chemistry of ASAs, involvement of sperm-specific T cells, the site and risk factors of ASA production, and the prevalence of ASAs in the different compartments of the body. Two other chapters on the occurrence of ASAs in women and the significance of sperm immobilizing ASAs are included. Section III addresses the clinical impact of ASAs. The chapters in this section discuss autoimmune infertility, tests for detection of sperm antibodies, impact of ASAs on male fertility and the role of assisted reproductive technologies and other methodologies to treat immunoinfertility. Section IV includes three chapters discussing the application of immune reactions to gametes and hormones in the development of novel immunocontraceptives for wildlife and humans.

In conclusion, this book is a unique and novel treatise in offering up-to-date information on ASA-mediated infertility. The authors of this book are expert investigators who are pioneers in their fields. This book will provide a model source of authentic, vital, and viable information on the latest scientific developments in the field of immunoinfertility and immunocontraception to clinicians, scientists, students, residents, and fellows working in the field of reproductive biology, obstetrics and gynecology, and urology.

Marburg, Germany   Walter K.H. Krause
Morgantown, WV, USA   Rajesh K. Naz

Contents

Contributors

A. Agarwal
Cleveland Clinic Lerner College of
Medicine and Case Western Reserve
University, 9500 Euclid Avenue,
Cleveland, OH 44195, USA
agarwaa@ccf.org

John R. Aitken
ARC Centre of Excellence in Biotechnology
and Development, School of Environmental
and Life Sciences, University of Newcastle
Callaghan, NSW 2308, Australia
john.aitken@newcastle.edu.au

Arcangelo Barbonetti
Department of Internal Medicine,
Andrologic Unit, University of L'Aquila,
Coppito, 67100 L'Aquila, Italy
arcangelobarbonetti@virgilio.it

Sudhanshu Bhushan
Department of Anatomy and Cell Biology,
Justus-Liebig-University of Giessen,
35385 Giessen, Germany;
sudhanshu.bhushan@anatomie.med.
uni-giessen.de

Jerome H. Check
Department of Obstetrics and Gynecology,
Division of Reproductive Endocrinology
& Infertility, The University of Medicine
and Dentistry of New Jersey,
Robert Wood Johnson Medical
School at Camden,
Cooper Hospital/University Medical Center,
Camden, NJ, USA
laurie@ccivf.com

Gary N. Clarke
Department of Obstetrics and Gynecology,
University of Melbourne
Andrology Unit, Royal Women's Hospital,
Melbourne, Australia
gary.clarke@thewomens.org.au

Monika Fijak
Department of Anatomy and
Cell Biology, Justus-Liebig-University
of Giessen,
35385 Giessen, Germany
monika.fijak@anatomie.med.uni-giessen.de

Felice Francavilla
Department of Internal Medicine,
Andrologic Unit, University of L'Aquila,
Coppito, 67100 L'Aquila, Italy
francavi@cc.univaq.it

B.M. Gadella
Departments of Biochemistry and Cell
Biology and of Farm Animal Health,
Utrecht University,
3584 CM Utrecht,
The Netherlands
B.M.Gadella@uu.nl

Jagdish Chandra Gupta
Talwar Research Foundation, E-8 Neb
Valley, Neb Sarai,
New Delhi-110068, India
jagdishgupta2@gmail.com

Akiko Hasegawa
Laboratory of Developmental Biology
and Reproduction, Advanced Medical
Sciences, Hyogo College of Medicine,
Japan
zonapel@hyo-med.ac.jp

John C. Herr
Health Science Center,
University of Virginia,
Charlottesville, VA 22908, USA
jch7k@virginia.edu

Michael Hertl
Department of Dermatology and
Allergology, Philipp University,
35033 Marburg, Germany
hertl@med.uni-marburg.de

Katarina Jewgenow
Leibniz Institute for Zoo and Wildlife
Research, PF 601103,
10252 Berlin, Germany
jewgenow@izw-berlin.de

Marzena Kamieniczna
Department of Reproductive Biology
and Stem Cells, Institute of Human
Genetics, Polish Academy of Sciences,
Strzeszynska 32, 60-479 Poznan, Poland
kaspmarz@man.poznan.pl

Koji Koyama
Department of Obstetrics and
Gynecology, Institute for Advanced
Medical Sciences, Hyogo College
of Medicine, 1-1 Mukogawa-cho,
Nishinomiya, Hyogo 6638501, Japan
kkoyama@hyo-med.ac.jp

Walter K. H. Krause
Klinik für Dermatologie und Allergologie,
Philipps-Universität,
35033 Marburg, Germany
krause@med.uni-marburg.de

Maciej Kurpisz
Department of Reproductive Biology and
Stem Cells, Institute of Human Genetics,
Polish Academy of Sciences,
Strzeszyńska 32, 60-479 Poznan, Poland
kurpimac@man.poznan.pl

M. Marconi
Department of Urology,
University of Chile,
Santos Dumont 999, Santiago, Chile
marcelomarconi@yahoo.es

Andrea Meinhardt
Department of Anatomy and Cell Biolog,
Justus-Liebig-University of Giessen,
35385 Giessen, Germany
andreas.meinhardt@anatomie.med.
uni-giessen.de

Rajesh K. Naz
Center for Research in Reproductive
Sciences (CRRS), West Virginia University,
School of Medicine, 2085 Robert C. Byrd
Health Sciences Center North,
Morgantown, WV 26506, USA
Rnaz@hsc.wvu.edu

Brett Nixon
School of Environmental and Life Sciences,
University of Newcastle, University Drive,
Callaghan, NSW 2308, Australia
brett.nixon@newcastle.edu.au

Shilpi Purswani
Talwar Research Foundation, E-8 Neb
Valley, Neb Sarai,
New Delhi-110068, India
dushtkt@gmail.com

T.M. Said
Andrology Laboratory and Reproductive
Tissue Bank, The Toronto Institute for
Reproductive Medicine, ReproMed
56 Aberfoyle Crescent, Toronto,
ON M8X2W4, Canada
tsaid@repromed.ca

Jagathpala Shetty
Center for Research in Contraceptive and
Reproductive Health, University of
Virginia Health Science Center,
Charlottesville, VA 22908, USA
Js4ed@virginia.edu

G.P. Talwar
Talwar Research Foundation, E-8 Neb
Valley, Neb Sarai,
New Delhi-110068, India
gptalwar@gmail.com

Z. Ulcová-Gallová
Department of Obstetrics and Gynecology,
Charles University, Alej Svobody 80,
Plzen-Lochotin, 326 00, Czech Republic
ulcova@fnplzen.cz

Hemant Kumar Vyas
Talwar Research Foundation, E-8 Neb
Valley, Neb Sarai,
New Delhi-110068, India
hemantkvyas@gmail.com

Wolfgang Weidner
Department of Urology and Pediatric
Urology, University Hospital Giessen
and Marburg GmbH,
Justus-Liebig-Universität,
Rudolf- Buchheim-Street 7,
35385 Gießen, Germany
W.weidner@chiru.med.uni-giessen.de

Section I

Sperm Antigens

Proteomics of Human Spermatozoa

1.1

Brett Nixon and R. John Aitken

1.1.1
Introduction

Interest in sperm function has greatly intensified for two reasons: first, it is becoming increasingly apparent that human infertility can be traced to male factors, including alterations in sperm proteins, and second, there is increasing empirical evidence that sperm provide essential elements, both nucleic acid- and protein-based, to early zygote development possibly beyond their role in fertilization. Nevertheless, despite their pivotal role in reproduction, we know surprisingly little about the overall molecular composition of this unique and highly specialized cell.

The production of spermatozoa represents the culmination of an extraordinary process of cytodifferentiation known as spermatogenesis that occurs within testes and involves dramatic cellular and functional changes. The process of spermatogenesis produces a highly compartmentalized spermatozoon with a number of defined intracellular domains and a mosaic surface architecture [1, 2]. Interestingly, spermatogenesis also results in the silencing of the male genome such that on leaving the testis, the spermatozoa are both transcriptionally and translationally inactive. In the absence of de novo protein synthesis, the functionality of these cells is largely, if not solely, dependent on posttranslational modifications to their protein complement. This applies equally to the maturation of these cells in the epididymis, and to their postejaculatory capacitation in the female reproductive tract. These features, combined with the relative ease of obtaining large numbers of purified spermatozoa that can be driven into different functional states, make the cell particularly amenable to proteomic analyses. Indeed, while modern genetic profiling methods including differential display [3, 4], SAGE [5] and microarray [6–9] technologies might be suitable for analyzing differentiating germ cells in the testes, they are of no value in characterizing the changes that confer functionality on the male gamete.

R. J. Aitken (✉)
ARC Centre of Excellence in Biotechnology and Development, School of Environmental and Life Sciences, University of Newcastle, Callaghan, NSW 2308, Australia
e-mail: john.aitken@newcastle.edu.au

W. K. H. Krause and R. K. Naz (eds.), *Immune Infertility*,
DOI: 10.1007/978-3-642-01379-9_1.1, © Springer Verlag Berlin Heidelberg 2009

Resolving the proteomic composition of various mammalian spermatozoa is being undertaken at a rapid pace as advances are made in protein and peptide separation, detection, and identification [10–13]. This resource will ultimately provide valuable insights into the posttranslational modifications that regulate the functionality of this highly specialized cell and the opportunity to identify potential contraceptive targets [14]. Herein, we review recent literature on the global proteomic analysis of human spermatozoa, assess the relative merits of the different methods used and discuss issues and future directions in the field.

1.1.2
Technologies Used for the Study of the Sperm Proteome

1.1.2.1
Two Dimensional Polyacrylamide Gel Electrophoresis

Until recently, 2D polyacrylamide gel electrophoresis (PAGE) represented the method of choice as the front end of large scale sperm proteomic analyses. The principal reasons for this include the fact that it can be used to visualize a very large number of proteins simultaneously, and can be used in a differential display format [15]. This ability to study complex biological systems in their entirety rather than as a multitude of individual components makes it far easier to discover the many complex relationships between proteins in functioning cells.

In 2D-PAGE, proteins are first separated by isoelectric focusing before being further resolved by SDS-PAGE in the second dimension. Separated proteins can then be visualized by numerous staining methods to produce a 2D image array that can contain thousands of proteins [15]. The identification of individual proteins from polyacrylamide gels, has traditionally been carried out using comigration with known proteins, immunoblotting, N-terminal sequencing or internal peptide sequencing. In recent years there has been a fundamental shift in the way such experiments are performed, principally due to the rapid growth of large-scale genomic databases. The current widely used method relies on excising spots from gels, proteolytically digesting the spots, and then extracting the peptides produced. The final stage involves analyzing these peptides by mass spectrometry (MS) or tandem mass spectrometry (MS/MS) and then correlating the mass spectral data derived from the peptides with information contained in either protein, genomic, or expressed sequence tag databases (ESTs).

The use of preparative 2D-PAGE analyses to identify human sperm proteins has been reported from several groups [16–29]. Early studies using careful analysis of multiple replicated samples, established a database (Human Sperm Protein Encyclopedia) of 1,397 protein spots [21]. Within this data set, at least 98 protein spots were accessible to both ^{125}I vectorial labeling and biotinylation, suggesting an association with the sperm surface. Furthermore, 22 protein spots were immunologically reactive to a phosphotyrosine antibody and clustered into five protein isoforms. Higher resolution 2D-PAGE maps of normozoospermic human sperm proteins have recently been generated using a series of overlapping, narrow pH ranges for the initial isoelectrofocusing step [30]. Although this approach cataloged a total of 3,872 different protein spots, only 16 protein identities were reported.

In an attempt to understand which proteins might be important for contraceptive purposes, Shetty et al. [26] have examined the distribution of immunodominant sperm antigens on 2D Western blots using antisperm antibodies (ASA) from patients' sera. In total, 98 sperm auto and isoantigenic protein spots were recognized by sera derived from infertile patients but not fertile controls. Of these antigens, six were identified that were possibly relevant to antibody-mediated immunoinfertility [26]. An additional seven basic protein spots uniquely recognized by infertile sera have recently been reported by this group using an alternative first dimension separation consisting of nonequilibrium pH gradient electrophoresis (NEPHGE) [24]. Similarly, Bohring and Krause [17] reported the presence of 18 antigens from isolated sperm membranes which could be identified after 2D electrophoresis by ASA from seminal plasma of infertile or vasectomized men. A similar study with a narrower focus on sperm-immobilizing antibodies, has identified four proteins as potential sperm antigens responsible for this activity [27].

These types of 2D electrophoresis-based studies have been valuable in cataloging the overall nature and complexity of sperm proteome and the features of some of those proteins targeted by the human immune system, in terms of molecular mass and isoelectric point. However, actual protein identifications have been difficult to secure with this technology, generally relying on Western blot procedures employing antibodies against defined antigens or, more recently, the use of matrix assisted laser desorption ionization–time of flight (MALDI–TOF) MS techniques to characterize protein spots excised from the gels. Using this approach Shetty et al. [25] were able to generate sequence data on several novel sperm proteins as well as an unambiguous positive identification of angiotensin converting enzyme. Interestingly, several protein spots (charge train isomers) generated the same amino acid sequence data, emphasizing the importance of posttranslational modifications to sperm proteins in creating the complex array of protein spots seen when extracts of these cells are analyzed by 2D-gel electrophoresis [25]. The most detailed MALDI–TOF analysis of the human sperm proteome generated to date has mapped over 1,000 spots on 2D gels and secured identifications on 131 different proteins, almost a quarter of which had not previously been recorded on human spermatozoa [31, 32]. Interestingly, in addition to the anticipated abundance of cytoskeletal, mitochondrial, flagellar and membrane proteins, these data also provided some surprising findings such as the presence of a large proportion of proteins involved in transcription, protein synthesis and turnover [31, 32].

Despite their value in establishing a database of expressed proteins, 2D electrophoresis strategies suffer from a number of technical limitations including: the time consuming nature of the technique, its limited dynamic range, the fact that it does not work well for hydrophobic proteins, has an inherent variability that often makes it difficult in identifying matching protein spots between gel images, and is essentially nonquantitative [15]. This latter problem, is a reflection of the nature of many of the widely used staining techniques, such as silver staining, which themselves suffer from a limited dynamic range, so that the intensity of less abundant spots is not linearly correlated to that of more abundant spots. Moreover, some types of proteins, especially those that are posttranslationally modified, can give quantitatively and qualitatively different staining in comparison to similar amounts of other proteins. However, the technique is amenable for the detection of the presence or absence of one or more spots within a gel and has been used successfully to compare sperm protein expression profiles from patients who experience failed fertilization at IVF with fertile controls. One recent study of this nature, conservatively reported 20 consistent differences in protein expression between infertile (six spots missing, three additional spots, four less abundant, seven more abundant) compared with the controls [33]. Two of the proteins that were more intense in the patients were identified as secretory actin-binding protein and outer dense fiber protein 2/2, thus inviting speculation that the cause of infertility may be related to structural defects in either the motility apparatus or the actin cytoskeleton [33].

1.1.2.2
Difference in Gel Electrophoresis

Comparative studies are now also being facilitated through the introduction of the latest generation of fluorescent protein stains. Specifically, comparisons of proteomic profiles based on intact proteins are now able to be conducted with the Ettan DIGE (2D difference in gel electrophoresis) system from GE Healthcare (Piscataway, NJ). This technology is based on the development of a number of size and charge-matched, spectrally resolvable dyes (CyDyes) that are used to label different protein preparations prior to their separation by 2D-gel-electrophoresis [34]. The differentially labeled protein mixtures are then combined and resolved on the same gel, thus eliminating any inherent intergel variability in electrophoretic migration patterns. Following separation, the migration of individual protein populations can be resolved by scanning the gel with lasers tuned to the excitation wavelengths of the corresponding CyDyes (typically Cy3 and Cy5) [35, 36]. This information can then be related to the migration of a differentially labeled (Cy2) internal standard protein preparation. DeCyder software is subsequently used to accurately map and compare the migration of individual proteins for each of the proteomes being compared. With this technology, statistically significant differences in the migration of individual protein spots can be ascertained with just six replicates [35–37], whereas conventional proteomic techniques require several times this number of replicates to be mapped before any differences could be identified with confidence [21].

Once protein spots have been identified that significantly change between one physiological state and another they can be excised from the 2D gel and identified by MS. Such DIGE technology is therefore readily amendable to the simultaneous assessment of global changes associated with sperm function, rather than measuring, for example, levels of a single marker protein [37]. Examples where this has been used to directly visualize physiologically relevant proteins include comparisons of the posttranslational changes that occur in mammalian spermatozoa as they engage the process of epididymal maturation [37]. This analysis revealed significant decreases in protein spots unambiguously identified as α-enolase, endoplasmin, lactate dehydrogenase 3, testis lipid binding protein and cytokeratin, while spots associated with the β-subunit of the F1 ATPase, heat shock protein 70 and phosphatidyl ethanolamine binding protein (PEBP) all increased during epididymal transit. The rise in PEBP was particularly dramatic, amounting to a 4.8-fold increase during transition from the caput to cauda epididymis. This protein is especially interesting because independent studies have identified PEBP as a key component of a decapacitation system that regulates the rate at which capacitation occurs in mature caudal epididymal spermatozoa [38, 39]. DIGE has also recently been applied to assess protein concentrations in different germ cell types to identify those proteins specifically or preferentially expressed at each stage of spermatogenesis [40] and to screen human seminal plasma as a potential source of biomarkers for disorders of the male reproductive system associated with male infertility [41]. Interestingly, the latter study identified four and one candidate markers for nonobstructive and obstructive azoospermia, respectively.

1.1.2.3
Chromatographic Separation Methods

While the analysis of intact proteins with DIGE is likely to continue to play an important role in comparative studies of the sperm proteome, recent technical developments have heralded a new era in proteomics where the emphasis is placed not on whole proteins but on peptides. By virtue of their smaller size, peptides are much more homogenous structures than proteins which can exhibit significant variation in physiochemical properties such as size, charge, and hydrophobicity as a consequence of posttranslational modifications such as glycosylation or proteolytic cleavage. As an average sized protein of around 30–50 kDa will produce approximately 50 tryptic peptides, the number of entities that have to be analyzed increases dramatically when attention shifts from proteins to peptides. However, the development of nanoscale chromatographic strategies to purify individual peptides, combined with improved MS systems has made the rapid, detailed analysis of large numbers of tryptic peptides, a realistic possibility [15].

The same purification techniques are available for peptide purification as are used for whole protein purification, and include size-exclusion chromatography, ion-exchange chromatography, and reversed-phase HPLC. It is the latter of these techniques that is most commonly used for peptide purification in proteomics. In reversed-phase HPLC the peptides are generally retained due to hydrophobic interactions with the stationary silica phase. Polar mobile phases, such as water mixed with methanol or acetonitrile, are subsequently used to elute the bound peptides in order of decreasing polarity (increasing hydrophobicity). While reversed phase chromatography can be used as the sole separation procedure for moderately complex peptide mixtures prior to tandem mass spectrometric analysis, it is generally considered to have insufficient resolution for the analysis of more complex mixtures. This reflects the fact that although an MS instrument can perform mass measurements on several co-eluting peptides, if many peptides co-elute the instrument cannot fragment them all and therefore valuable information is likely to be irretrievably lost.

The first comprehensive analysis of the human sperm proteome utilizing an LC-MS/MS approach recorded the identification of greater than 1,760 proteins [13]. In this study, spermatozoa from a single fertile individual were fractionated into detergent-soluble and detergent-insoluble fractions and resolved by SDS–PAGE. The gel was then separated into 35 slices and digested with trypsin. Of the 1,760 proteins identified by nano LC-MS/MS of these gel sections, 1,350 proteins were uniquely present in the soluble fraction, 719 in the insoluble fraction, and 309 in both fractions. However, the individual proteins identified were not reported [13]. Using a similar approach, a more recent study reported the identification of 1,056 unique gene products in human spermatozoa [12]. Interestingly, approximately 8% of these proteins had not previously been characterized [12]. Similar experimental strategies in which the sperm samples were first enzymatically digested and focused in IPG strips before being run through a nanoflow reversed-phase column coupled to a linear IT, provided identifications of 858 and 829 unique gene products in the mature spermatozoa of mouse and rat respectively [10, 11]. In the latter species, bioinformatics demonstrated that at least 60 of these proteins were specifically expressed in the genitourinary tract, including: pyruvate dehydrogenase 1, ropporin, testis-specific serine kinase 4, testis-specific transporter, and retinol dehydrogenase 14.

Furthermore, since peptides are inherently less variable than proteins, they constitute a more reliable basis for quantitative proteomic comparisons. Indeed the peptide profile of a given cell type seems to be so robust that it can be used as the basis for comparing complex proteomic mixtures without the need for differential labeling of each protein population, as is the case with DIGE. Such peptide-based comparisons have been facilitated by the introduction of DecyderMS software that automatically detects, matches, and analyzes peptides from multiple LC-MS/MS experiments [42, 43]. This analysis platform creates a virtual 2D image of the MS survey scan by plotting retention time against mass:charge ratio, then statistically evaluates which peptides have changed position during a process such as epididymal maturation or capacitation. Once a change has been identified, the specific nature of the modification can then be resolved down to the level of posttranslational modifications on single amino acids [14]. As such, this technique that was formerly best suited to rapidly building a proteomic database rather than being applied in a differential display proteomic assay, is now becoming a viable alternative to 2DE for the analysis of certain complex mixtures [42, 43]. This approach is clearly going to become increasingly attractive as a means of not only extracting as much information as possible from a protein sample but also generating a short-list of the gene products that are functionally important. One of the ways in which such information can be generated is through comparative proteomics. For example, the proteomic profiles of spermatozoa from the caput and cauda epididymis, could be compared to identify which posttranslational modifications are relevant to sperm maturation. Similarly, comparative analyses of spermatozoa before and after capacitation or from normal fertile donors and infertile patients should also shed light on those elements of the proteome that are likely to be of functional relevance.

The main disadvantages of this approach are concerned with postexperimental data processing. The extremely large volume of data collected in an MS experiment presents a significant problem in terms of both the time required to collate and assemble the data into a useable format and the computing power needed to complete database searching. This problem may eventually be alleviated as mass spectrometric instrumentation, sequencing algorithms and the performance of computing resources, continue to improve and become more affordable. These improvements, coupled with the increasing stringency of data requirements of journals are helping to make results more transparent and address the burden of erroneous identification of proteins that appear in many published proteomes [44]. One other disadvantage of this approach is that it is generally limited to use with organisms that have complete genome sequence data available for searching. However, complete genomic sequence data will likely be available for all the major research organisms at some point in the future and therefore this will no longer represent a problem. There is also considerable scope for improvement in this technology, as it could, for example, be combined with specific peptide or protein enrichment strategies, such as immobilized metal affinity chromatography [45, 46], to reduce sample complexity and focus on phosphorylation and/or alternative forms of posttranslational protein modification required to achieve changes in sperm function.

In this context, recent reports have begun to characterize important sub-proteomes associated with sperm capacitation. For instance, Lefievre et al. [47] have recently provided a valuable insight into the role of nitric oxide in human sperm physiology by identifying targets for S-nitrosylation using the biotin switch assay coupled with MS/MS analyzes. This study reported the identification of 240 S-nitrosylated proteins including established substrates for S-nitrosylation such as tubulin, glutathione S-transferase and heat shock proteins, in addition to novel physiologically significant proteins not previously reported in other cells including A-kinase anchoring protein types 3 and 4, voltage-dependent anion-selective channel protein 3 and semenogelin 1 and 2. Similarly, the phosphoproteome of capacitated human spermatozoa has also been studied using phosphopeptide enrichment coupled with MS/MS [48]. In this study, greater than 60 phosphorylated sequences were mapped by MS/MS and identified targets for capacitation-associated tyrosine phosphorylation included: valosin-containing protein, a homolog of the SNARE-interacting protein NSF, and A-kinase anchoring protein types 3 and 4.

Furthermore, protein enrichment through strategies of subcellular fractionation has also been reported, including such recent examples as the proteomic characterizations of sperm regions that mediate sperm–egg interactions [49–51]. In their study, Stein et al. [52] analyzed the protein composition of three subcellular fractions from the head of mouse spermatozoa including: acrosomal contents, plasma membrane and outer acrosomal membrane. Within the three subcellular compartments, a total of 114 distinct proteins were identified that met their criteria for a potential role in oocyte interactions. Approximately 25% of the cell surface fraction proteins were previously uncharacterized and several others were identified that were not previously known to be on the sperm surface. In a complementary study designed to exclusively study proteins involved in primary zona binding, van Gestel et al. [51] isolated highly purified preparations of apical plasma membranes from the head of boar spermatozoa. These fractions were then solubilized, affinity purified with native zona pellucida ghosts and analyzed by LC-MS/MS. Indicative of the involvement of multiple sperm proteins in zona pellucida binding, several persistently bound proteins were identified including: isoforms of spermadhesin AQN-3, P47, fertilin beta and peroxiredoxin 5. Such studies therefore provide an important insight into the events of sperm–zona interactions and fertilization and warrant further investigation in human spermatozoa.

1.1.3
Conclusions

Simultaneous advances in MS design, computing power, and the availability of genomic sequence data for a variety of organisms have fuelled rapid growth in the field of proteomic analysis and served to enhance the utility and applicability of proteomic analyzes for the study sperm function. Ambitious, large-scale, mass-spectrometry-based proteomic analyzes have identified complex inventories comprising thousands of sperm proteins with a dynamic range of abundance of several orders of magnitude. In fact, obtaining mass-spectrometry data has already ceased to be the limiting step in sperm proteomics. Instead, the main challenge that lies ahead is to exploit this valuable resource in order to define which specific elements of the proteome are of functional significance and understand the cascade of posttranslational modifications involved in generating a functional spermatozoon. Ultimately the success of such studies will be measured by our progress in understanding the molecular mechanisms that may be targeted for contraceptive purposes or implicated in the etiology of defective sperm function.

References

1. Gadella BM, Lopes-Cardozo M, van Golde LM, Colenbrander B, Gadella TWJ (1995) Glycolipid migration from the apical to the equatorial subdomains of the sperm head plasma membrane precedes the acrosome reaction. Evidence for a primary capacitation event in boar spermatozoa. J Cell Sci 108:935–946
2. Phelps BM, Primakoff PK, Koppel DE, Low MG, Myles DG (1988) Restricted lateral diffusion of PH-20, a PI-anchored sperm membrane protein. Science 240:1780–1782
3. Anway MD, Li Y, Ravindranath N, Dym M, Griswold MD (2003) Expression of testicular germ cell genes identified by differential display analysis. J Androl 24:173–184
4. Catalano RD, Vlad M, Kennedy RC (1997) Differential display to identify and isolate novel genes expressed during spermatogenesis. Mol Hum Reprod 3:215–221
5. O'Shaughnessy PJ, Fleming L, Baker PJ, Jackson G, Johnston H (2003) Identification of developmentally regulated genes in the somatic cells of the mouse testis using serial analysis of gene expression. Biol Reprod 69:797–808
6. Aguilar-Mahecha A, Hales BF, Robaire B (2001) Expression of stress response genes in germ cells during spermatogenesis. Biol Reprod 65:119–127
7. Almstrup K, Nielsen JE, Hansen MA, Tanaka M, Skakkebaek NE, Leffers H (2004) Analysis of cell-type-specific gene expression during mouse spermatogenesis. Biol Reprod 70:1751–1761
8. Guo R, Yu Z, Guan J, Ge Y, Ma J, Li S, Wang S, Xue S, Han D (2004) Stage-specific and tissue-specific expression characteristics of differentially expressed genes during mouse spermatogenesis. Mol Reprod Dev 67:264–272
9. Yu Z, Guo R, Ge Y, Ma J, Guan J, Li S, Sun X, Xue S, Han D (2003) Gene expression profiles in different stages of mouse spermatogenic cells during spermatogenesis. Biol Reprod 69:37–47
10. Baker MA, Hetherington L, Reeves G, Muller J, Aitken RJ (2008) The rat sperm proteome characterized via IPG strip prefractionation and LC-MS/MS identification. Proteomics 8:2312–2321
11. Baker MA, Hetherington L, Reeves GM, Aitken RJ (2008) The mouse sperm proteome characterized via IPG strip prefractionation and LC-MS/MS identification. Proteomics 8:1720–1730
12. Baker MA, Reeves G, Hetherington L, Muller J, Baur I, Aitken RJ (2007) Identification of gene products present in Triton X-100 soluble and insoluble fractions of human spermatozoa lysates using LC-MS/MS analysis. Proteomic Clin Appl 1:524–532
13. Johnston DS, Wooters J, Kopf GS, Qiu Y, Roberts KP (2005) Analysis of the human sperm proteome. Ann NY Acad Sci 1061:190–202
14. Aitken RJ, Baker MA (2008) The role of proteomics in understanding sperm cell biology. Int J Androl 31:295–302
15. Hunter TC, Andon NL, Koller A, Yates JR, Haynes PA (2002) The functional proteomics toolbox: methods and applications. J Chromatogr B Analyt Technol Biomed Life Sci 782:165–181

16. Bhande S, Naz RK (2007) Molecular identities of human sperm proteins reactive with antibodies in sera of immunoinfertile women. Mol Reprod Dev 74:332–340

17. Bohring C, Krause W (1999) The characterization of human spermatozoa membrane proteins – surface antigens and immunological infertility. Electrophoresis 20:971–976

18. Kritsas JJ, Schopperle WM, DeWolf WC, Morgentaler A (1992) Rapid high resolution two-dimensional electrophoresis of human sperm proteins. Electrophoresis 13:445–449

19. Morgentaler A, Schopperle WM, Crocker RH, DeWolf WC (1990) Protein differences between normal and oligospermic human sperm demonstrated by two-dimensional gel electrophoresis. Fertil Steril 54:902–905

20. Naaby-Hansen S (1990) Electrophoretic map of acidic and neutral human spermatozoal proteins. J Reprod Immunol 17:167–185

21. Naaby-Hansen S, Flickinger CJ, Herr JC (1997) Two-dimensional gel electrophoretic analysis of vectorially labeled surface proteins of human spermatozoa. Biol Reprod 56:771–787

22. Primakoff P, Lathrop W, Bronson R (1990) Identification of human sperm surface glycoproteins recognized by autoantisera from immune infertile men, women, and vasectomized men. Biol Reprod 42:929–942

23. Shen SL, Luo Y, Ning L, He DL (2007) Differential analysis of two-dimensional gel electrophoresis profiles of spermatozoal protein in human normal semen and idiopathic asthenospermia. Zhong Hua Nan Ke Xue 13:50–52

24. Shetty J, Bronson RA, Herr JC (2008) Human sperm protein encyclopedia and alloantigen index: mining novel allo-antigens using sera from ASA-positive infertile patients and vasectomized men. J Reprod Immunol 77:23–31

25. Shetty J, Diekman AB, Jayes FC, Sherman NE, Naaby-Hansen S, Flickinger CJ, Herr JC (2001) Differential extraction and enrichment of human sperm surface proteins in a proteome: identification of immunocontraceptive candidates. Electrophoresis 22:3053–3066

26. Shetty J, Naaby-Hansen S, Shibahara H, Bronson R, Flickinger CJ, Herr JC (1999) Human sperm proteome: immunodominant sperm surface antigens identified with sera from infertile men and women. Biol Reprod 61:61–69

27. Shibahara H, Sato I, Shetty J, Naaby-Hansen S, Herr JC, Wakimoto E, Koyama K (2002) Two-dimensional electrophoretic analysis of sperm antigens recognized by sperm immobilizing antibodies detected in infertile women. J Reprod Immunol 53:1–12

28. Xu C, Rigney DR, Anderson DJ (1994) Two-dimensional electrophoretic profile of human sperm membrane proteins. J Androl 15:595–602

29. Yoshii T, Kuji N, Komatsu S, Iwahashi K, Tanaka Y, Yoshida H, Wada A, Yoshimura Y (2005) Fine resolution of human sperm nucleoproteins by two-dimensional electrophoresis. Mol Hum Reprod 11:677–681

30. Li LW, Fan LQ, Zhu WB, Nien HC, Sun BL, Luo KL, Liao TT, Tang L, Lu GX (2007) Establishment of a high-resolution 2-D reference map of human spermatozoal proteins from 12 fertile sperm-bank donors. Asian J Androl 9:321–329

31. de Mateo S, Martinez-Heredia J, Estanyol JM, Domiguez-Fandos D, Vidal-Taboada JM, Ballesca JL, Oliva R (2007) Marked correlations in protein expression identified by proteomic analysis of human spermatozoa. Proteomics 7:4264–4277

32. Martinez-Heredia J, Estanyol JM, Ballesca JL, Oliva R (2006) Proteomic identification of human sperm proteins. Proteomics 6:4356–4369

33. Pixton KL, Deeks ED, Flesch FM, Moseley FL, Bjorndahl L, Ashton PR, Barratt CL, Brewis IA (2004) Sperm proteome mapping of a patient who experienced failed fertilization at IVF reveals altered expression of at least 20 proteins compared with fertile donors: case report. Hum Reprod 19:1438–1447

34. Tonge R, Shaw J, Middleton B, Rowlinson R, Rayner S, Young J, Pognan F, Hawkins E, Currie I, Davison M (2001) Validation and development of fluorescence two-dimensional differential gel electrophoresis proteomics technology. Proteomics 1:377–396

35. Friedman DB (2007) Quantitative proteomics for two-dimensional gels using difference gel electrophoresis. Methods Mol Biol 367:219–239
36. Friedman DB, Lilley KS (2008) Optimizing the difference gel electrophoresis (DIGE) technology. Methods Mol Biol 428:93–124
37. Baker MA, Witherdin R, Hetherington L, Cunningham-Smith K, Aitken RJ (2005) Identification of post-translational modifications that occur during sperm maturation using difference in two-dimensional gel electrophoresis. Proteomics 5:1003–1012
38. Gibbons R, Adeoya-Osiguwa SA, Fraser LR (2005) A mouse sperm decapacitation factor receptor is phosphatidylethanolamine-binding protein 1. Reproduction 130:497–508
39. Nixon B, MacIntyre DA, Mitchell LA, Gibbs GM, O'Bryan M, Aitken RJ (2006) The identification of mouse sperm-surface-associated proteins and characterization of their ability to act as decapacitation factors. Biol Reprod 74:275–287
40. Rolland AD, Evrard B, Guitton N, Lavigne R, Calvel P, Couvet M, Jegou B, Pineau C (2007) Two-dimensional fluorescence difference gel electrophoresis analysis of spermatogenesis in the rat. J Proteome Res 6:683–697
41. Yamakawa K, Yoshida K, Nishikawa H, Kato T, Iwamoto T (2007) Comparative analysis of interindividual variations in the seminal plasma proteome of fertile men with identification of potential markers for azoospermia in infertile patients. J Androl 28:858–865
42. Johansson C, Samskog J, Sundstrom L, Wadensten H, Bjorkesten L, Flensburg J (2006) Differential expression analysis of *Escherichia coli* proteins using a novel software for relative quantitation of LC-MS/MS data. Proteomics 6:4475–4485
43. Kaplan A, Soderstrom M, Fenyo D, Nilsson A, Falth M, Skold K, Svensson M, Pettersen H, Lindqvist S, Svenningsson P, Andren PE, Bjorkesten L (2007) An automated method for scanning LC-MS data sets for significant peptides and proteins, including quantitative profiling and interactive confirmation. J Proteome Res 6:2888–2895
44. Steen H, Mann M (2004) The ABC's (and XYZ's) of peptide sequencing. Nat Rev Mol Cell Biol 5:699–711
45. Li Y, Lin H, Deng C, Yang P, Zhang X (2008) Highly selective and rapid enrichment of phosphorylated peptides using gallium oxide-coated magnetic microspheres for MALDI-TOF-MS and nano-LC-ESI-MS/MS/MS analysis. Proteomics 8:238–249
46. Schilling M, Knapp DR (2008) Enrichment of phosphopeptides using biphasic immobilized metal affinity-reversed phase microcolumns. J Proteome Res 7:4164–4172
47. Lefievre L, Chen Y, Conner SJ, Scott JL, Publicover SJ, Ford WC, Barratt CL (2007) Human spermatozoa contain multiple targets for protein S-nitrosylation: an alternative mechanism of the modulation of sperm function by nitric oxide? Proteomics 7:3066–3084
48. Ficarro S, Chertihin O, Westbrook VA, White F, Jayes F, Kalab P, Marto JA, Shabanowitz J, Herr JC, Hunt DF, Visconti PE (2003) Phosphoproteome analysis of capacitated human sperm. Evidence of tyrosine phosphorylation of a kinase-anchoring protein 3 and valosin-containing protein/p97 during capacitation. J Biol Chem 278:11579–11589
49. Nixon B, Bielanowicz A, McLaughlin EA, Tanphaichitr N, Ensslin MA, Aitken RJ (2009) Composition and significance of detergent resistant membranes in mouse spermatozoa. J Cell Physiol 218:122–134
50. Sleight SB, Miranda PV, Plaskett NW, Maier B, Lysiak J, Scrable H, Herr JC, Visconti PE (2005) Isolation and proteomic analysis of mouse sperm detergent-resistant membrane fractions: evidence for dissociation of lipid rafts during capacitation. Biol Reprod 73:721–729
51. van Gestel RA, Brewis IA, Ashton PR, Brouwers JF, Gadella BM (2007) Multiple proteins present in purified porcine sperm apical plasma membranes interact with the zona pellucida of the oocyte. Mol Hum Reprod 13:445–454
52. Stein KK, Go JC, Lane WS, Primakoff P, Myles DG (2006) Proteomic analysis of sperm regions that mediate sperm–egg interactions. Proteomics 6:3533–3543

Methods of Analysis of Sperm Antigens Related to Fertility

1.2

Jagathpala Shetty and John C. Herr

1.2.1
Introduction

The discovery of sperm antigens involved in fertilization requires a comprehensive under-standing of the composition of the sperm plasma membrane as well as the membranes involved in sperm–egg plasma membrane interaction. The plasma membrane of the sperm contacts the outer investments of the oocyte including the corona radiate and zona pellucida (ZP) and subsequently undergoes the acrosome reaction. Following the acrosome reaction the anterior aspect of the sperm head is remodeled and the inner acrosomal membrane (IAM) becomes the limiting membrane on the anterior two-thirds of the sperm head. The mem-brane overlying the equatorial segment of the acrosome is believed to be the initial site of fusion with the egg plasma membrane [1]. Knowledge of the molecular composition of the sperm plasma membrane and the structural domains involved in various sperm functions leading to fertilization may be employed to design contraceptive vaccines, "intelligent sper-micides" that target surface receptors, or contraceptive antagonists. Toward these applied endpoints a target discovery strategy should be employed that identifies those sperm anti-gens that are unique, germ cell specific, immunogenic, and accessible to antibodies or antag-onists at the cell surface. Although conventional gene profiling methods, including differential display [2, 3], serial analysis of gene expression [4] and microarray [5–8] technologies, are suitable for profiling relative levels of messenger RNAs in precursor germ cells such as spermatogonia, spermatocytes, or spermatids, these "transcriptomic" techniques can only be complimentary to understanding the comprehensive proteomic composition of fully differ-entiated spermatozoa. Proteomics can verify the presence of a target protein, provide an estimate of its relative abundance, and provide evidence of its immunogenicity. In this con-text, spermatozoa are in some respects ideal cells for proteomic analyses since they can be easily purified in large numbers and pharmacologically manipulated to drive into different physiological states such as capacitation and acrosome reaction. With recent developments

J. Shetty (✉)
Center for Research in Contraceptive and Reproductive Health, University of Virginia Health Science Center, Charlottesville, VA, USA
e-mail: Js4ed@virginia.edu

W. K. H. Krause and R. K. Naz (eds.), *Immune Infertility*,
DOI: 10.1007/978-3-642-01379-9_1.2, © Springer Verlag Berlin Heidelberg 2009

in protein microsequencing by mass spectrometry, along with the wealth of information now available from the genome projects, technologies are at hand to readily determine amino acid sequences of a protein spot on a two-dimensional (2D) gel or from a complex mixture of enriched proteins. The peptide sequence can be used to deduce and synthesize a set of gene-specific oligonucleotides which can then be used to PCR amplify or hybridization clone and sequence a corresponding cDNA, leading to characterization of genes and proteins of hitherto unknown sperm components, particularly those associated with the acrsosome, plasma membrane and acrosomal membrane domains. This chapter reviews several proteomic methods of analysis that are currently being employed to identify and characterize sperm antigens that are relevant to sperm function and fertility.

1.2.2
Two-Dimensional Gel Electrophoresis

The functionality of spermatozoal proteins is significantly influenced by posttranslational modifications that may take place during spermiogenesis, during the maturation of spermatozoa in the epididymis, during the postejaculatory capacitation processes in the female reproductive tract, or following the acrosome reaction. Two-dimensional gel electrophoresis offers a classical proteomic tool to dissect the molecular transformations that spermatozoa undergo in various functional states through a comparison of 2D gel images from various experimental conditions. The pioneering innovation of O'Farrell [9] led to the development of 2D gel electrophoresis. Proteins are resolved in two dimensions: the first dimension separates proteins in a pH gradient according to their isoelectric point (pI) by isoelectric focusing (IEF), while in the second dimension the proteins are separated according to their molecular weight by SDS-PAGE. Since its introduction IEF has undergone several advances. The first dimension may be carried out in polyacrylamide gel rods that are formed in glass tubes and contain ampholytes that form a pH gradient in an electric field. The introduction of immobilized pH gradients (IPGs) by Bjellqvist et al. [10] had a significant impact on the use of IEF to separate complex mixtures over a wide pH range. The IPGs enable the formation of stable and reproducible pH gradients capable of focusing acidic and basic proteins on a single gel prepared with broad pH gradients. Once a broad pH gradient gel is stained with a reagent that allows the repertoire [encyclopedia] of proteins to be resolved (e.g., silver stain), a narrow pH gradient gel may then be employed to expand particular pI regions of the protein encyclopedia. This approach can increase the separation between protein spots of interest, especially as an antecedent to coring spots for microsequencing.

Two dimensional electrophoresis followed by Western blotting is widely applied as a tool to study sperm–antibody interactions or other protein–protein interactions [as in Far-Western analysis of receptor–ligand interactions] and to analyze proteins from different domains of the sperm. A critical requirement of proteomic research is high quality separation of cellular constituents, usually referred to as protein resolution. Two-dimensional gel electrophoresis may be preceded by various methods of subcellular fractionation, isolation, and enrichment of proteins to generate a proteome of particular subcellular compartments.

1.2.2.1
Vectorial Labeling of Surface Proteins

Molecules exposed on the cell surface represent key targets for both understanding the complex processes of differentiation and function of the spermatozoa and offer candidate contraceptive vaccinogens (CV) or receptors for drug agonists or antagonists. Surface labeling of the proteins exposed on the spermatozoa may be achieved by labeling with radioactive ^{125}I (radioiodination) or biotin (biotinylation). Radioiodination involves the introduction of radioactive iodine into certain amino acids, usually tyrosines in proteins and peptides. The iodo-bead iodination method [11] is a convenient, gentle and efficient method for vectorial iodination of membrane bound proteins. Identification of the iodinated cell surface proteins is achieved by performing an autoradiograph of the proteins after resolution by 2D gel electrophoresis. Surface labeling with biotin may be accomplished using the reagent sulfo-NHS-LC-biotin which reacts with primary amines exposed at the sperm surface. The biotinylated proteins along with non-biotinylated proteins may be subsequently fractionated by 2D gel electrophoresis and the biotinylated proteins can be identified by avidin blotting, using peroxidase conjugated avidin followed by enhanced chemiluminescence [12].

Naaby Hansen et al. [11] identified a repertoire of proteins exposed on the surface of ejaculated human spermatozoa by utilizing high resolution 2D gel system using both IEF and nonequilibrium pH gradient electrophoresis (NEPHGE). A total of 181 surface protein spots were identified by radiolabeling the intact sperm with ^{125}I, while 228 protein spots were biotinylated out of 1,397 total protein spots that were digitized and cataloged from silver-stained gels. The protein spots labeled with ^{125}I and biotin constituted a "sperm surface protein index." In a later study, Shetty et al. [12] reported surface labeling the sperm with sulfo-NHS-LC-biotin, which has an additional sulfur group which restricts the penetration of the biotin reagent through the cell membrane during surface labeling. Use of this improved biotinylating reagent limited the number of biotinylated proteins detected to 68 and enabled identification of eight novel sperm molecules.

D'Cruz et al. [13] identified target antigens recognized by clinically important complement-fixing antisperm antibodies (ASA) by indirect immunoprecipitation after surface biotinylation of motile sperm with ASA-positive sera from autoimmune, isoimmune, and vasectomized patients. Paradowska et al. [14] applied the same technique to identify human ASA reactive mouse sperm surface proteins. Stein et al. [15] used sulfo-NHS-LC-biotin to biotinylate mouse sperm surface proteins. Biotinylated proteins were further isolated using monomeric avidin beads and microsequenced after fractionating the proteins by SDS-PAGE. Pasten et al. [16] made use of sperm surface biotinylation experiments to determine the presence of proteasomes on the sperm surface and their possible role in fertilization. In an experiment on the rearrangement of macaque hyluronidase PH-20, Yudin et al. [17] demonstrated this protein's localization on the surface by surface-labeling with biotin.

In our experience, even though biotinylation with the sulfo-NHS-LC-biotin improved the quality of surface labeling, and verification of labeling of known surface molecules such as angiotensin-converting enzyme (ACE), PH-20 and SAGA1 served as useful positive controls, the subsequent cloning and characterization of two unknown biotinylated protein spots yielded novel acrosomal membrane proteins namely SAMP14 [18] and SAMP32 [19]. This suggests that acrosomal membrane proteins may also be biotinylated by this procedure, possibly because of their exposure following spontaneous acrosome reaction among a subset of sperm. Another possible drawback of the procedure was the inability to visualize several of the biotinylated proteins on a silver stained gel, probably due to their low abundance. The avidin step, which amplifies reaction products and may provide higher sensitivity, resulted in spots on the Western blot that are but not visible on the silver stained gel.

1.2.2.2
Identification of Fertility Related Sperm Antigens by Naturally Occurring Antisperm Antibodies

The occurrence of ASA in association with many cases of unexplained infertility has shown that fertilization can be blocked at various stages by ASA, causing sperm aggluti- nation and/or immobilization, or interfering in the process of sperm–oocyte interaction [20, 21]. The presence of ASA does not exert in most cases any harmful effect on patients, except for their infertility. For this reason, identification of the cognate sperm antigens in these cases has been seen as a route to candidate CVs. ASA are found in 9–12.8% of infertile couples. However, these antibodies are also present in approximately 1–2.5% of fertile men [22, 23] and in 4% of fertile women. The presence of ASA in the fertile popu- lation suggests that not all ASA cause infertility [24–26]. This observation requires con- sideration in the design of a discriminating method to identify the cognate antigens relevant to infertility utilizing sera or seminal plasma containing ASA. Another aspect to be con- sidered is the accessibility of an antibody to its cognate sperm antigen. Sperm interact with their surroundings through their surfaces within the male and female tracts and it is through the plasma membrane that the sperm contacts the egg investments. Hence a strategy that identifies sperm surface antigens that elicit immune responses in humans might offer a particularly attractive subset of sperm proteins for contraceptive targeting. An extensive literature has emerged on the subject of identification of sperm antigens recognized by systemic and/or local auto and iso-antibodies from infertile individuals using immunob- lotting techniques (see reviews from Chamley et al. [27] and Lombardo et al. [28]). Most of the cited studies used uni-dimensional gel electrophoresis for the separation of sperm proteins and as a result the molecular weights of relevant sperm antigens were conflicting, probably due to differences in methodology or in the immunodominant repertoires of ASA-positive individuals. Shetty et al. [29] employed a 2D proteomic approach coupled with immunoblotting, vectorial labeling and computer aided 2D gel analysis to target sperm surface proteins relevant to fertility while screening the sperm proteins with sera from infertile men and women. A subset of six auto- and iso-antigens was identified as possibly relevant to antibody-mediated infertility. The serum samples were initially screened for the presence of ASA by immunobead binding test (IBT) [20] and only those sera showing significant reactivity for the presence of ASA were utilized to identify immunodominant antigens. By monitoring bead binding to the sperm surface, the IBT test offers an opportunity to identify and prescreen patients with autoantibodies to surface exposed epitopes. In order to have a comprehensive overview of the repertoire of immu- noreactive sperm proteins recognized by serum samples from fertile and infertile subjects of both sexes, the blots were serially incubated with five serum samples from each group of subjects. Figure 1.2.1 shows one such experiment [29]. Serum samples from the infertile subjects were selected based on their high immunoreactivity, heterogeneity in the immunoreactivity and unique recognition of certain protein spots following individual Western blot analysis of the sera. Comparison of Western blots probed with sera from fertile (Fig. 1.2.1a, b) and infertile subjects (Fig. 1.2.1c, d) demonstrated that several discrete sperm antigens were recognized by sera from infertile patients (arrows). Sperm antigens unique to infertile patients were identified by excluding those antigens recognized by serum samples from clinically fertile subjects using the software Bio Image "2D Analyzer" to compare 2D immunoblots. A database of 2D gel images of silver stained proteins and a data base of vectorially labeled sperm surface proteins (sperm surface index) [11] allowed the definition of a subset of sperm surface antigens relevant to antibody-mediated infertility. These immunogens were microsequenced, cloned and characterized. Examples are ESP [30, 31] SAMP32 [19], SAMP14 [18, and unpublished data] and CABYR [32]. Among these antigens ESP, SAMP32 and SAMP14 are intra-acrosomal proteins and become exposed on the sperm surface following the acrosome reaction. CABYR, in

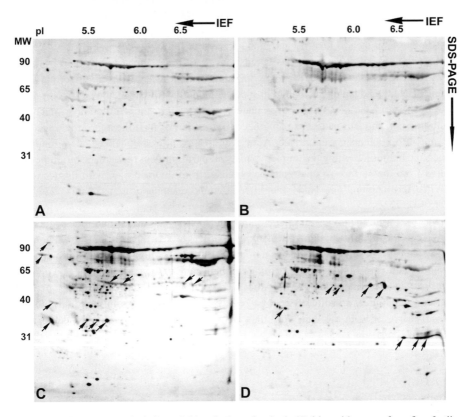

Fig. 1.2.1 2D Western analysis by serial incubation of a single 2D blot with serum from five fertile males (**a**) and fertile females (**b**) compared with those from five infertile males (**c**) and infertile females (**d**) (dilution: 1:2,000). Note major auto- and isoantigens (*arrows*) that are uniquely recognized by the infertile subjects. [29]

contrast, is primarily localized to the fibrous sheath of the principal piece of the sperm tail [32]. Vectorial labeling of CABYR with ^{125}I suggests this protein may be released and exposed even with gentle handling of sperm, or perhaps a subset of CABYR molecules are surface exposed since the single copy CABYR gene undergoes remarkable alternative splicing resulting in protein microheterogeneity.

Other studies employing 2D immunoblotting led to the identification of discrete specific sperm proteins recognized by sperm immobilizing sera [33]; immuno-infertile female sera containing ASA [34], and seminal plasma containing ASA [35]. A well-known risk factor for the development of ASA in the male is disruption of the vas deferens, which is achieved during vasectomy for sterilization. Failure to restore the fertility in several cases of vasectomy reversal is attributed to the development of ASA following vasectomy [36]. Sera from vasectomized male subjects can be useful reagents to identify fertility related sperm antigens [37, 38]. Employing a battery of such sera Shetty et al. [39], identified potential fertility related antigens unique to sera collected following vasectomy by comparing immunoreactivity of serum samples from pre- and postvasectomy with a 2D Western blot approach. Domagala et al. [40] employed a similar approach in identifying six novel antigens; four of which were recognized by the ASA positive infertile males, one recognized by a vasectomized man and one recognized by ASA positive seminal plasma.

Another approach to identify antigens involved in fertility is by probing 2D Western blots with antibodies that were recovered from the surface of sperm obtained from the ejaculate of infertile men [as opposed to using circulating antisperm antibody]. Such studies have the advantage of potentially detecting antigens identified by antibodies that transudate from the serum or are produced locally within the reproductive mucosae, including iso- and auto-antigens recognized by secretory IgA, if the appropriate secondary anti-IgA reagents are employed. Auer et al. [41] employed enhanced chemiluminescence and immumoblotting techniques to analyze sperm antigens recognized by antibodies eluted from the surface of spermatozoa obtained from infertile men with unsuccessful in vitro fertilization. The study identified immuno-reactive proteins from 37/36 and 19/18 kDa zones.

Naz [42] used the powerful phage display technology to identify peptide sequences that were specifically recognized by immunoinfertile sera with a long-term goal of identifying sperm peptide sequences that might find applications in the specific diagnosis and treatment of immuno-infertility in humans, and in the development of a contraceptive vaccine. The study led to the identification of seven dodecamer peptide sequences that were specifically recognized by the immuno-infertile sera. This technical approach aided in the discovery of a novel peptide sequence that was designated YLP12 [43, 44].

1.2.2.3
Differential Extraction

Differential extraction of sperm proteins involves various solubilization methods to preferentially enrich peripheral membrane proteins, hydrophobic membrane associated proteins or hydrophilic proteins. One of the well-known and powerful techniques to enrich the membrane associated hydrophobic protein is temperature-induced phase partitioning in TX-114 [45], which allows the separation of hydrophobic integral membrane proteins from the hydrophilic proteins. The technique is based on the ability of the nonionic detergent TX-114 to partition into two distinct phases above 23°C: a detergent-rich phase and a detergent-depleted or aqueous phase. Amphipathic membrane proteins, whether anchored to a lipid by a glycosylphosphatidylinositol (GPI) moiety or a hydrophobic polypeptide, partition predominantly into the detergent-rich phase, whereas hydrophilic proteins partition predominantly into the aqueous phase [46]. Shetty et al. [12] exploited this technique to identify sperm membrane associated proteins. The sperm surface proteins were labeled before extraction using sulfo-NHS-LC-biotin and the proteins were resolved on large format 2D gels capable of high resolution. Surface localized proteins were identified by avidin blotting of the biotinylated proteins transferred to nitrocellulose membranes. Figure 1.2.2 demonstrates the identification of several membrane associated sperm surface localized proteins by 2D gel analysis and avidin blotting [12]. The method facilitated the identification of eight novel sperm proteins in addition to several known membrane proteins. For example, two acrosomal membrane proteins: SAMP14 [18], a GPI anchored Ly6/uPAR superfamily protein and SAMP32 [19], an autoantigenic protein, emerged from this approach. Antibodies against recombinant human SAMP14 and SAMP32 inhibited both the binding and the fusion of human sperm to zona free hamster eggs, suggesting that these molecules may have a role in sperm–egg interaction. Triton X-114 phase partitioning is routinely applied to characterize a protein or to check the presence or absence of a known hydrophobic protein under various experimental conditions [47–49].

Salt Extraction: Peripheral membrane proteins are known to be extracted by relatively mild treatments. One of the ways to isolate a soluble form of an extrinsic membrane protein

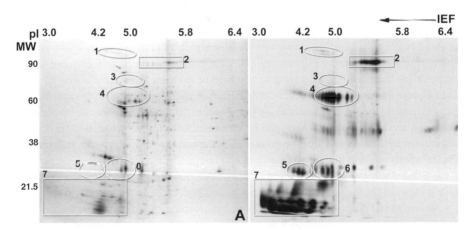

Fig. 1.2.2 Analysis of surface biotinylated, TX-114 phase partitioned sperm proteins. A silver stained 2D gel from the detergent phase extract enriched for membrane associated proteins (**a**) is matched with an avidin-ECL blot from the same phase (**b**). Clusters of biotinylated putative surface protein spots are circled or boxed in the avidin blot and their corresponding location on the silver stained gel is indicated [12]

is by treatment with high ionic strength solution (1M NaCl or 1M KCl). The procedure aims at the disruption of weak electrostatic interactions and hydrogen bonds, and, occasionally, weak hydrophobic interactions in order to break the interactions between the extrinsic proteins and the membrane [50]. Johnson et al. [51] were able to extract an adenylate cyclase-activating factor from bovine sperm by treating the sperm with various salts such as NH_4HCO_3, NaCl and Na acetate. Combining vectorial labeling and 2D gel electrophoresis, Shetty et al. [12] identified several surface labeled, peripheral membrane proteins and obtained a novel peptide sequence by mass spectrometry using mild treatment with NaCl (1M).

1.2.2.4
Subcellular Fractionation of the Sperm

Detergent-resistant membrane domains (lipid rafts): Lipid rafts are plasma membrane microdomains which are defined as small, heterogeneous, highly dynamic regions that serve to compartmentalize cellular processes [52]. A multiplicity of cellular functions have been associated with these lipid microdomains, such as membrane trafficking, cellular signal transduction, viral entry and fertilization [53]. The lipid content contributes to the hydrophobic nature of raft domains and leads to two inherent biochemical properties: insolubility at 4°C in Triton X-100 (TX-100) detergent, and light buoyant-density after centrifugation in a sucrose density gradient. These properties are used to isolate detergent-resistant membrane (DRM) as a biochemical correlate of lipid rafts [54].

Initial evidence for raft formation in male germ cells came from identification of the raft protein, caveolin-1, in the head and flagellum of mouse and guinea pig sperm, implicating these structures in the regulation of both motility and sperm–zona interaction [55]. In order to determine alteration of the protein composition in DRMs following capacitation, Sleight et al. [56] performed a proteomic analysis of mouse sperm proteins isolated in the light buoyant-density fraction. The immunoglobulin superfamily protein Izumo, a well-known sperm–egg fusion protein [57] was also one of the predominant protein enriched in the preparation. Thaler et al. [58] made a similar kind of study and reported that several individual proteins became enriched or depleted in DRM fractions following capacitation. Studies done on the pig [59] and boar [60] support the hypothesis that capacitation induced increased levels of sperm DRMs, with an enhanced ZP affinity. Nixon et al. [61] have shown that DRMs isolated from spermatozoa possessed the ability to selectively bind to the ZP of unfertilized, but not fertilized, mouse oocytes. Collectively, these data provide compelling evidence that mouse spermatozoa possess membrane microdomains that provide a platform for the assembly of key recognition molecules on the sperm surface.

An alternative method for the enrichment and isolation of sperm membrane proteins involves preparation of membranes through hypoosmotic swelling, homogenization and sonication [62]. Membranes are further isolated by differential centrifugation steps. Purified human sperm membrane proteins can be separated by 2D gel electrophoresis and further analysis of the sperm antigens can be achieved.

Oko's group [63] has devised a methodology to obtain a sperm head fraction consisting solely of the IAM bound to the detergent-resistant perinuclear theca. On the exposed IAM surface of this fraction, they defined an electron dense protein layer that was termed IAM extracellular coat (IAMC). Their approach has led to the identification of a novel inner acrosomal protein IAM38 from bovine sperm with a demonstrated role in sperm–egg interaction [63].

1.2.2.5
Use of Polyclonal and Monoclonal Antibodies

Polyclonal or monoclonal antibodies may also be used for the identification, isolation and characterization of sperm antigens that are relevant to fertility. A number of sperm antigens have been identified by means of monoclonal antibodies [47, 57, 64–72]. Among the most significant findings was the discovery of the immunoglobulin superfamily protein Izumo, by using monoclonal antibody OBF13, which interfered with sperm–egg interaction [57]. Izumo was shown to localize within the acrosome and to have a definitive role in sperm–egg fusion during fertilization. Izumo was identified by separation of the crude extracts from mouse sperm by 2D gel electrophoresis and subsequent immunoblotting with the monoclonal antibody.

1.2.2.6
Identification of GPI Anchored Proteins

In mammals, more than 200 cell surface proteins with various functions, such as hydroxylation, cellular adhesion and receptor activity are anchored to the membrane by a covalently attached GPI moiety [73–75]. GPI deficiency causes developmental abnormalities, failure of skin barrier formation and female infertility in mice indicating that GPI anchor is essential for cell integrity [76, 77].

A few GPI-anchored proteins discovered from sperm are CD59, CD52, TESP5, PH20 [hyaluronidase] and SAMP14. PH-20 is proposed to have multiple functions involved in cell signaling and serve as a receptor for the ZP, in addition to its hyaluronidase activity [78]. The recent discovery that a testicular isoform of angiotensin ACE is a GPI anchored protein releasing factor which is crucial for fertilization [79] has shown the importance of GPI-anchored proteins in the fertilization process.

A standard method to isolate GPI-anchored molecule from the cell surface is, treatment of the cells with GPI-specific phospholipase C (PI-PLC) that cleaves GPI anchors specifically, leaving the lipid moiety in the membrane, and releasing the protein with a terminal cyclic phosphoinositol [80]. Even though there is no single report on the identification of GPI-anchored molecules from the sperm surface on a global scale, an experiment carried out on oocytes by Coonrod et al. [81] investigated human sperm-hamster oocyte interactions and determined that PI-PLC cleavable GPI-anchored proteins are involved in sperm–egg binding and fusion. 2D electrophoresis was then utilized to visualize proteins released from hamster oocytes following PI-PLC treatment. The authors demonstrated that treatment of hamster oocytes with PI-PLC inhibits sperm–egg interaction and releases a 25–40 kDa protein cluster (pI 5–6) from the oolemma suggesting that this released protein cluster represents an oolemmal GPI-linked surface protein(s) which is involved in human sperm-hamster egg interaction. A comprehensive search for all the GPI anchored molecules in spermatozoa by proteomic analysis may be needed to identify the full repertoire of molecules that are directly involved in fertilization.

1.2.2.7
Two-Dimensional Differential in-Gel Electrophoresis (2D-DIGE)

The recent development of 2D-DIGE [82] is beginning to have an impact on the field of reproductive immunology assisting in the identification and characterization of potential fertility related proteins. This technology is based on the creation of a family of size and charge-matched spectrally resolvable dyes that are used to label different protein preparations prior to 2D gel electrophoresis, allowing up to three distinct protein mixtures to be separated within a single 2D PAGE gel. By running such differentially labeled protein mixtures on the same gel, between-gel differences in electrophoretic migration patterns can be entirely eliminated. Baker et al. [83] used this technique to isolate and characterize those proteins that undergo processing in rat spermatozoa as they transit the epididymal tract. The technique can be effectively applied to determine post-translational modifications of the sperm at various functional states (non-capacitated, capacitated and acrosome reacted) and also to identify fertility related proteins by using sperm proteins from healthy fertile specimens vs. infertile specimens. Since so few genes related to human infertility are now known, this method may open up the field of male infertility genetics by "back-tracking" into the genome from the proteomes of affected individuals compared to fertile controls.

1.2.2.8
Identification of Phosphoproteins and Glycoproteins

In addition to the proteomic methods described above, several other strategies being employed to identify interesting sperm proteins include identification of phosphoproteins and glycoproteins. It is well established that capacitation, a prerequisite event for fertilization requires a cyclic AMP-dependent increase in tyrosine phosphorylation. One of the approaches employed to target phosphoproteins involved in the capacitation event is 2D gel analysis coupled to antiphosphotyrosine immunoblots and tandem mass spectrometry [84]. The glycoproteins on the other hand may be identified by lectin blotting coupled to 2D gel electrophoresis [31].

1.2.2.9
Identification and Mining of Low Abundant Proteins

An important challenge in most of the proteomic methods described above is the identification and mining of antibody reactive, low abundant proteins. Prefractionation of the proteins by continuous elution preparative electrophoresis (using PrepCell from Bio-Rad) and preparative IEF (using Rotofor from Bio-rad) are useful methods of choice for enriching these low abundant proteins.

1.2.2.10
Coring of Protein Spots for Microsequencing and Cloning of Novel Genes

In excising proteins from a 2D gel it is essential to precisely define the boundaries of individual protein spots to obtaining pure proteins for microsequencing. Figure 1.2.3 demonstrates exceptionally useful tools for coring spots of interest from a silver stained 2D gel. These custom-made coring tools consist of hollow cylindrical steel tubes with specialized tips milled to a razor sharp edge. Different bore sizes range from a diameter of 0.5–5 mm and each coring tool holds a solid piston within the tube for expulsing gel plugs. A tube of appropriate diameter is chosen to just encompass an individual protein spot and the acrylamide plug is precisely drawn into the tube by placing the tube vertically on the center of the spot with the coring tip down and applying gentle pressure. The piston is used to extrude the gel piece into a sample tube. Use of these precision coring tools has resulted in a high incidence of unique and novel peptide sequence resulting from mass spectrometry. Such sequences may match an Expressed Sequence Tag (EST) sequence which may then be used to clone the corresponding gene by PCR. In the absence of any known sequence in the data

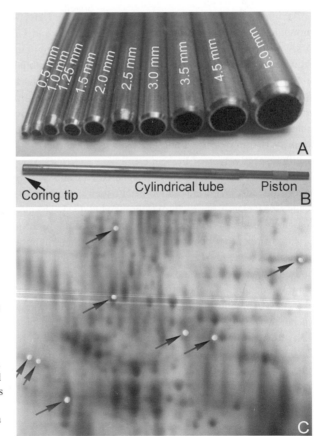

Fig. 1.2.3 Technique for protein spot excision from 2D gels using finely milled coring tools of various bores. (**a**) The sharpened end of several coring tools. (**b**) A lateral view of a single coring tool showing the cylindrical tube with a solid piston used to extrude the cored gel plug from the tube. (**c**) Portion of a silver stained 2D gel showing various spots cored for protein digestion and microsequencing using a 1.5 mm bore coring tool

base, the gene can be cloned by using a completely degenerate deoxyinosine-containing sense primer and adaptor primer, and performing a 5′ and 3′ rapid amplification of cDNA ends (RACE) PCR [32].

1.2.3
cDNA Library Screening

This strategy combines recombinant DNA technology with the experimental approach as described by Hjort and Griffin [85]. Typically a testis lambda expression library is used in this strategy and is plated with a chosen strain of E.coli as host bacterium. After growth at 42°C and induction with isopropyl-β-thiogalactoside (IPTG), the nitrocellulose filters are screened with the sperm antibody of interest. Bound recombinant protein is detected by use of an isotype specific secondary antibody coupled to horse-radish peroxidase. The cDNA insert of the positive clone is utilized again to reprobe the testis lambda cDNA library to confirm the sequence of the identified clone and also to identify any additional clones.

Wright et al. [86] identified the SP-10 cDNA (ARCV1 gene) using the MHS-10 monoclonal antibody with this method. Diekman and Goldberg [87] used sera from ASA-positive infertile patients and vasectomized men to identify an antigen, designated AgX, expressed by recombinant bacteriophage in a human testis library. Later studies used similar methods to identify additional sperm/testis antigens [88, 89]. In another study, the FA-1 mAb was used for a screening of murine testis lambda gt11 cDNA expression library [90] and the novel sperm protein discovered was named FA-1 for its potential role in fertilization. A similar strategy was employed by the same group to identify two more sperm antigens NZ-1 [91] and NZ-2 [92] from mouse and human origin respectively.

Two monoclonal antibodies, designated S71 and S72 (by World Health Organization workshop on ASA), were used to isolate their corresponding cDNA clones from a human testis λZAP cDNA library by Westbrook et al. [71]. The cloned gene was named SPAN-X for sperm protein associated with the nucleus on the X chromosome.

In an attempt to identify peptide sequences that might be involved in ZP binding Naz et al. [44] screened FliTrx random phage display library with solubilized human ZP. A novel dodecamer sequence, designated as YLP_{12}, was identified that is involved in sperm-ZP recognition/binding. A subtractive cDNA hybridization technology was employed by Naz et al. [93] to obtain sperm specific antigens that could be targeted as potential contraceptive vaccines. The ^{32}P-labeled single stranded cDNA of human testis, subtracted with poly(A)$^+$ RNA of human peripheral white blood cells, was used to screen the human testis cDNA-ZAP II library. The putative positive clones were further screened for binding with the solubilized human oocyte ZP preparation. The procedure allowed the discovery of a novel testis-specific antigen named CV. In vitro studies with the CV antibodies showed inhibition of human sperm from penetration of zona-free hamster oocytes and human sperm binding to human ZP.

cDNA library screening techniques can also be used as a strategy to isolate the complete cDNA for an unknown candidate molecule when a small region of the cDNA corresponding to the gene is known (e.g., through EST data base). Shetty et al. [18] applied the technique to clone the full-length cDNA for SAMP14 using a PCR amplified partial cDNA (derived from EST) clone from human testis as a probe to screen a λDR2 cDNA library. A similar strategy was used earlier by Wolkowicz et al. [94] to clone the full-length cDNA for a human sperm flagellar protein tectin-B1.

The identification of a candidate molecule is followed by experiments to determine its localization, tissue specificity and functional assays to elucidate its possible role in fertilization. This generally requires expression of a recombinant protein in bacteria or in a host of choice to produce sufficient protein to generate antibodies and for functional assays.

1.2.4
Summary

An integration of several methods of protein isolation, enrichment, and identification provide powerful tools to dissect the molecular architecture of spermatozoa. For example combining vectorial labeling with phase partitioning and immunoblotting has the potential to enrich for and readily identify a subset of hydrophobic membrane associated auto-antigens. Figure 1.2.4 depicts an overview of the different methods that can be employed to identify and characterize sperm antigens that are functionally relevant for fertilization and events leading to fertilization. Even though 2D electrophoresis technology has its limitations, it still remains a stalwart approach when coupled with mass spectrometry for the methodical characterization of proteomes. Currently one of the major challenges in identifying functionally relevant sperm antigens is to devise methodologies to isolate and enrich the molecules from subdomains of the sperm involved in the fertilization event, so that a careful analysis of all the molecules including the low abundant ones can be made. The use of naturally occurring ASA remains an attractive approach for the identification of immunoreactive antigens for immunocontraceptive purposes and for defining the autoantigens associated with immunoinfertility. We predict that more sperm auto-antigens will be defined by the methods discussed above as the full protein repertoire recognized by mankind's immune diversity is resolved. We envision a future time when 2D immunoblots and databases of 2D gels may become a standard clinical assay for the differential diagnosis of immuno-infertility. Protein arrays containing the major immunodominant proteins recognized by the human immune response may in the future offer simple diagnostic tests for determining patients with antibodies to sperm surface antigens essential for fertilization.

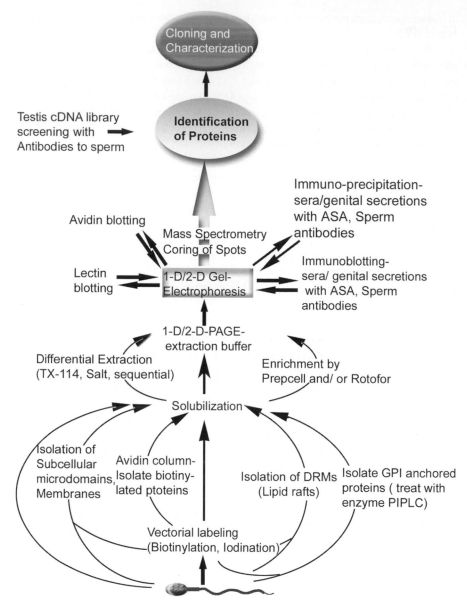

Fig. 1.2.4 An outline of molecular approaches applied to the sperm cell that are useful in the identification of sperm antigens involved in fertilization

References

1. Yanagimachi R (1994) Mammalian fertilization. In: Knobil E, Neill JD (eds) The physiology of reproduction. New York, Raven, pp 189–317
2. Anway MD, Li Y, Ravindranath N et al (2003) Expression of testicular germ cell genes identified by differential display analysis. J Androl 24:173–184
3. Catalano RD, Vlad M, Kennedy RC (1997) Differential display to identify and isolate novel genes expressed during spermatogenesis. Mol Hum Reprod 3:215–221
4. O'Shaughnessy PJ, Fleming L, Baker PJ et al (2003) Identification of developmentally regulated genes in the somatic cells of the mouse testis using serial analysis of gene expression. Biol Reprod 69:797–808
5. Aguilar-Mahecha A, Hales BF, Robaire B (2001) Expression of stress response genes in germ cells during spermatogenesis. Biol Reprod 65:119–127
6. Almstrup K, Nielsen JE, Hansen MA et al (2004) Analysis of cell-type-specific gene expression during mouse spermatogenesis. Biol Reprod 70:1751–1761
7. Guo R, Yu Z, Guan J et al (2004) Stage-specific and tissue-specific expression characteristics of differentially expressed genes during mouse spermatogenesis. Mol Reprod Dev 67:264–272
8. Yu Z, Guo R, Ge Y et al (2003) Gene expression profiles in different stages of mouse spermatogenic cells during spermatogenesis. Biol Reprod 69:37–47
9. O'Farrell P (1975) High resolution two-dimensional electrophoresis of proteins. J Biol Chem 250:4007–4021
10. Bjellqvist B, Ek K, Righetti PG et al (1982) Isoelectric focusing in immobilized pH gradients: principle, methodology and some applications. J Biochem Biophys Methods 6:317–339
11. Naaby-Hansen S, Flickinger CJ, Herr JC (1997) Two-dimensional electrophoretic analysis of vectorially labeled surface proteins of human spermatozoa. Biol Reprod 56:771–787
12. Shetty J, Diekman AB, Jayes FC et al (2001) Differential extraction and enrichment of human sperm surface proteins in a proteome: identification of immunocontraceptive candidates. Electrophoresis 22:3053–3066
13. D'Cruz OJ, Haas GG Jr, Lambert H (1993) Heterogeneity of human sperm surface antigens identified by indirect immunoprecipitation of antisperm antibody bound to biotinylated sperm. J Immunol 151:1062–1074
14. Paradowska A, Bohring C, Krause E et al (2006) Identification of evolutionary conserved mouse sperm surface antigens by human antisperm antibodies (ASA) from infertile patients. Am J Reprod Immunol 55:321–330
15. Stein KK, Go JC, Lane WS et al (2006) Proteomic analysis of sperm regions that mediate sperm–egg interactions. Proteomics 6:3533–3543
16. Pasten C, Morales P, Kong M (2005) Role of the sperm proteasome during fertilization and gamete interaction in the mouse. Mol Reprod Dev 71:209–219
17. Yudin AI, Cherr GN, Vandevoort CA et al (1988) Rearrangement of the PH-20 protein on the surface of macaque spermatozoa following exposure to anti-PH-20 antibodies or binding to zona pellucida. Mol Reprod Dev 50:207–220
18. Shetty J, Wolkowicz MJ, Digilio LC et al (2003) SAMP14, a novel, acrosomal membrane-associated, glycosylphosphatidylinositol-anchored member of the Ly-6/urokinase-type plasminogen activator receptor superfamily with a role in sperm-egg interaction. J Biol Chem 278:30506–30515
19. Hao Z, Wolkowicz MJ, Shetty J et al (2002) SAMP32, a testis-specific, isoantigenic sperm acrosomal membrane-associated protein. Biol Reprod 66:735–744
20. Bronson R, Cooper G, Rosenfeld D (1984) Sperm antibodies: their role in infertility. Fertil Steril 42:171–183

21. Isojima S, Li TS, Ashitaka Y (1968) Immunologic analysis of sperm-immobilizing factor found in sera of women with unexplained sterility. Am J Obstet Gynecol 101:677–683
22. Ayvaliotis B, Bronson R, Rosenfeld D et al (1985) Conception rates in couples where autoimmunity to sperm is detected. Fertil Steril 43:739–742
23. Collins JA, Burrows EA, Yeo J et al (1993) Frequency and predictive value of antisperm antibodies among infertile couples. Hum Reprod 8:592–598
24. Heidenreich A, Bonfig R, Wilbert DM et al (1994) Risk factors for antisperm antibodies in infertile men. Am J Reprod Immunol 31:69–76
25. Omu AE, Makhseed M, Mohammed AT et al (1997) Characteristics of men and women with circulating antisperm antibodies in a combined infertility clinic in Kuwait. Arch Androl 39:55–64
26. Sinisi AA, Di Finizio B, Pasquali D et al (1993) Prevalence of antisperm antibodies by SpermMARtest in subjects undergoing a routine sperm analysis for infertility. Int J Androl 16:311–314
27. Chamley LW, Clarke GN (2007) Antisperm antibodies and conception. Semin Immunopathol 29:169–184
28. Lombardo F, Gandini L, Dondero F et al (2001) Antisperm immunity in natural and assisted reproduction. Hum Reprod Update 7:450–456
29. Shetty J, Naaby-Hansen S, Shibahara H et al (1999) Human sperm proteome: immunodominant sperm surface antigens identified with sera from infertile men and women. Biol Reprod 61:61–69
30. Wolkowicz MJ, Digilio L, Klotz K et al (2008) Equatorial segment protein (ESP) is a human alloantigen involved in sperm–egg binding and fusion. J Androl 29:272–282
31. Wolkowicz MJ, Shetty J, Westbrook A et al (2003) Equatorial segment protein defines a discrete acrosomal subcompartment persisting throughout acrosomal biogenesis. Biol Reprod 69:735–745
32. Naaby-Hansen S, Mandal A, Wolkowicz MJ et al (2002) CABYR, a novel calcium-binding tyrosine phosphorylation-regulated fibrous sheath protein involved in capacitation. Dev Biol 242:236–254
33. Shibahara H, Sato I, Shetty J et al (2002) Two-dimensional electrophoretic analysis of sperm antigens recognized by sperm immobilizing antibodies detected in infertile women. J Reprod Immunol 53:1–12
34. Bhande S, Naz RK (2007) Molecular identities of human sperm proteins reactive with antibodies in sera of immunoinfertile women. Mol Reprod Dev 74:332–340
35. Bohring C, Krause E, Habermann B et al (2001) Isolation and identification of sperm membrane antigens recognized by antisperm antibodies, and their possible role in immunological infertility disease. Mol Hum Reprod 7:113–118
36. Marmar JL (1991) The status of vasectomy reversals. Int J Fertil 36:352–357
37. Naaby-Hansen S (1990) The humoral autoimmune response to vasectomy described by immunoblotting from two-dimensional gels and demonstration of a human spermatozoal antigen immunochemically crossreactive with the D2 adhesion molecule. J Reprod Immunol 17:187–205
38. Primakoff P, Lathrop W, Bronson R (1990) Identification of human sperm surface glycoproteins recognized by autoantisera from immune infertile men, women, and vasectomized men. Biol Reprod 42:929–942
39. Shetty J, Bronson RA, Herr JC (2008) Human sperm protein encyclopedia and alloantigen index: mining novel allo-antigens using sera from ASA-positive infertile patients and vasectomized men. J Reprod Immunol 77:23–31
40. Domagala A, Pulido S, Kurpisz M et al (2007) Application of proteomic methods for identification of sperm immunogenic antigens. Mol Hum Reprod 13:437–444
41. Auer J, Senechal H, Desvaux FX et al (2000) Isolation and characterization of two sperm membrane proteins recognized by sperm-associated antibodies in infertile men. Mol Reprod Dev 57:393–405

42. Naz RK (2005) Search for peptide sequences involved in human antisperm antibody-mediated male immunoinfertility by using phage display technology. Mol Reprod Dev 72:25–30
43. Naz RK, Chauhan SC (2001) Presence of antibodies to sperm YLP(12) synthetic peptide in sera and seminal plasma of immunoinfertile men. Mol Hum Reprod 7:21–26
44. Naz RK, Zhu X, Kadam AL (2000) Identification of human sperm peptide sequence involved in egg binding for immunocontraception. Biol Reprod 62:318–324
45. Bordier C (1981) Phase separation of integral membrane proteins in Triton X-114 solution. J Biol Chem 256:1604–1607
46. Hooper NM, Turner AJ (1988) Ectoenzymes of the kidney microvillar membrane. Aminopeptidase P is anchored by a glycosyl-phosphatidylinositol moiety. FEBS Lett 229:340–344
47. Diekman AB, Westbrook-Case VA, Naaby-Hansen S et al (1997) Biochemical characterization of sperm agglutination antigen-1, a human sperm surface antigen implicated in gamete interactions. Biol Reprod 57:1136–1344
48. Westbrook-Case VA, Winfrey VP, Olson GE (1994) Characterization of two antigenically related integral membrane proteins of the guinea pig sperm periacrosomal plasma membrane. Mol Reprod Dev 39:309–321
49. Young GP, Koide SS, Goldstein M et al (1988) Isolation and partial characterization of an ion channel protein from human sperm membranes. Arch Biochem Biophys 262:491–500
50. Ohlendieck K (2003) Extraction of membrane proteins. In: Protein purification protocols. Methods in molecular biology, vol 244, pp 283–293
51. Johnson RA, Jakobs KH, Schultz G (1985) Extraction of the adenylate cyclase-activating factor of bovine sperm and its identification as a trypsin-like protease. J Biol Chem 260:114–121
52. Pike LJ (2006) Rafts defined: a report on the keystone symposium on lipid rafts and cell function). J Lipid Res 47:1597–1598
53. Mishra S, Joshi PG (2007) Lipid raft heterogencity: an enigma. J Neurochem 103:135–142
54. Brown DA, Rose JK (1992) Sorting of GPI-anchored proteins to glycolipid-enriched membrane subdomains during transport to the apical cell surface. Cell 68:533–544
55. Travis AJ, Merdiushev T, Vargas LA et al (2001) Expression and localization of caveolin-1, and the presence of membrane rafts, in mouse and guinea pig spermatozoa. Dev Biol 240:599–610
56. Sleight SB, Miranda PV, Plaskett NW et al (2005) Isolation and proteomic analysis of mouse sperm detergent-resistant membrane fractions: evidence for dissociation of lipid rafts during capacitation. Biol Reprod 73:721–729
57. Inoue N, Ikawa M, Isotani A et al (2005) The immunoglobulin superfamily protein Izumo is required for sperm to fuse with eggs. Nature 434:234–238
58. Thaler CD, Thomas M, Ramalie JR (2006) Reorganization of mouse sperm lipid rafts by capacitation. Mol Reprod Dev 73:1541–1549
59. Bou Khalil M, Chakrabandhu K, Xu H et al (2006) Sperm capacitation induces an increase in lipid rafts having zona pellucida binding ability and containing sulfogalactosylglycerolipid. Dev Biol 290:220–235
60. van Gestel RA, Brewis IA, Ashton PR et al (2005) Capacitation-dependent concentration of lipid rafts in the apical ridge head area of porcine sperm cells. Mol Hum Reprod 11:583–590
61. Nixon B, Bielanowicz A, McLaughlin EA et al (2009) Composition and significance of detergent resistant membranes in mouse spermatozoa. J Cell Physiol 218:122–134
62. Bohring C, Krause W (1999) The characterization of human spermatozoa membrane proteins–surface antigens and immunological infertility. Electrophoresis 20:971–976
63. Yu Y, Xu W, Yi YJ et al (2006) The extracellular protein coat of the inner acrosomal membrane is involved in zona pellucida binding and penetration during fertilization: characterization of its most prominent polypeptide (IAM38). Dev Biol 290:32–43
64. Anderson DJ, Johnson PM, Alexander NJ et al (1987) Monoclonal antibodies to human trophoblast and sperm antigens: report of two WHO-sponsored workshops, June 30, 1986, Toronto, Canada. J Reprod Immunol 10:231–257

65. Herr JC, Flickinger CJ, Homyk M et al (1990) Biochemical and morphological characterization of the intra-acrosomal antigen SP-10 from human sperm. Biol Reprod 42:181–193
66. Hsi BL, Yeh CJ, Fénichel P et al (1988) Monoclonal antibody GB24 recognizes a trophoblast-lymphocyte cross-reactive antigen. Am J Reprod Immunol Microbiol 18:21–27
67. Isojima S, Kameda K, Tsuji Y et al (1987) Establishment and characterization of a human hybridoma secreting monoclonal antibody with high titers of sperm immobilizing and agglutinating activities against human seminal plasma. J Reprod Immunol 10:67–78
68. Naz RK, Morte C, Garcia-Framis V et al (1993) Characterization of a sperm-specific monoclonal antibody and isolation of 95-kilodalton fertilization antigen-2 from human sperm. Biol Reprod 49:1236–1244
69. Neilson LI, Schneider PA, Van Deerlin PG et al (1999) cDNA cloning and characterization of a human sperm antigen (SPAG6) with homology to the product of the Chlamydomonas PF16 locus. Genomics 60:272–280
70. Primakoff P, Hyatt H, Myles DG (1985) A role for the migrating sperm surface antigen PH-20 in guinea pig sperm binding to the egg zona pellucida. J Cell Biol 101:2239–2244
71. Westbrook VA, Diekman AB, Klotz KL et al (2000) Spermatid-specific expression of the novel X-linked gene product SPAN-X localized to the nucleus of human spermatozoa. Biol Reprod 63:469–481
72. Yan YC, Wang LF, Koide SS (1987) Properties of a monoclonal antibody interacting with human sperm. Arch Androl 18:245–254
73. Ikezawa H (2002) Glycosylphosphatidylinositol (GPI)-anchored proteins. Biol Pharm Bull 25:409–417
74. Kinoshita T, Ohishi K, Takeda J (1997) GPI-anchor synthesis in mammalian cells: genes, their products, and a deficiency. J Biochem 122:251–257
75. Nozaki M, Ohishi K, Yamada N et al (1999) Developmental abnormalities of glycosylphosphatidylinositol-anchor-deficient embryos revealed by Cre/loxP system. Lab Invest 79:293–299
76. Alfieri JA, Martin AD, Takeda J, Kondoh G et al (2003) Infertility in female mice with an oocyte-specific knockout of GPI-anchored proteins. J Cell Sci 116:2149–2155
77. Tarutani M, Itami S, Okabe M et al (1997) Tissue-specific knockout of the mouse Pig-a gene reveals important roles for GPI-anchored proteins in skin development. Proc Natl Acad Sci U S A 94:7400–7405
78. Cherr GN, Yudin AI, Overstreet JW (2001) The dual functions of GPI-anchored PH-20: hyaluronidase and intracellular signaling. Matrix Biol 20:515–525
79. Kondoh G, Tojo H, Nakatani Y et al (2005) Angiotensin-converting enzyme is a GPI-anchored protein releasing factor crucial for fertilization. Nat Med 11:160–166
80. Griffith OH, Volwerk JJ, Kuppe A (1991) Phosphatidylinositol-specific phospholipases C from *Bacillus cereus* and *Bacillus thuringiensis*. Methods Enzymol 197:493–502
81. Coonrod S, Naaby-Hansen S, Shetty J et al (1999) PI-PLC releases a 25–40 kDa protein cluster from the hamster oolemma and affects the sperm penetration assay. Mol Hum Reprod 5:1027–1033
82. Unlü M, Morgan ME, Minden JS (1997) Difference gel electrophoresis: a single gel method for detecting changes in protein extracts. Electrophoresis 18:2071–2077
83. Baker MA, Witherdin R, Hetherington L et al (2005) Identification of post-translational modifications that occur during sperm maturation using difference in two-dimensional gel electrophoresis. Proteomics 5:1003–1012
84. Ficarro S, Chertihin O, Westbrook VA et al (2003) Phosphoproteome analysis of capacitated human sperm. Evidence of tyrosine phosphorylation of a kinase-anchoring protein 3 and valosin-containing protein/p97 during capacitation. J Biol Chem 278:11579–11589
85. Hjort T, Griffin PD (1985) The identification of candidate antigens for the development of birth control vaccines. An international multi-centre study on antibodies to reproductive tract antigens, using clinically defined sera. J Reprod Immunol 8:271–278

86. Wright RM, John E, Klotz K et al (1990) Cloning and sequencing of cDNAs coding for the human intra-acrosomal antigen SP-10. Biol Reprod 42:693–701
87. Diekman AB, Goldberg E (1994) Characterization of a human antigen with sera from infertile patients. Biol Reprod 50:1087–1093
88. Liang ZG, O'Hern PA, Yavetz B et al (1994) Human testis cDNAs identified by sera from infertile patients: a molecular biological approach to immunocontraceptive development. Reprod Fertil Dev 6:297–305
89. Liu QY, Wang LF, Miao SY et al (1996) Expression and characterization of a novel human sperm membrane protein. Biol Reprod 54:323–330
90. Zhu X, Naz RK (1997) Fertilization antigen-1: cDNA cloning, testis-specific expression, and immunocontraceptive effects. Proc Natl Acad Sci U S A. 94:4704–4709
91. Naz RK, Zhu X (1997) Molecular cloning and sequencing of cDNA encoding for a novel testis-specific antigen. Mol Reprod Dev 48:449–457
92. Zhu X, Naz RK (1998) Cloning and sequencing of cDNA encoding for a human sperm antigen involved in fertilization. Mol Reprod Dev 51:176–183
93. Naz RK, Zhu X, Kadam AL (2001) Cloning and sequencing of cDNA encoding for a novel human testis-specific contraceptive vaccinogen: role in immunocontraception. Mol Reprod Dev 60:116–127
94. Wolkowicz MJ, Naaby-Hansen S, Gamble AR et al (2002) Tektin B1 demonstrates flagellar localization in human sperm. Biol Reprod 66:241–250

Sperm Surface Proteomics

1.3

B. M. Gadella

1.3.1
Introduction

1.3.1.1
The Sperm Surface

The sperm is a highly polarized cell with a minimum of cytosol and organelles [1, 2]. The sperm head has two organelles namely the nucleus that houses the male haploid genome which is highly condensed to protamines and a large secretory granule called the acrosome, which is oriented over the anterior area of the sperm nucleus. At the distal part of the sperm head the flagellum sprouts. In the mid-piece of this flagellum mitochondria are spiraled around the microtubules of the flagellum. In the tail part, specific cytoskeletal elements surround the microtubules of the flagellum. The surface of the head, midpiece, and tail parts of the sperm is heterogeneous [3, 4] and reflects the polar distributed organelles that lie under the surface. Especially the sperm head surface is heterogeneous and at least different regions can be distinguished with separate functions in the fertilization process. In general, the sperm of fertile men has lost many somatic cell features, doesn't house an endoplasmic reticulum, Golgi, lysosomes, or peroxisomes, and has lost ribosomes. As a result, the sperm has lost the potential for gene expression (both transcription and translation processes are completely silenced [5]). The sperm also has lost almost the entire cytoplasm. The cell has a typical ordering of the remaining organelles and cytoskeletal elements and probably this polar ordering is reflected into the lateral ordering of the sperm's surface domain [6].

B. M. Gadella
Departments of Biochemistry and Cell Biology and of Farm Animal Health, Utrecht University, 3584 CM, Utrecht, The Netherlands
e-mail: B.M.Gadella@uu.nl

W. K. H. Krause and R. K. Naz (eds.), *Immune Infertility*,
DOI: 10.1007/978-3-642-01379-9_1.3, © Springer Verlag Berlin Heidelberg 2009

1.3.1.2
Function of Sperm Membrane Domains at Fertilization

Especially the subdomains of the sperm head area have diversified functions in the series of processes that are involved in fertilization. The apical ridge area of the sperm head specifically recognizes and binds to the zona pellucida (the extracellular matrix of the oocyte) [7] while a larger area of the sperm head surface (the pre-equatorial domain) is involved in the acrosome reaction, which results in the release of acrosome components required for zona penetration [2, 8]. The equatorial segment of the sperm head remains intact after the acrosome reaction and is the specific area that recognizes and fuses with the oolemma (the egg's plasma membrane) in order to fertilize the oocyte [9]. Although the mid-piece and the tail surfaces of the sperm cell are also heterogeneous, the functions of these surface specializations are not yet understood [10]. It is well possible that they are involved in organization of optimal sperm motility characteristics. When studying the sperm surface proteins, the researcher has to keep in mind that a rather complex surface is under study and especially for studying the processes of fertilization in which the sperm head surface is involved (zona binding, acrosome reaction, and fertilization) this specific surface area needs first to be separated and purified.

1.3.1.3
Sperm Surface Dynamics Before Fertilization

The surface domain of the sperm is already apparent in spermatids before spermination in the seminiferous tubules of the testis [1]. The molecular dynamics, involved in the establishment of surface specialization upon spermatogenesis, is largely unknown. Moreover, once liberated in the lumen of the seminiferous tubule the sperm will start its travel through the male and female genital tract and will meet a sequence of different environments. During this voyage, surface remodeling takes place most likely at any site of the two genital tracts at the following instances: (1) upon somatic maturation in the epididymis [11], (2) by re- and decoating events induced by the accessory fluids combined at ejaculation, probably stabilizing the sperm for its further journey in the female genital tract [12, 13], (3) after their deposition in the female genital tract which is followed with the removal of extracellular glycoprotein coating (release of decapacitation factors) and further remodeling by (cervical) uterine; oviduct secretions are activating the sperm to meet the oocyte (in vivo capacitation) [14, 15], and (4) the sperm also interacts with cumulus cells, remaining follicular fluid components surrounding and impregnating the zona pellucida [16, 17], and with components even in the peri-vitellin space (i.e., the fluid filled space between the zona pellucida and the oolemma) [18]. All these changing environments may cause surface remodeling of the sperm and therefore, may influence its potential to fertilize the oocyte.

The possible mechanisms of altering the sperm surface are reviewed earlier [19] and are schematically drawn in Fig. 1.3.1. It is very difficult to study the above described sperm surface alterations in situ. However, for many mammalian species, including human, specific sperm handling and incubation media have been optimized for

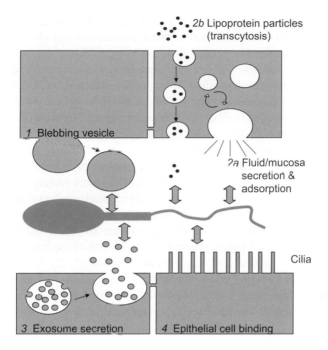

Fig. 1.3.1 Possible alterations at the surface of sperm because of somatic modifications in the lumen of the male and female genital tracts (adapted from [19]). Possible interactions of male and female genital tract components with the sperm surface: (1) From the diverse epithelia of the male and female genital tracts blebbing vesicles containing cytosol may be released into the genital fluids. Such vesicles may interact and exchange surface components with sperm. It is highly unlikely that such vesicles fuse with sperm as this would dramatically increase the volume of sperm (which has been reduced maximally in order to obtain an ergonomically designed cell optimally suited for fertilization). (2a) Serum components can be released into the genital fluids by transcytosis [80]. Interestingly lipoprotein particles may invade the surroundings of sperm and may facilitate exchange of larger particles and the sperm surface. (2b) Fluid phase secretion and adsorption of either fluid or mucosa may directly alter the ECM of sperm. (3) Apocrine secretion of exosomes has been suggested to alter the sperm surface and sperm functioning. Exosomes have been demonstrated to be secreted by the epididymis (epididymosomes) and by the prostate (prostasomes) [81, 82] but likely are also secreted throughout the female genital tract. Interestingly exosomes may provide sperm with tetraspanins, a group of membrane proteins involved in tethering of proteins into protein complexes. Recently the addition of CD9 onto the sperm surface by membrane particles has been described to occur even when sperm reaches the perivitellin space [18]. (4) Sperm interacts with ciliated epithelial cells; this has been observed in the oviduct [83], and probably has a physiological role during in situ capacitation. Sperm interactions with other ciliated epithelial cells of the female and male genital tract have not been studied extensively. It is possible that such interactions are important for sperm surface remodeling and for sperm physiology

efficient in vitro fertilization purposes. In general, mammalian sperm are activated in a medium that compares with the oviduct in that it contains the capacitation factors such as high concentrations of bicarbonate, free calcium ions, and lipoproteins such as albumin [8]. In some species specific glycoconjugates [20] or phosphodiesterase inhibitors are added for extra sperm activation [21]. All strategies are designed to evoke capacitation in vitro. This implies that the researcher can observe the relevant sperm surface reorganization primed under in vitro condition for fertilization. The membrane composition as well as ordering of membrane components can be compared with control conditions (media without the capacitation factors) or with the membrane ordering of the sperm at collection time. The sperm can be collected at ejaculation for humans, boars, stallions, and bulls, but it needs to be aspirated from the cauda epididymis for murine species (rat, mouse Guinea pig) which can also be the case under certain clinical conditions from male subfertile patients in the IVF clinic. Especially the surface reordering of membrane proteins and lipids in the sperm head has been studied extensively under in vitro capacitation conditions (for recent reviews see [8, 22]). It is important to stress the importance of the sperm surface reordering and changes in composition of membrane components because of diverse extracellular factors. The induced lateral redistribution of membrane components appears also to be instrumental for the assemblage of a functional sperm protein complex involved in sperm–zona binding, as well as for the zona-induction of the acrosome reaction [7, 23, 24]. Therefore, the researcher interested in the surface proteome of sperm needs, beyond understanding the composition of the sperm surface proteins, to consider how these proteins are organized and whether they are functionally complexed for their physiological role in fertilization.

1.3.2
Isolation of Sperm Surface Proteins

Membrane proteins can be classified as integral membrane proteins and peripheral proteins. Most integral membrane proteins have an extracellular domain and a transmembrane domain (often an alpha helix region with the hydrophobic part exposed to the fatty acid moieties of the phospholipid bilayer); however, other integral membrane proteins interact by covalent lipid anchors such as GPI, or by processes such as acylation[25]. Peripheral proteins have electrostatic interactions with the integral membrane proteins or with the lipids of the membrane. Discrimination between these two membrane proteins can be done by treating membrane preparations with high salt concentration, which destabilizes the electrostatic interaction and leads to the release of peripheral membrane proteins while the integral membrane proteins remain in the insoluble membrane fraction. In general, to study the sperm surface proteins one has to isolate the sperm membrane from soluble proteins and insoluble nonmembrane material (such as cytoskeleton components and the condensed nuclear chromatin). Furthermore, the researchers need to pay attention to indirect interactions of nonsurface material with the membrane extract.

To isolate the membrane fraction, end specific sperm disruption methods such as ultrasonication and nitrogen cavitation have been designed [26]. Sonication gives less pure and less defined membrane fraction [27]. After sperm disruption differential centrifugation techniques need to be employed to isolate sperm membranes from insoluble cellular debris and soluble components. The researcher needs to consider that the disruption method, as well as the isolation protocol, is really delivering sperm plasma membrane and also intracellular membranes. This is especially relevant for studying proteins involved in zona recognition. When the plasma membrane preparation also contains acrosomal contamination one can be sure that secondary (intra-acrosomal) zona binding proteins will be identified and they will possibly overwhelm the amount of primary (plasma membrane) zona binding proteins [7, 28]. To this end, the specific abundance of marker proteins or specific activities of marker enzymes of plasma membrane and intracellular membranes need to be quantified. The relative purification is necessary for the purity of the membrane fraction of surface proteins. In our hands an optimized nitrogen cavitation method turned out to yield a 200 times enriched plasma membrane fraction over possible contaminating membranes with a yield of approximately 30% of the sperm's surface [26]. Moreover, ultrastructural analysis of this membrane fraction and of disrupted sperm showed that the isolated plasma membrane fraction contained resealed plasma membrane vesicles. The vesicles were so called right-side outside unilamellar vesicles implicating that the outer and inner sides of the vesicle membranes had the same protein topology as in the intact plasma membrane of the sperm and that the resealed plasma membrane vesicles had not encapsulated intracellular membranes. This membrane preparation turned out to be instrumental to study protein–protein interactions relevant for the sperm–zona binding [7] and for the redistribution of membrane microdomains believed to represent lipid rafts [29].

Human sperm surface preparations are usually made after a hypo-osmotic incubation followed by sonication and differential centrifugation (see for instance [30]). The purity of such membrane preparations for sperm plasma membrane material is not well documented and contamination with intracellular membranes is likely (see Sect. 1.3.2).

Another method to isolate surface proteins is to make use of lectins immobilized to form beads. Lectins can bind to specific sugar residues at the extracellular domain of integral membrane proteins. Some marker lectins exclusively bind to the sperm plasma membrane. Therefore, affinity chromatography using immobilized lectins can be used to extract surface proteins [31]. This method can also be employed on nitrogen cavitated and solubilized sperm plasma membrane material.

Finally membrane raft isolation procedures can be employed to isolate microdomains from sperm [32, 33]. Most methods use detergents at low temperature (4°C) to isolate the detergent resistant membrane (DRM) fraction. Our group has found that this DRM fraction after capacitation becomes highly enriched in GPI anchored proteins and in proteins involved in zona binding and the acosrosome reaction [24, 29]. With the use of phosphatidylinositol specific phospholipase C, GPI anchored proteins can be cleaved of the DRM (enriched in these proteins) in untreated sperm [34]. We have preliminary data suggesting that DRM from the entire sperm contains besides surface membrane material also intercellular (acrosomal) membrane material. The DRM fraction of the whole sperm contains components that could be labeled with marker lectins for the outer acrosomal membrane. DRMs from purified plasma membranes did not show any labeling with this lectin. The best explanation for these results is that the outer acrosomal membrane also contains lipid rafts, which may explain the results of [35].

1.3.3
Detection of Sperm Surface Proteins

1.3.3.1
Tagging of Sperm Proteins and Peptides

In the previous chapter a number of protein separation and mass spectrometric techniques were mentioned, which are of relevance for detecting and identifying amino acid sequences of peptides and proteins of sperm samples [36, 37]. Here, the strategies for proteomic analysis of surface sperm specific proteins will be specified. First of all, a number of proteomic protocols for studying differential expression of proteins in biological specimen under experimentally manipulated conditions cannot be used on the sperm. Those techniques make use of the fact that cells are fed with amino acids that are used for translation (amino acid coded tagging AACT [38, 39]). Control cells are fed with normal amino acids while the experimentally conditioned cells are fed with amino acids having stable isotope label tags (SILAC; most commonly used are the deuterium labeled amino acids $^2H_3$-Leu, $^2H_4$-Lys, $^2H_3$-Met, $^2H_2$-Tyr, $^2H_3$-Ser, and $^2H_2$-Gly; other labeled acids used are ^{15}N-enriched amino acids, $^{13}C_6$-Lys or –Arg, and ^{18}O labeled amino acids; for review see [40]). Most of these techniques can also be used to detect translational capacities of cell extracts in vitro. The use of isotopically labeled amino acids is not applicable for the sperm as the translational machinery has shut down in the last phase of spermatogenesis [5]. This implies that variations in the sperm surface protein composition are either due to the changing environments the sperm faces en route to fertilizing the oocyte (Sect. 1.3.3) or due to aberrations in the sperm formation process in the testis.

A number of sperm surface labeling techniques have been used to for proteomic analysis of sperm surface proteins. In human sperm for instance, ^{125}I labeling of sperm surface proteins or biotinylation of surface proteins has been employed to detect immunodominant sperm surface antigens [41, 42]. This method turned out to be not completely "membrane proof" as intracellular proteins became iodinated with this.

Another important technique is to use isotope-coded affinity tagging of protein mixtures. With this technique cystein containing proteins are tagged with either a light isotope tag or with a heavy coded tag. The tag includes a biotin group, an acid cleavable linker (TFA is used for cutting the biotin group), an isotope coded tag ($C_{10}H_{17}N_3O_3$ with either nine ^{13}C or nine ^{12}C atom) and a protein reactive group (iodoacetamine allowing covalent linking to Cys) [43]. The ICAT technology can be used on the isolated and solubilized membrane protein fractions and may be useful to detect changes in protein composition of sperm surface under various physiological and in vitro conditions (for instance the release of decapacitation factors during in vitro fertilization treatment, or alterations of the sperm surface proteins of sperm collected at different regions of the epididymis). The limitation of this technique is that only cystein containing proteins are tagged and therefore, only a relatively small subproteome can be detected. The labeled proteins are trypsinized and the resulting peptides are analyzed with LC and MS/MS technology. Another labeling technique useful to detect changes in the protein composition of the sperm surface is iTRAQ [44]. The big difference with ICAT (described above) is that in

ITRAQ the tag is covalently linked to peptides and not to proteins. The tag is isobaric and has an amino-specific protein reactive group which will label all peptide fragments. The isobaric tag consists of a reporter and a balance group, and in between a MS/MS fragmentation side. When the reporter group is a heavier isotope, the balance group is a lighter isotope so that together they form an isobaric group. This principle allows multiplex comparative analysis of peptide mixtures from more than two samples. Recently the technique has been upgraded and eight different experimental conditions can be compared. The big advantage is that ITRAQ is tagging all peptides of a given sample and that more than two samples can be compared with one another in one LC-MS/MS run.

Posttranslational changes of the sperm surface membrane can also be detected [45]. In this study 2D gel electrophoresis followed by western blot for protein phosphorylation was used to obtain protein spots of phosphorylated proteins. The matching spots from corresponding 2D gels were plugged and trypsinized followed by MS/MS detection. This approach provided valuable information on up and down regulation of protein phosphorylation at the individual protein level. However, the use of a Fe^{3+}-immobilized metal affinity chromatography column (IMAC) can be employed to trypsinized sperm surface protein samples. The peptides containing phosphoamino residues can be isolated. Identification of the phosphorylated peptides has led to a map of protein phosphorylation changes in human sperm [45–47]. Similarly a biotin-switch assay has been employed to detect protein S-nitrosylation in human sperm [48] which provided fundamental new insights in NO mediated sperm signaling under in vitro capacitation conditions. The modifications of these proteins take place intracellularly and only a surface specific membrane protein preparation can provide insights into surface post translational protein (see also Sect. 1.3.3.2).

1.3.3.2
Surface Specific Considerations for Sperm Proteomics

Section 1.3.3.1 deals with the applicability of a number of proteomic strategies to study sperm proteins. However, a number of additional considerations have to be taken into account when studying sperm surface proteomics. The researcher should be sure about the surface topology of the proteins under investigation. A first step in this direction is to isolate the membrane of interest (see Sect. 1.3.2). However, additional scrutiny needs to be involved in ruling out the high amount of proteins that interact only indirectly with the sperm surface as they become easily co-isolated and identified. To this end, the sperm can be labeled with membrane impermeable tags prior to membrane subfractionation. Most commonly a biotinylated tag is used which is covalently bound to the sperm surface proteins [49–51]. A streptavidin immobilized affinity column can be used to isolate the biotinylated proteins. After isolation, the tag can be cleaved enzymatically and the proteins can be digested for conversion into peptides for MS/MS analysis. Importantly this technique has some drawbacks, as one has to be sure that only surface oriented proteins are labeled. If sperm cells deteriorate during biotinylation, intracellular proteins will become biotinylated because they are accessible to the tag. For extracellular matrix components, this will always be the case even for intact sperm. Moreover, the sperm does contain a certain portion of endogenously biotinylated proteins. Finally, nonlabeled proteins may interact with the biotinylated proteins and thus may also be immobilized into the streptavidin columns. Indeed many studies using immuno-purified surface labeled membrane samples report the identification of a large number of nonmembrane proteins. There are many ways to reduce the amount of this contamination. For recent reviews on this topic see [25]. Besides the two steps mentioned here (labeling of the sperm surface and subsequent membrane isolation) the resulting preparations need to be treated with high salt media to get rid of adhering extracellular matrix and cytosolic components. The resulting membrane sample is highly enriched in integral membrane proteins.

Another important issue for integral membrane proteins, i.e., with (multiple) alpha helices spanning the membrane or with beta sheet barrels, is that such proteins have high hydrophobic domains. This property of a major portion of membrane proteins prevents easy solubilization which normally is required for (2D) gel-electrophoresis. Recent reviews provide an excellent overview of techniques that can be employed to identify these integral membrane proteins [25, 52]. For sperm surface proteomics, one should realize that the (2D) gel electrophoresis approaches fail to detect a large number of integral membrane proteins. The proposed experimental approach (either ICAT or ITRAQ described in the previous paragraph) overcomes this limitation by digesting a specific isolated sperm surface protein fraction and analyzing the derived peptides with LC-MS/MS.

The author would recommend combining a sperm surface protein labeling method (Sect. 1.3.3.1) with a surface membrane isolation method (Sect. 1.3.2) prior to immobilized affinity column steps. The resulting protein sample preferably is directly digested and, after ITRAQ labeling, analyzed in a full LC-MS/MS platform or alternatively, it is first subjected to ICAT and then digested for LC-MS/MS. The advantage of this approach is that peptides are obtained from membrane proteins without any gel electrophoretic step, allowing full range coverage of the sperm surface proteins.

1.3.4
Comparison of Surface Proteomics of Human Sperm with Those of Mouse and Porcine or Bovine Sperms

In Sects. 1.3.1–1.3.3 of this chapter, a number of considerations for studying the sperm surface proteome have been summarized. They need to be carefully considered in order to make proteomic databases of sperm surface protein composition more useful or meaningful. In this section more emphasis is put on how existing sperm proteomic libraries should be interpreted and where appropriate some comments will be made on suitability or originality of approaches used to decipher protein compositions of the sperm surface.

A number of groups have successfully analyzed the proteome of sperm (reviewed in Chap. 1.2 of this book). When browsing through the data generated, one needs to be critical of how the protein samples were prepared in order to understand how meaningful the proteomic libraries generated actually are for the sperm surface: (1) Sperm membranes are often isolated by the method of [30] in which sperms are first incubated in a hypo-osmotic environment followed by sonication and differential centrifugation. However, the purification for plasma membrane marker proteins from possible contaminating intracellular membranes is not tested convincingly for human sperm. (2) Indirect reacting proteins, for instance from the extracellular matrix or the cytoskeleton, may also be identified when the isolated membrane preparations were not subjected to high concentration of salt [25]. (3) Other groups use surface modification techniques to study sperm surface membrane proteins [41]. The labeled proteins are supposed to originate from the sperm surface but this approach has led to the iodination or biotinylation of many intracellular proteins. (4) The isolated or labeled proteins are routinely solubilized and subsequently separated using protein gel-electrophoresis. The drawback of this technique is that an important group of integral membrane proteins, because of their hydrophobic properties, are not suitable for PAGE [25] and off-gel peptide fractionation would become the method of choice for full surface proteome coverage [53].

These points of attention are valid for sperm surface proteomic studies independently of the mammalian species under study. However, there are also a number of species specific advantages and disadvantages in studying the human, mouse, and porcine or bovine sperm surface which will be dealt with in the next sections.

1.3.4.1
Human Sperm Proteomics

Some specific limitations intrinsic to human sperm need to be considered when studying the sperm surface proteome: (1) Humans (and some primate species) produce semen with a rather high content of abnormal sperm (immature, deteriorated, or morphologically aberrant) [84]. Even in the ejaculate of fertile men, the proportion of deteriorated sperm is >40% [54, 55], whereas the ejaculate of a fertile boar (male porcine) has only <5% aberrant sperm [56]. When assessing human sperm with the strict Tijgerberg criteria, semen with only 15% morphologically normal sperm turned out to be fertile with normal fertilization rates and morphology scores were rarely higher than 30% for most fertile men [57]; in porcine sperm this morphology score is rarely below 85% [56]. The problem with human sperm is that the surface of aberrant sperm are also labeled and/or isolated following the above mentioned methods (Sects. 1.3.2 and 1.3.3). Therefore, the resulting protein mixtures will contain more proteins from malfunctional sperm and intracellular labeled proteins when compared to porcine or mouse sperm. On the other hand the relative abundance of abnormal sperm in ejaculates from males with reduced fertility characteristics is of use for diagnostic proteomic comparisons [58]. With respect to the theme of this book, sperm antigens have been detected and characterized by comparing sperm proteins from healthy and infertile men. (2) For proper sperm surface isolation one needs to have large amounts of sperm cells. This is not the case for the commonly used method to isolate total sperm membranes using the hypo-osmotic treatment followed by sonication and differential centrifugation. For sperm cavitation and subfractionation of sperm membranes one needs much more starting material. However, the amount of sperm released in a human ejaculate (from a healthy fertile donor) is less than 200 million sperms [59] while for porcine (and bovine) sperm, this number is approximately 100–200 times higher [60, 61]. (3) As we are more interested in the genomics and proteomics of our own species than that of domestic animals, complete genome and proteome maps can be found in databases [62]. This allows identification of all proteins and peptides isolated or labeled.

1.3.4.2
Mouse Sperm Proteomics

Also proteomic data obtained from mouse sperm needs to be taken with some extra care: (1) When mouse sperms are collected by (electro stimulated) ejaculation, they will almost immediately deteriorate because of the spermicidal coagulation plug in which the sperms become entrapped during collection (in contrast to the in vivo situation where the sperms remain separated from the coagulation plug). Therefore, mouse sperms for IVF purposes or for studying sperm surface are routinely obtained by aspirating the epididymis [63]. Obviously this influences the quality of such specimen as epididymal sperm may not be fully maturated and the amount of sperm collected is not sufficient for proper membrane subfractionation studies. (2) Specific problems to sperm surface isolation are related to the hook shaped morphology of the mouse sperm head. Probably related to this, only one attempt has been described to strip the plasma membrane from mouse sperm with nitrogen cavitation [64] without data on the purification degree of the cavitate. The other sperm surface isolation method by blunt hypotonic sonication resulted in only low purity of mouse sperm plasma membranes, 4–10 times less [27]. (3) Obviously the mouse species also has specific advantages over human and porcine species for the sperm surface proteomics. Like for humans, the complete genome and proteome of mouse are available [65]. (4) Because the mouse is an important laboratory animal model, species specific genetic breeding lines are available. When compared to humans (also valid to some extent for porcine samples [31]), the advantage is that within a specific breeding line relatively low biodiversity exists which will result in much more repeatable data [66]. (5) Of course the mouse is also a model of choice for generating genetic knock out or silencing phenotypes for validating the function of certain translation products identified in proteomics [67, 68]. Because of the fact that the mouse gives birth to nests (multiple off-springs) and has a relatively short generation time, this laboratory species is very well suited for obtaining fertility data that can be related to proteomic data bases to verify the functionality of certain proteins in fertilization. Genotypic manipulation of humans is of course not permitted.

1.3.4.3
Porcine and Bovine Sperm Proteomics

The major potentials of porcine and bovine sperm: (1) Each ejaculate contains an overwhelming amount of mature and morphologically intact functional sperm [60, 61]. (2) Moreover, for both species a reliable method has been described for purification of the apical plasma membrane (or further subfractionation to obtain surface specific to membrane microdomains) [28, 69]. Therefore, much more reliable surface membrane protein samples can be obtained from these species than from humans and mouse. (3) Both in porcine and bovine species mostly the off-spring is produced by artificial insemination. In the last decade, all large AI-industries have set up huge fertility data sets of individual male animals, sperm collection time, female animals inseminated, nonreturn rate, birth rate, and litter size (for pigs). The enormous amounts of data for each sperm producing animal can be used to get very relevant correlations between sperm characteristics and fertility potential. In collaboration with the AI industries these data sets can become accessible to correlate the presence of certain sperm surface proteins in the sperm sample from a boar or bull to the fertility performance of the animal [70, 71]. To a lesser extent this is also possible for equine sperm [72]. (4) The equine and bovine species are mono-oestrus and therefore have a reproductive physiology that resembles the human reproductive physiology more than that of the laboratory animals or pigs which are poly-oestrus mammals [73, 74]. (5) Unfortunately the genome-annotation for the proteome of those species is not yet completed. However, the incomplete proteome at this moment hampers complete identification of proteins (our attempt to identify zona binding proteins resulted in the identification of 55% of the proteins whereas 45% of the proteins were not identified in proteomic data lists [7]. This disadvantage is only temporary as the complete pig genome is expected to be published in January 2010 (Curcher, personal communication); the bovine and equine genomes are also nearly completed and will become accessible to the public. (6) Porcine and bovine breeding is performed on a very large scale worldwide. The off-spring is of course relevant in the context of using those animals for delivery of milk for dairy products and for our need of animal derived materials. Sometimes, animals will be slaughtered to harvest these materials. For veterinary scientists it is possible to obtain fresh materials from those animals at the slaughterline continuously. This enables the researcher to obtain materials of >6,000 animals per day. In our setting, we were, for instance, able to isolate 5,000 ovaries with ovulatory follicles from adult pigs in one collection session [26]. From this material we isolated 500,000 oocytes with a mature diameter size and a functional zona pellucida. We were able to isolate zona ghosts that were not contaminated with other proteins as was verified on solubilized zona material by 2D IEF-SDS-PAGE [7]. This zona material was used to identify isolated apical plasma membrane proteins. A number of integral membrane proteins originating from the testis (such as fertilin beta) and GPI anchored proteins attached to the sperm surface, when traveling through the epididymis (spermadhesins), were identified [33]. Although a number of proteins were not identified, this direct primary zona binding approach could not have been carried out with mouse or human material as such an amount of purified, mature, and prefertilization zona ghost material cannot be prepared from these species. In addition, because of their larger size farm animals are easier to approach for internal genital tract processing of the sperm surface. Examples are of epididymal surface remodeling or of in vitro manipulation of the sperm surface in the oviduct [75–77]. (7) Although technically possible it is very expensive to perform genotypic silencing of farm animal species. This is due to the larger size of these animals compared to laboratory animals; both the housing of animals and the relatively long generation time in larger animals make these types less suitable for studies. We should note here that fertility data from molecular manipulated mouse experiments can only to a limited manner be extrapolated to other mammalian species. This is because proteins involved in reproduction show a very rapid evolutionary diversification. There is a lot of redundancy in proteins within one species (in porcine sperm there are >10 zona binding proteins;[7]) and between species completely different sets of proteins are involved in the same processes related to fertilization because of rapid evolutionary diversification of proteins [78, 79]. For this reason phenotypically altered mice may not always provide insights to understand the role of sperm surface proteins identified in other mammalian species.

1.3.5
Conclusions

Antigens at the surface of sperm are of considerable interest when compared to intracellular antigens as the latter are accessible for immuno-responses only when the integrity of sperm is compromised. When immune responses are elicited from the sperm surface also intact functional sperms are recognized. The fertilization potential of such sperms may be altered by the immune response. Therefore, proteomic studies that focus exclusively on the sperm surface material are very relevant for immune infertility studies. A number of factors have been considered to ensure that only the proteins of sperm surface membranes are isolated or labeled. Moreover, the fact that an important class of integral membrane proteins is not suitable for protein gel electrophoretic separation steps needs to be considered when studying the sperm surface proteome. A complete off gel system for complete coverage of membrane proteins needs to be used. It is difficult to compare the surface proteomes of humans, mouse, and farm animals as the sperm surface proteome is highly species specific and each mammalian species has its own drawbacks and advantages for studying the sperm surface proteome. The functional relevance of genotypic silencing experiments of mouse sperm proteins for human reproduction is therefore up to a certain degree questionable. The major drawbacks for studying the human surface proteome are the limited amount of material that is present in an individual ejaculate and the high incidence of aberrant sperm (both are no issues for farm animal species). Another drawback is that genetic manipulation of the human being is not permitted (this is not an issue for murine species, while it is possible but very expensive and time consuming for farm animals). Finally, in many studies the specificity of labeling methods and that of sperm surface separation from intracellular and extracellular components have not been analyzed or at least not with high enough scrutiny. For functional sperm surface proteomics it will be of fundamental interest to have specific sperm surface protein preparations. Also the interacting structures should be purified satisfactorily. The researcher should realize that sperms have no changes in translation (which is silenced already in late spermatids). Somatic cells and fluids from the male and female genital tract are involved in the relevant surface modifications to achieve fertilization. Finally the complex and domain-dynamic organization of the sperm surface needs to be considered when studying the protein composition of the fertile surface of the sperm. In this respect it is noteworthy that the sperm membrane proteins form complexes at different places on the sperm surface with specific functions in mammalian fertilization.

References

1. Eddy EM, O'Brien DA (1994) The spermatozoon. In: Knobil E, Neild JD (eds) The physiology of reproduction. Raven, New York, pp 29–78
2. Yanagimachi R (1994) Mammalian fertilization. In: Knobil E, Neild JD (eds) The physiology of reproduction. Raven, New York, pp 29–78

3. Gadella BM, Lopes-Cardozo M, van Golde LM, Colenbrander B, Gadella TW Jr (1995) Glycolipid migration from the apical to the equatorial subdomains of the sperm head plasma membrane precedes the acrosome reaction. Evidence for a primary capacitation event in boar spermatozoa. J Cell Sci 108:935–946

4. Phelps BM, Primakoff P, Koppel DE, Low MG, Myles DG (1988) Restricted lateral diffusion of PH-20, a PI-anchored sperm membrane protein. Science 240:1780–1782

5. Boerke A, Dieleman SJ, Gadella BM (2007) A possible role for sperm RNA in early embryo development. Theriogenology 68:147–155

6. Gadella BM, Tsai PS, Boerke A, Brewis IA (2008) Sperm head membrane reorganisation during capacitation. Int J Dev Biol 52:473–480

7. van Gestel RA, Brewis IA, Ashton PR, Brouwers JF, Gadella BM (2007) Multiple proteins present in purified porcine sperm apical plasma membranes interact with the zona pellucida of the oocyte. Mol Hum Reprod 13:445–454

8. Flesch FM, Gadella BM (2000) Dynamics of the mammalian sperm plasma membrane in the process of fertilization. Biochim Biophys Acta 1469:197–235

9. Vjugina U, Evans JP (2008) New insights into the molecular basis of mammalian sperm–egg membrane interactions. Front Biosci 13:462–476

10. Kan FW, Pinto da Silva P (1987) Molecular demarcation of surface domains as established by label-fracture cytochemistry of boar spermatozoa. J Histochem Cytochem 35:1069–1078

11. Gatti JL, Castella S, Dacheux F, Ecroyd H, Metayer S, Thimon V, Dachuex JL (2004) Posttesticular sperm environment and fertility. Anim Reprod Sci 82–83:321–339

12. Girouard J, Frenette G, Sullivan R (2008) Seminal plasma proteins regulate the association of lipids and proteins within detergent-resistant membrane domains of bovine spermatozoa. Biol Reprod 78:921–931

13. Gwathmey TM, Ignotz GG, Mueller JL, Manjunath P, Suarez SS (2006) Bovine seminal plasma proteins PDC-109, BSP-A3, and BSP-30-kDa share functional roles in storing sperm in the oviduct. Biol Reprod 75:501–507

14. Rodriguez-Martinez H (2007) Role of the oviduct in sperm capacitation. Theriogenology 68:138–146

15. Suarez SS, Pacey AA (2006) Sperm transport in the female reproductive tract. Hum Reprod Update 12:23–37

16. Getpook C, Wirotkarun S (2007) Sperm motility stimulation and preservation with various concentrations of follicular fluid. J Assist Reprod Genet 24:425–428

17. Gil PI, Guidobaldi HA, Teves ME, Uñats DR, Sanchez R, Giojalas LC (2008) Chemotactic response of frozen-thawed bovine spermatozoa towards follicular fluid. Anim Reprod Sci 108:236–246

18. Barraud-Lange V, Naud-Barriant N, Bomsel M, Wolf JP, Ziyyat A (2007) Transfer of oocyte membrane fragments to fertilizing spermatozoa. FASEB J 21:3446–3449

19. Gadella BM (2008) The assembly of a zona pellucida binding protein complex in sperm. Reprod Domest Anim 43(5):12–19

20. Mahmoud AI, Parrish JJ (1996) Oviduct fluid and heparin induce similar surface changes in bovine sperm during capacitation: a flow cytometric study using lectins. Mol Reprod Dev 43:554–560

21. Barkay J, Bartoov B, Ben-Ezra S, Langsam J, Feldman E, Gordon S, Zuckerman H (1984) The influence of in vitro caffeine treatment on human sperm morphology and fertilizing capacity. Fertil Steril 41:913–918

22. Gadella BM, Visconti PE (2006) Regulation of capacitation. In: De Jonge C, Barratt C (eds) The sperm cell: production, maturation, fertilization, regeneration. Cambridge Unversity Press, Cambridge, pp 134–169

23. Ackermann F, Zitranski N, Heydecke D, Wilhelm B, Gudermann T, Boekhoff I (2008) The Multi-PDZ domain protein MUPP1 as a lipid raft-associated scaffolding protein controlling the acrosome reaction in mammalian spermatozoa. J Cell Physiol 214:757–768

24. Tsai PS, De Vries KJ, De Boer-Brouwer M, Garcia-Gil N, Van Gestel RA, Colenbrander B, Gadella BM, Van Haeften T (2007) Syntaxin and VAMP association with lipid rafts depends on cholesterol depletion in capacitating sperm cells. Mol Membr Biol 24:313–324

25. Dormeyer W, van Hoof D, Mummery CL, Krijgsveld J, Heck AJ (2008) A practical guide for the identification of membrane and plasma membrane proteins in human embryonic stem cells and human embryonal carcinoma cells. Proteomics 8:4036–4053

26. Flesch FM, Voorhout WF, Colenbrander B, van Golde LM, Gadella BM (1998) Use of lectins to characterize plasma membrane preparations from boar spermatozoa: a novel technique for monitoring membrane purity and quantity. Biol Reprod 59:1530–1539

27. Baker SS, Cardullo RA, Thaler CD (2002) Sonication of mouse sperm membranes reveals distinct protein domains. Biol Reprod 66:57–64

28. Flesch FM, Wijnand E, van de Lest CH, Colenbrander B, van Golde LM, Gadella BM (2001) Capacitation dependent activation of tyrosine phosphorylation generates two sperm head plasma membrane proteins with high primary binding affinity for the zona pellucida. Mol Reprod Dev 60:107–115

29. van Gestel RA, Brewis IA, Ashton PR, Helms JB, Brouwers JF, Gadella BM (2005) Capacitation-dependent concentration of lipid rafts in the apical ridge head area of porcine sperm cells. Mol Hum Reprod 11:583–590

30. Bohring C, Krause W (1999) The characterization of human spermatozoa membrane proteins–surface antigens and immunological infertility. Electrophoresis 20:971–976

31. Runnebaum IB, Schill WB, Töpfer-Petersen E (1995) ConA-binding proteins of the sperm surface are conserved through evolution and in sperm maturation. Andrologia 27:81–90

32. Asano A, Selvaraj V, Buttke DE, Nelson JL, Green KM, Evans JE, Travis AJ (2009) Biochemical characterization of membrane fractions in murine sperm: identification of three distinct subtypes of membrane rafts. J Cell Physiol 218:537–548

33. Boerke A, Tsai PS, Garcia-Gil N, Brewis IA, Gadella BM (2008) Capacitation-dependent reorganization of microdomains in the apical sperm head plasma membrane: functional relationship with zona binding and the zona-induced acrosome reaction. Theriogenology 70:1188–1196

34. Hutchinson TE, Rastogi A, Prasad R, Pereira BM (2005) Phospholipase-C sensitive GPI-anchored proteins of goat sperm: possible role in sperm protection. Anim Reprod Sci 88: 271–286

35. Olson GE, Winfrey VP, Bi M, Hardy DM, NagDas SK (2004) Zonadhesin assembly into the hamster sperm acrosomal matrix occurs by distinct targeting strategies during spermiogenesis and maturation in the epididymis. Biol Reprod 71:1128–1134

36. Aitken RJ, Nixon B (2009) Proteomics of human sperm. In: Immune infertility (this book)

37. Shetty J, Herr JC (2009) Methods of analysis of sperm antigens related to fertility. In: Immune infertility (this book)

38. Gu S, Du Y, Chen J, Liu Z, Bradbury EM, Hu CA, Chen X (2004) Large-scale quantitative proteomic study of PUMA-induced apoptosis using two-dimensional liquid chromatography-mass spectrometry coupled with amino acid-coded mass tagging. J Proteome Res 3:1191–1200

39. Gu S, Liu Z, Pan S, Jiang Z, Lu H, Amit O, Bradbury EM, Hu CA, Chen X (2004) Global investigation of p53-induced apoptosis through quantitative proteomic profiling using comparative amino acid-coded tagging. Mol Cell Proteomics 3:998–1008

40. Chen X (2008) An isotope-coding strategy for quantitative proteomics. In: O'Connor CD, Hames BD (eds) proteomics. Scion, Bloxham, pp 17–32

41. Shetty J, Bronson RA, Herr JC (2008) Human sperm protein encyclopedia and alloantigen index: mining novel allo-antigens using sera from ASA-positive infertile patients and vasectomized men. J Reprod Immunol 77:23–31

42. Shetty J, Naaby-Hansen S, Shibahara H, Bronson R, Flickinger CJ, Herr JC (1999) Human sperm proteome: immunodominant sperm surface antigens identified with sera from infertile men and women. Biol Reprod 61:61–69

43. Patton WF, Schulenberg B, Steinberg TH (2002) Two-dimensional gel electrophoresis; better than a poke in the ICAT? Curr Opin Biotechnol 13:321–328
44. Zieske LR (2006) A perspective on the use of iTRAQ reagent technology for protein complex and profiling studies. J Exp Bot 57:1501–1508
45. Ficarro S, Chertihin O, Westbrook VA, White F, Jayes F, Kalab P, Marto JA, Shabanowitz J, Herr JC, Hunt DF, Visconti PE (2003) Phosphoproteome analysis of capacitated human sperm. Evidence of tyrosine phosphorylation of a kinase-anchoring protein 3 and valosin-containing protein/p97 during capacitation. J Biol Chem 278:11579–11589
46. Asquith KL, Baleato RM, McLaughlin EA, Nixon B, Aitken RJ (2004) Tyrosine phosphorylation activates surface chaperones facilitating sperm–zona recognition. J Cell Sci 117:3645–3657
47. Platt MD, Salicioni AM, Hunt DF, Visconti PE (2009) Use of differential isotopic labeling and mass spectrometry to analyze capacitation-associated changes in the phosphorylation status of mouse sperm proteins. J Proteome Res 8(3):1431–1440
48. Lefièvre L, Chen Y, Conner SJ, Scott JL, Publicover SJ, Ford WC, Barratt CL (2007) Human spermatozoa contain multiple targets for protein S-nitrosylation: an alternative mechanism of the modulation of sperm function by nitric oxide? Proteomics 7:3066–3084
49. Holt WV, Elliott RM, Fazeli A, Satake N, Watson PF (2005) Validation of an experimental strategy for studying surface-exposed proteins involved in porcine sperm-oviduct contact interactions. Reprod Fertil Dev 17:683–692
50. Shetty J, Wolkowicz MJ, Digilio LC, Klotz KL, Jayes FL, Diekman AB, Westbrook VA, Farris EM, Hao Z, Coonrod SA, Flickinger CJ, Herr JC (2003) SAMP14, a novel, acrosomal membrane-associated, glycosylphosphatidylinositol-anchored member of the Ly-6/urokinase-type plasminogen activator receptor superfamily with a role in sperm–egg interaction. J Biol Chem 278:30506–30515
51. Stein KK, Go JC, Lane WS, Primakoff P, Myles DG (2006) Proteomic analysis of sperm regions that mediate sperm–egg interactions. Proteomics 6:3533–3543
52. Tan S, Tan HT, Chung MC (2008) Membrane proteins and membrane proteomics. Proteomics 8:3924–3932
53. Ernoult E, Gamelin E, Guette C (2008) Improved proteome coverage by using iTRAQ labelling and peptide OFFGEL fractionation. Proteome Sci 6:27
54. Hendin BN, Falcone T, Hallak J, Nelson DR, Vemullapalli S, Goldberg J, Thomas AJ Jr, Agarwal A (2000) The effect of patient and semen characteristics on live birth rates following intrauterine insemination: a retrospective study. J Assist Reprod Genet 17(5):245–252
55. Keel BA (2004) How reliable are results from the semen analysis? Fertil Steril 82:41–44
56. Gadella BM, Colenbrander B, Lopes-Cardozo M (1991) Arylsulfatases are present in seminal plasma of several domestic mammals. Biol Reprod 45:381–386
57. Kruger TF, Menkveld R, Stander FS, Lombard CJ, Van der Merwe JP, van Zyl JA, Smith K (1986) Sperm morphologic features as a prognostic factor in in vitro fertilization. Fertil Steril 46:1118–1123
58. Domagała A, Pulido S, Kurpisz M, Herr JC (2007) Application of proteomic methods for identification of sperm immunogenic antigens. Mol Hum Reprod 13:437–444
59. Lenau H, Gorewoda I, Niermann H (1980) Relationship between sperm count, serum gonadotropins and testosterone levels in normo-, oligo- and azoospermia. Reproduction 4:147–156
60. Brito LF, Silva AE, Rodrigues LH, Vieira FV, Deragon LA, Kastelic JP (2002) Effects of environmental factors, age and genotype on sperm production and semen quality in Bos indicus and Bos taurus AI bulls in Brazil. Anim Reprod Sci 70:181–190
61. Levis DG, Reicks DL (2005) Assessment of sexual behavior and effect of semen collection pen design and sexual stimulation of boars on behavior and sperm output–a review. Theriogenology 63:630–642
62. Hober S, Uhlén M (2008) Human protein atlas and the use of microarray technologies. Curr Opin Biotechnol 19:30–35

63. Si W, Men H, Benson JD, Critser JK (2009) Osmotic characteristics and fertility of murine spermatozoa collected in different solutions. Reproduction 137:215–223
64. Lopez LC, Shur BD (1987) Redistribution of mouse sperm surface galactosyltransferase after the acrosome reaction. J Cell Biol 105:1663–1670
65. Kasukawa T, Katayama S, Kawaji H, Suzuki H, Hume DA, Hayashizaki Y (2004) Construction of representative transcript and protein sets of human, mouse, and rat as a platform for their transcriptome and proteome analysis. Genomics 84:913–921
66. Kasai K, Teuscher C, Smith S, Matzner P, Tung KS (1987) Strain variations in anti-sperm antibody responses and anti-fertility effects in inbred mice. Biol Reprod 36:1085–1094
67. Cooper TG, Wagenfeld A, Cornwall GA, Hsia N, Chu ST, Orgebin-Crist MC, Drevet J, Vernet P, Avram C, Nieschlag E, Yeung CH (2003) Gene and protein expression in the epididymis of infertile c-ros receptor tyrosine kinase-deficient mice. Biol Reprod 69:1750–1762
68. Okabe M, Cummins JM (2007) Mechanisms of sperm–egg interactions emerging from gene-manipulated animals. Cell Mol Life Sci 64:1945–1958
69. Lalancette C, Dorval V, Leblanc V, Leclerc P (2001) Characterization of an 80-kilodalton bull sperm protein identified as PH-20. Biol Reprod 65:628–636
70. Boe-Hansen GB, Christensen P, Vibjerg D, Nielsen MB, Hedeboe AM (2008) Sperm chromatin structure integrity in liquid stored boar semen and its relationships with field fertility. Theriogenology 69:728–736
71. Parkinson TJ (2004) Evaluation of fertility and infertility in natural service bulls. Vet J 168:215–229
72. Vidament M, Dupere AM, Julienne P, Evain A, Noue P, Palmer E (1997) Equine frozen semen: freezability and fertility field results. Theriogenology 48:907–917
73. Distl O (2007) Mechanisms of regulation of litter size in pigs on the genome level. Reprod Domest Anim 42:10–16
74. May PC, Finch CE (1987) Aging and responses to toxins in female reproductive functions. Reprod Toxicol 1:223–228
75. Dacheux JL, Castella S, Gatti JL, Dacheux F (2005) Epididymal cell secretory activities and the role of proteins in boar sperm maturation. Theriogenology 63:319–341
76. Ignotz GG, Cho MY, Suarez SS (2007) Annexins are candidate oviductal receptors for bovine sperm surface proteins and thus may serve to hold bovine sperm in the oviductal reservoir. Biol Reprod 77:906–913
77. Suarez SS (2008) Regulation of sperm storage and movement in the mammalian oviduct. Int J Dev Biol 52:455–462
78. Herlyn H, Zischler H (2008) The molecular evolution of sperm zonadhesin. Int J Dev Biol 52:781–790
79. Turner LM, Hoekstra HE (2008) Causes and consequences of the evolution of reproductive proteins. Int J Dev Biol 52:769–780
80. Cooper TG, Yeung CH, Bergmann M (1988) Transcytosis in the epididymis studied by local arterial perfusion. Cell Tissue Res 253:631–637
81. Gatti JL, Métayer S, Belghazi M, Dacheux F, Dacheux JL (2005) Identification, proteomic profiling, and origin of ram epididymal fluid exosome-like vesicles. Biol Reprod 72:1452–1465
82. Thimon V, Frenette G, Saez F, Thabet M, Sullivan R (2008) Protein composition of human epididymosomes collected during surgical vasectomy reversal: a proteomic and genomic approach. Hum Reprod 23:1698–1707
83. Sostaric E, Dieleman SJ, van de Lest CH, Colenbrander B, Vos PL, Garcia-Gil N, Gadella BM (2008) Sperm binding properties and secretory activity of the bovine oviduct immediately before and after ovulation. Mol Reprod Dev 75:60–74
84. Ford JJ, McCoard SA, Wise TH, Lunstra DD, Rohrer GA (2006) Genetic variation in sperm production. Soc Reprod Fertil 62:99–112

Sperm Functions Influenced by Immune Reactions

1.4

Walter K. H. Krause

1.4.1
Sperm Agglutination

The first investigation of cognate antigens binding sperm agglutinating ASA was published by Koide et al. [1]. The ASA were obtained from the blood serum of infertile women or were monoclonal antibodies (mAb) raised in the mouse and active against human sperm proteins. Among the antigens identified were the following:

1. YWK-II mAb recognized as a cognate antigen of a molecular mass between 60 and 72 kDa, immune localized in the equatorial sector of the human sperm head. The cDNA of YWK-II antigen has been mapped to chromosome locus 11q24-25; the polypeptide belongs to the APP protein family. Proteins of this family are also found in plaques of Alzheimer disease, and therefore, it is also named as APLP2 [2].
2. rSMP-B, a sperm tail component with 72 kDa, recognized by ASA from the serum of infertile women. The gene was expressed only in spermatids. The human analog (hSMP-1, see below) is coded by the HSD-I gene, which is located on human chromosome 9, region p12–p13 [3].
3. Calpastatin, a 17.5-kDa protein,is localized by immune staining with polyclonal antibodies in the acrosomal region and slightly on the tail. The cDNA consisted of 758 bp having 99.7% homology with the gene coding calpastatin. The gene was found to be transcribed only in spermatids. Calpastatin binds calpain, a Ca-dependent cysteine endopeptidase (see below).
4. A 75-kDa protein was found with no homology of the nucleotide sequence to any other DNA.

A mouse mAb A36 induced extensive "tangled" sperm agglutination. The mAb A36 cognate sperm surface antigen is a GPI/NLK-like protein involved in sperm agglutination [4].

W. Krause
Klinik für Dermatologie und Allergologie, Philipps-Universität, Marburg, Germany
e-mail: krause@med.uni-marburg.de

W. K. H. Krause and R. K. Naz (eds.), *Immune Infertility*,
DOI: 10.1007/978-3-642-01379-9_1.4, © Springer Verlag Berlin Heidelberg 2009

A polyclonal antibody from the rabbit against the human c-kit peptide was able to inhibit acrosome reaction in human sperm and to increase sperm agglutination. By immune fluorescence, the localization of the c-kit peptide in the acrosomal region was demonstrated, but the staining was absent in acrosome-reacted sperm. Thus the c-kit peptide may be involved in acrosome reaction [5; Fig. 1.4.1].

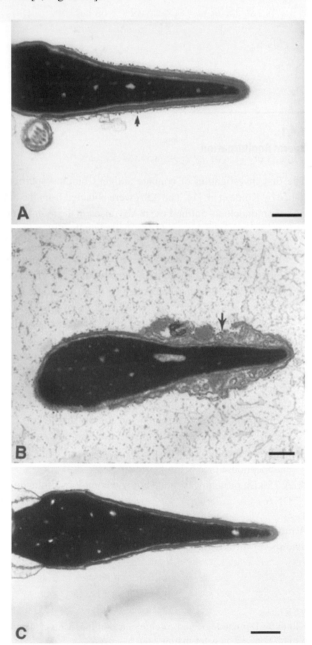

Fig. 1.4.1 Immunolocalization of c-kit receptor in human spermatozoa by electron microscopy. (**a**) The immunogold particles were located on the plasma membrane (PM) surface (*arrows*) of the acrosomal regions in the acrosome-intact spermatozoa. (**b**) After the acrosome reaction, gold particles remained associated with the acrosomal vesicles (*arrows*), presumably in the PM components of the vesicles. (**c**) No gold label was observed on the acrosome-intact spermatozoa incubated with normal rabbit serum sperm. Bar 0.5 mm (from Feng et al. [5], with permission)

Norton et al. [6] engineered a recombinant single-chain variable fragment (scFv) antibody binding to a tissue-specific carbohydrate epitope located on human sperm agglutination antigen-1 (SAGA-1), the sperm glycoform of CD52. The recombinant antisperm antibody (RASA) was expressed in E. coli HB2151 cells. RASA aggregated human spermatozoa in a tangled (head-to-head, head-to-tail, tail-to-tail) pattern of agglutination [7].

Bandivdekar et al. [8] described a human sperm-specific antigen of about 80 kDa, which agglutinated epididymal spermatozoa. The nature of the antigen was not further elucidated.

1.4.2
Sperm Apoptosis

Several proteins of the signal transduction pathways of apoptosis are present on the sperm surface, e.g., the externalization of phosphatidylserin, CD95, and some caspases [9]. On the other hand, spermatozoa do not stain with Fas protein antibodies [10]; therefore, it is questionable whether the complete instruments of apoptosis are present in spermatozoa and whether these proteins are functionally active.

In particular, cryopreservation of sperm induces mechanisms of apoptosis [11–13]. Also the damage to spermatozoa in consequence of co-incubation with *Chlamydia trachomatis* lipopolysaccharide (LPS) was triggered by a caspase-mediated apoptosis-like mechanism [14].

Reports on the binding of ASA to functional proteins involved in apoptosis are scarce in the literature. The binding of ASA to the inactive form of caspase-3 and to HSP70 as cognate antigens was demonstrated by our group [15]. The pathophysiologic significance of these ASA was unclear at that time.

1.4.3
Sperm Motility

Immobilization of sperm by ASA is a special feature. The ASA were demonstrated exclusively in the sera of infertile women. They appear to activate the complement system; their presence is frequently associated with impaired penetration of the cervical mucus.

The literature describing these antibodies is nearly exclusively from Japanese authors. In the study of Tsuji et al. [16] the presence of sperm immobilizing antibodies was found to be associated with the HLA-DRB1*0901 and HLA-DQB1*0303 types, which are characteristically prevalent among Japanese. This association may account for the high prevalence of sperm immobilizing antibodies in Japanese people. In rare cases, sperm immobilizing antibodies were found also in male sera [17].

Isojima [18], the discoverer of this type of impairment of sperm function, characterized the chemical structure of an antigen epitope corresponding to human monoclonal antibody H6-3C4; it was found to consist of internally repetitive, unbranched *N*-acetyllactosamine (blood type I antigen). Ejaculated human sperm appeared to be densely covered with sialyl blood type I antigen and sialyl branched internally repetitive *N*-acetyllactosamine (sialyl blood type I antigen). Later, this antigen was identified as human CD52 antigen, which is inserted into the sperm membrane during the epididymal passage [19, 20]. CD52 is a glycosylphosphatidylinositol (GPI) anchor protein occurring in lymphocytes, the epididymis, seminal plasma, and on ejaculated sperm surface. The biological function of CD52 in mature sperm is not well understood. It is possibly active in depressing the complement activity. It appears obvious that this carbohydrate molecule is highly antigenic to females, as a similar antigen does not exist in a female organism.

In general, it is difficult to explain how other ASA will interfere with sperm motility, as it is likely that ASA bind to antigens of sperm membranes, while sub-cellular structures will not be reached by ASA in the living cell.

Neilson et al. [21] used serum from an infertile male with high titers of ASA to identify novel human sperm antigens by screening of a testis expression library. The human gene encodes 1.8 and 2.8 kb mRNAs are highly expressed in testis but not in other tissues tested. The deduced amino acid sequence of the full-length cDNA revealed striking homology to the product of the Chlamydomonas reinhardtii PF16 locus, which encodes a protein localized to the central pair of the flagellar axoneme. Antibodies raised against the peptide sequences localized the protein to the tails of permeabilized human sperm.

The results of Inaba et al. [22] using immune electron microscopy suggested that flagellar movement of sperm is also modulated by proteasomes, which regulate the activity of outer dynein arm by cAMP-dependent phosphorylation of the 22-kDa dynein light chain. Complement regulatory proteins such as C1-INH, CD55, CD46, and CD59 were expressed on sperms [23]. IgG antibodies to these proteins significantly reduced sperm motility in general and other motion parameters.

A cation channel protein (CATSPER1) was shown to be expressed in spermatids and ejaculated spermatozoa by Li et al. (2006). The mRNA of this protein was also shown to be present in the cells. Application of antibodies to CATSPER1 was able to inhibit total motility and progressive motility. The mechanism of this inhibition remains unclear up to now.

1.4.4
Cervix Mucus Penetration

ASA concentrations in the cervix mucus are generally low. A frequency of 3.2% in infertile women, compared to 10.4% of seminal samples of infertile men, is described in [24]. In particular, women with immobilizing antibodies may display different titers also in the cervix mucus, which inhibit sperm migration [25] and result in poor post-coital test and reduced fertility.

However, the impairment of sperm penetration into the cervical mucus appears mostly to be independent of the cognate antigens of ASA. It appears to be a consequence of two mechanisms: firstly, the activation of the complement cascade by immunoglobulins attached to the sperm surface; secondly, as a consequence of cell lysis and initiation of the phagocytotic process. The complement-induced cell lysis depends on the immunoglobulin class of the antibody; IgM is far more effective than IgG, while some IgA subclasses are unable to interact with the early complement components.

Activation of complement components in cervical mucus has been carefully studied. Complement activating ASA may be effective only in the mucus, because the seminal plasma contains complement inhibitors. During their residence in the cervical mucus, spermatozoa are exposed to complement activity. The complement activity in cervical mucus is approximately 12% of that of serum [26].

Another mechanism explaining the impairment of cervical mucus penetrating ability of sperm and the induction of the shaking phenomenon by ASA, in particular that of the IgA class appears to be mediated through the Fc portion of the IgA (Jager et al. 1981; [27]). Sperm recovered after mucus penetration displayed a reduced binding to IgA immuno-beads [28]. Experimentally, Bronson [29] showed that IgA bound to the sperm surface, which was degraded by an IgA protease from *Neisseria gonorrhoeae*, did no longer inhibit mucus permeation.

1.4.5
Acrosome Reaction

The loss of the acrosome along with the release of the acrosomal content in order to enable the spermatozoa to permeate through the zona pellucida(ZP) is called acrosome reaction. Most ASA increase the number of acrosome-reacted spermatozoa. In our group we showed that a number of spontaneously occurring ASA were able to enhance the number of acrosome-reacted sperm [30], but none of them was able to inhibit acrosome reaction in vitro. In our study, all patients whose ASA were bound to the acrosome region of the donor sperm, showed abnormal acrosin activity in their own spermatozoa, indicating a functional relevance of the cognate antigens.

When seminal plasma samples containing ASA or spermatozoa loaded with ASA were adsorbed with fertilization antigen-1 (FA-1), the percentage of immunobead-free swimming sperm increased on an average of 50% [31]. The rate of spermatozoa undergoing acrosome reaction as induced by the calcium ionophore A23187 showed improvement in 78% of the sperm samples after FA-1 adsorption.

There is a large data pool on antigens involved in acrosome reaction and antibodies to these antigens. Calpastatin, a 17.5-kDa protein, is an integral part of the acrosomal cytoplasma. Using polyclonal antibodies to calpastatin, immunostaining was seen over the acrosomal region and slightly on the tail. The cDNA consists of 758 bp. The gene was found to be transcribed only in spermatids. The inhibition of calpastatin leads to a premature acrosome reaction [1]. Calpastatin binds calpain, a Ca-dependent cysteine endopeptidase. Antibodies to calpains bind to the region between the plasma membrane (PM) and the outer acrosomal membrane of sperm. After the acrosome reaction, all of the anticalpain antibodies labeled the acrosomal shroud presenting acrosomal contents.

CD46 is a membrane complement regulator, which has an impact on T cell activation as well as on spermatozoa–egg interactions. After induction of antibodies to CD46, the incubation of spermatozoa with immune sera caused deposition of immunoglobulin and

C3b in an acrosome pattern and reduced motility. Testis sections from immune rats revealed no immunoglobulin deposition on CD46-positive sperm precursors, suggesting that acrosomal CD46 was inaccessible in this location, but spermatozoa became positive for antibody binding after acrosome reaction [32].

Auer et al. [33] isolated a protein P36 as a cognate antigen of ASA, which was found to be a glycolytic enzyme. P36 was not detectable at the surface of live non-acrosome-reacted sperm cells. It was characterized as human triosephosphate isomerase (TPI), which catalyzes the interconversion of dihydroxyacetone phosphate and D-glyceraldehyde 3-phosphate. Its functional role in the sperm function is not clear; it may be independent of the catalytic activity, as demonstrated already for other sperm enzymes.

Cheng et al. [34] found ASA from an infertile female patient to be specific for a human sperm membrane protein (hSMP-1), a testis-specific protein. Polyclonal antibodies against a fragment of the mouse protein homologue showed intense hSMP-1 immune reactivity on the acrosome of human sperm. In the mouse, anti-rhSMP-1 antibodies significantly inhibited the acrosome reaction of spermatozoa and decreased the average number of sperms bound to each oocyte.

Some studies have suggested that ASA may somewhat modify sperm PM integrity. Rossato et al. [35] demonstrated that sperm with ASA bound to their PMs showed low HOS test scores. It appeared possible that ASA modify sperm PM permeability or fluidity, leading to low fertilizing potential.

Feng et al. [36] analyzed ASA from a woman who was found immune infertile by indirect immunobead test (IBT). Immunobead binding was shown by 79% of spermatozoa, but after acrosome reaction induced by calcium ionophore, no binding was further visible. The antibodies reacted with 35-, 40-, 47-, and 65-kDa proteins extracted from acrosome-intact donor sperm.

Triphan et al. [37] identified voltage-dependent anion channels (VDAC) , which are highly conserved, pore-forming proteins in the acrosomal region, by the use of specific antibodies. The staining in immune fluorescence increased with time in acrosome-reacted spermatozoa, indicating that the antigens are liberated during acrosome reaction. There is, however, no clear evidence to date that VDAC participate in the physiological course of the acrosome reaction.

Wang et al. [38] described the sperm lysozyme-like protein 1 (SLLP-1), which is a unique nonbacteriolytic, c-lysozyme-like protein and is present in the acrosome of human spermatozoa. Antisera to SLLP1 were shown to block binding of sperm to hamster oocytes. The occurrence of ASA binding to this antigen has not been described up to now.

Chiu et al. [39] described two men with high concentrations of ASA, which bound to a novel protein localized in the acrosome called SPRASA. They were able to determine the peptide sequence of the protein by MALDI-MS and could show that it was a theoretical protein, XP-085564 encoded by the lysozyme/alpha-lactalbumine gene family. Only ASA from infertile men react with SPRASA, suggesting that this novel protein may be important in the processes of fertility.

A neuronal glycine receptor/Cl(−) channel (GlyR) was detected on the PM of mammalian sperm. Pharmacological studies suggested that this receptor/channel is important for initiation of acrosome reaction by the ZP. A mAb against GlyR completely blocked ZP initiation of AR in normal mouse sperm. These findings indicate that sperm GlyR plays an essential role in the AR as initiated by the ZP [40].

Another protein of the acrosome is the 57 kDa fertility associated sperm antigen (FASA-57), defined by monoclonal antibodies [41]. FASA-57 was found to be localized on the acrosome of nonacrosome-reacted human spermatozoa and on the equatorial region after the acrosome reaction. It was found also in the spermatozoa from several other mammalian species. In a mouse model, a monoclonal antibody against FASA-57 inhibited sperm–egg binding and fusion in a dose-dependent manner with half-maximal inhibition. A rabbit anti-57 kDa antibody was able to inhibit acrosome reaction in a dose-dependent manner. The molecular nature of this protein has not yet been described.

FASA-57 has similar properties as the human sperm-associated antigen 9 (hSPAG9). It is not only restricted to a specific region (domain) of the acrosome but also undergoes relocation to the equatorial region in a stage-specific manner during acrosome reaction [42].

A very interesting protein localized in the acrosome reaction is sperm protein 17 (Sp17). It is a highly conserved protein localized in the testis and in the head and tail of ejaculated spermatozoa, as well as in other cilia within the fibrous sheath, which contains A-kinase anchoring proteins (AKAP) 3 and 4 (Fig. 1.4.2). Sp17 was additionally localized in human neoplastic cell lines; therefore, it is designated as a cancer testis antigen [43]. Sp17 was sequenced and cloned from human sperm [44], and from baboon, mice, rabbit, and rat sperm [45, 46]. There is a high degree of homology within these species. It is a three-domain protein that contains (1) a highly conserved N-terminal domain that is 45% identical to the human type II alpha regulatory subunit (RII alpha) of protein kinase A (PKA); (2) a central sulfated carbohydrate-binding domain; and (3) a C-terminal Ca^{++}/calmodulin (CaM) binding domain.

Sp17 is a cognate antigen to naturally occurring ASA. Lea et al. [47] constructed an ELISA using recombinant human Sp17 for the determination of Sp17-ASA in the serum of men following vasectomy. Additionally, the B cell epitopes of Sp17 were determined. The sera from men after vasectomy contained ASA against Sp17 and the linear B cell epitopes were found to be amino acids 52–79 and 124–136. In an ELISA, 11 % of infertile men and women displaying sperm antibodies (ASA) were positive for anti-SP17 antibodies [48].

1.4.6
Zona Binding

The binding of the sperm to the ZP occurs via specific receptors localized over the head region of the spermatozoa. ZP binds at two different receptors in the sperm membrane. One is a G_i-coupled receptor that activates β_1-phoshporlipase C and the other one is a tyrosine kinase receptor coupled to γ-phospholipase C [49].

Immunologic characterization of binding proteins is available in the literature. Mahony et al. [50] observed patients expressing ASA in their sera that bound to the sperm surface, most specifically at the head region and reduced ZP tight binding of spermatozoa as assessed by the hemizona assay (HZA). The responsible protein was not characterized. Liu et al. [51] described similar results. In their study they confirmed that ASA interfered predominantly with sperm–ZP binding. They concluded from their observations that the inhibition of oolemma binding may not be the major cause of failed fertilization involving sperm autoimmunity.

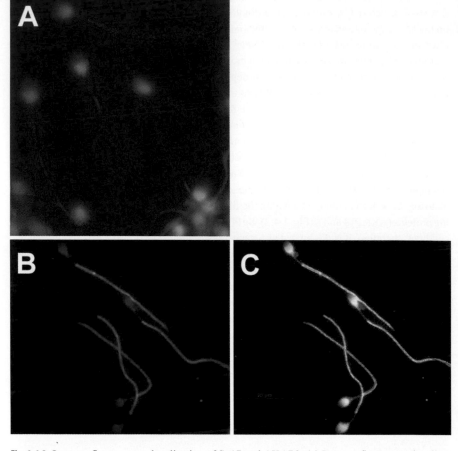

Fig. 1.4.2 Immunofluorescence localization of Sp17 and AKAP3. (**a**) Immunofluorescent localization of Sp17 in human spermatozoa. Sp17 is found in the principal piece, middle piece and in scattered patches throughout the head region. The nuclei are DAPI stained. (**b**) Immunofluorescent localization of AKAP3 in human spermatozoa. AKAP3 is located predominantly in the principal piece of the flagella. The nuclei are DAPI stained. (**c**) Co-localization of Sp17 and AKAP3 in human spermatozoa. AKAP3 (*green*), located in the principal piece, co-localizes with Sp17 in some areas (*yellow*) of the principal piece but not in others. Sp17 (*red*) is also located in the middle piece of the tail and head regions. The nuclei are DAPI stained. Scale bar is 20 μm for A, B and C (from Lea et al. [44], with permission)

One of the possible antigens involved in zona penetration is PH-20, a glycerolphosphatidyl-inositol-linked hyaluronidase. In the guinea pig, two regions of this enzyme (res. 94–119 and res. 424–444) were highly immunogenic. As PH-20 is present in many species and also in humans, it may be a cognate antigen of ASA in humans [52].

Mollova et al. [53] described a protein (Ag 1F10) composed of a single peptide chain with a relative molecular mass of 68/70 kDa and an isoelectric point of 3.5 in human sperm membranes. The zona binding activity of spermatozoa pre-incubated in the presence of a mAb to this protein was significantly inhibited both in porcine and human in vitro fertilization (IVF) systems. Naz et al. [54] described a dodecamer sequence, designated as YLP(12) that is involved in sperm—ZP recognition/binding. Anti-YLP(12) Fab' antibodies of naturally occurring ASA recognized a protein band of approximately 72 ± 2 kDa only in the lane of testis homogenates.

In mice, a sperm antigen designated as fertilization antigen 1 (FA-1) was identified [55]. The authors cloned and sequenced the cDNA and were able to translate a protein, which was a novel protein not included in protein databases up to that time. The protein specifically reacted with zona protein 3 (ZP3) of oocyte ZP. When polyclonal antibodies were generated, they completely blocked sperm-ZP interaction in mice. Similar results were found in the human system.

Zayas-Pérez et al. [56] described the binding of an antiserum to a 55-kDa protein of spermatozoa. It was located preferentially at the apical edge of the head in capacitated sperm but not in acrosome-reacted sperm. The binding to the ZP was totally inhibited by this antibody. Unfortunately, the molecular nature of the 55-kDa protein is not described.

Human sperm membrane protein (hSMP-1, PubMed locus U12978), a testis-specific protein expressed during human development, was immunologically localized in the acrosome. Naturally occurring antibodies against hSMP-1 were found in the sera of infertile women. The treatment of mice with antibodies against a recombinant protein significantly decreased the average number of sperms bound to each egg in the process of fertilization. These observations indicated the role of hSMP-1 in zona binding [34].

1.4.7
Oolemma Binding and Sperm–Egg Fusion

Several proteins are involved in the process of sperm–egg fusion. The knowledge on these proteins mainly originates from the experimental binding of human spermatozoa to zona-free hamster oocytes.

Francavilla et al. [57] studied the effect of ASA on the hamster egg penetration assay (HEPA). They added ASA from patients to motile donor sperm, but they did not find ASA with the ability to reduce the rate of acrosome-reacted sperm or to reduce the hamster egg penetration rate.

Noor et al. [58] constructed monoclonal antibodies that bound to various regions of the sperm head and inhibited fertilization. One of these specifically inhibited sperm–egg fusion in a concentration-dependent manner, while sperm–oolemma binding and sperm motility remained unaffected. This mAb exclusively recognized an epitope in the equatorial segment, the expression of which increased after capacitation and acrosome reaction.

A 20-kDa glycoprotein (GP20) was isolated from human sperm by Focarelli et al. [59]. An anti-gp20 antibody intensely stained the head and mid-piece; after acrosome reaction the antibody binding was restricted to a small band in the equatorial region. The antibody did not bind to sperm precursor cells in the testis or to epididymal epithelial cells. Therefore, it seems to be a protein added to the sperm membrane in the epididymis and represents one of the sperm coating antigens.

Gabriele et al. [60] described a human sperm protein with a molecular mass of 65 kDa, which bound D-mannose coupled to albumin (DMA) in presence of cations at a neutral pH. The binding of human spermatozoa to zona-free hamster eggs was reduced by DMA in a dose-dependent manner, suggesting that DMA-binding sites in human spermatozoa are involved in sperm–egg fusion.

Hamatani et al. [61] isolated and characterized SP-10, a sperm intra-acrosomal protein, which is produced specifically in the testis, but expressed in human spermatozoa only after acrosome reaction. A mAb to this protein inhibited sperm–oolemma binding in the zona-free hamster egg penetration test, but it did not inhibit sperm-zona binding in the HZA.

The presence of a CD46 (membrane cofactor protein of complement) isoform was demonstrated in human spermatozoa by means of monoclonal antibodies. Experiments showed that it is associated with the sperm–egg interaction. The expression of CD46 in other cells confers resistance to complement-mediated injury. Nomura et al. [62] found three infertile subjects with no expression of CD46 isoform on their spermatozoa when screening 542 idiopathic male infertile patients. All three patients, however, expressed normal CD46 isoforms on their lymphocytes and granulocytes. Thus, the loss of CD46 was sperm-specific, probably due to testicular germ cell-specific regulation of CD46 production. The analysis of the CD46 gene in the patients revealed no abnormality in 3′ and 5′ regions of the CD46 genome.

The complement fraction C1q is known to participate in many cellular events in addition to its role in the classical complement pathway. C1q and its receptors also play a role in gamete interactions leading to fertilization and it promotes the binding of human spermatozoa to the oolemma of zona-free hamster eggs in a concentration-dependent manner. Antibodies to this molecule mainly bound to spermatozoa after capacitation [63].

SP-10, a highly conserved intra-acrosomal sperm protein, is believed to play a role in egg–sperm binding. Human SP-10 has been demonstrated to be initially exposed on the sperm surface after acrosome reaction. MAb to peptides of Sp-10 did not inhibit sperm–zona binding, but inhibited sperm–oolemma binding in the zona-free hamster oocyte. The ligands of SP-10 have not yet been clarified. They are not the integrins [25, 26].

Koyama et al. [19] constructed a mAb against human CD52 antigen, a highly glycosylated molecule with an unusually small core peptide exclusively expressed on lymphocytes and mature sperm. The mAb strongly inhibited penetration of human spermatozoa into zona-free hamster oocytes. This observation indicates a role for CD52 in sperm–oocyte fusion.

Testicular protein Tpx-1, also known as CRISP-2, is a cysteine-rich secretory protein specifically expressed in the male reproductive tract. After in vitro capacitation and ionophore-induced AR, TPX1 is demonstrable in the equatorial segment of the acrosome. When a hamster oocyte penetration test is performed in the presence of anti-TPX1, the percentage of penetrated hamster oocytes is decreased, without affecting sperm motility [64].

A most interesting protein is the Izumo protein, a specific integral part of spermatozoa, which was shown to be the first sperm membrane protein essential for fusion. Inoue et al. [65] identified a new antigen by separation of the crude extracts from mouse sperm by 2D gel electrophoresis and subsequent immunoblotting with a mAb that specifically inhibited the sperm–oocyte fusion process. It was a testis (sperm)-specific 56.4-kDa antigen; the corresponding protein in humans had a size of 37.2 kDa. They termed the antigen "Izumo" after a Japanese shrine dedicated to marriage. The registered DNA sequence was confirmed by sequencing after polymerase chain reaction with reverse transcription (RT–PCR) with total RNA prepared from the testis. A human homologue was found as an unverified gene in the NCBI database (accession number BC034769). The gene encodes a novel immunoglobulin superfamily (IgSF), type I membrane protein with an extracellular immunoglobulin domain. By immunofluorescence, the Izumo protein was not detectable on the surface of fresh sperm, and only after the acrosome reaction it was detectable. When a polyclonal antihuman Izumo polyclonal antibody was added, no fusion of human spermatozoa to zona-free hamster eggs was observed.

The relevance of the Izumo protein for fertilization was underlined by the experiments of Naz [66], who was able to show that immunization of female mice with peptides derived from Izumo and other sperm-specific proteins could induce antibodies exerting a long-term contraceptive effect.

Genetic defects of the Izumo protein could not be verified in humans up to now. Hayasaka et al. [67] could demonstrate that none of the infertile patients with severe oligozoospermie failed to express this protein on sperm and Granados-Gonzalez et al. [68] could not demonstrate significant mutations in the Izumo gene 9 coding exons sequence in patients with fertilization failure by conventional IVF.

1.4.8
Pronucleus Formation

Oocytes fertilized with ASA bound sperm demonstrated abnormal cleavage of the embryos. The antigens involved had low molecular weights of 14, 18, and 22 kDa [69].

At gamete fusion the sperm tail is incorporated into the ooplasm, and the centriolar region forms the sperm aster. ASA against proteins of the centrioles may be responsible for mitotic arrest [70].

The human nuclear autoantigenic sperm protein (NASP) is a testicular histone-binding protein of 787 amino acids to which most vasectomized men develop ASA. In a study using recombinant deletion mutants spanning the entire protein coding sequence, 20/21 sera had ASA to one or more of the NASP fusion proteins. These may be the cognate antigens of ASA in vasectomized men. The clinical relevance of this antigen, as well as of their antibodies, remains unclear [71, 72].

1.4.9
Conclusions

As practical consequences of the research on ASA related sperm proteomic, those ASA will be identified, which decrease male fertility by inhibiting sperm functions that are essential for fertilization. The presence of antibodies in a biological substrate (serum, seminal plasma) that binds to specific antigens may be visualized by an ELISA or a RIA. However, in contrast to the earlier immunoassays, the sperm antigens used will be known proteins or peptides. As ASA of an individual patient bind to up to ten different proteins,

Table 1.4.1 Defined antigens of naturally occurring human ASA

Antigen	Localisation	Effect of ASA
YWK-II mAb	Equatorial sector of the human sperm head	Agglutination
hSMP-1	Acrosome	Agglutination
Calpastatin	Acrosomal region, tail	Agglutination
YLP(12), a 50±5 kDa membrane protein	Sperm surface	Agglutination
Caspase-3	Sperm surface	Apoptosis
HSP70	Sperm surface	Apoptosis
Human CD52 antigen	Sperm surface, inserted into the sperm membrane during the epididymal passage	Inhibition of motility
1.8- and 2.8 kb mRNAs highly and specifically expressed in testis	Tails of permeabilized human sperm	Inhibition of motility
FSA-1	Sperm surface	Inhibition of acrosome reaction
SPRASA	Acrosomal region	Inhibition of acrosome reaction
Calpastatin	Plasma membrane and the outer acrosomal membrane of sperm	Inhibition of acrosome reaction
Protein P36	Acrosome-reacted sperm	Inhibition of acrosome reaction
hSMP-1	Acrosome	Inhibition of acrosome reaction
FASA-57	Acrosome of non acrosome-reacted sperm, equatorial region after acrosome reaction	Inhibition of acrosome reaction
Sperm protein 17 (Sp17), highly conserved	Testis, head and tail of ejaculated spermatozoa	Inhibition of acrosome reaction
PH-20, a glycerolphosphatidyl-inositol-linked hyaluronidas	Sperm surface	Inhibition of zona binding
55-kDa protein of spermatozoa	Apical edge of the head in capacitated sperm	Inhibition of zona binding
Ag 1F10		Inhibition of zona binding
Fertilization antigen 1 (FA-1)	Specifically reacted with zona protein 3 (ZP3)	Inhibition of zona binding
hSMP-1	Sperm surface	Inhibition of zona binding
hSMP-1, PubMed locus U12978	Acrosome	Inhibition of zona binding
Human nuclear autoantigenic sperm protein (NASP)	Vasectomized men develop ASA to NASP	Unknown
SP-10, a highly conserved intra-acrosomal sperm protein	Sperm surface after acrosome reaction	Inhibition of sperm–oocyte fusion
YLP(12)	Sperm surface	Inhibition of zona binding
Acrin-1	Acrosomal	Ihibtion of acrosome reaction

in a patient with a significantly positive MAR test or IBT up to ten different ELISAs have to be performed in order to decide whether the patient suffers from immune infertility.

The identification of functionally relevant antigens is a prerequisite for treatment options (Table 1.4.1). At present, no antibody specific treatment of autoimmune diseases is possible, but the treatment is on the basis of the suppression of antibody production in general. Increasingly, however, the use of mAb in autoimmune diseases is described. It may be speculated that this procedure also may be adapted to the treatment of autoimmune infertility.

The analysis of the cognate antigens of ASA involved in the process of fertilization is important from another point of view: it improves the identification of immunogenic proteins which are candidates for immune contraception, i.e., which allow the artificial induction of antibodies in male or female inhibiting fertilization. Many groups have described approaches to this topic, but their quotation is outside the scope of this chapter.

References

1. Koide SS, Wang L, Kamada M (2000) Antisperm antibodies associated with infertility: properties and encoding genes of target antigens. Proc Soc Exp Biol Med 224:123–132
2. Yin X, Ouyang S, Xu W, Zhang X, Fok KL, Wong HY, Zhang J, Qiu X, Miao S, Chan HC, Wang L (2007) YWK-II protein as a novel G(o)-coupled receptor for Müllerian inhibiting substance in cell survival. J Cell Sci 120(Pt 9):1521–1528
3. Kuang Y, Yan YC, Gao AW, Zhai YM, Miao SY, Wang LF, Koide SS (2000) Immune responses in rats following oral immunization with attenuated *Salmonella typhimurium* expressing human sperm antigen. Arch Androl 45:169–180
4. Yakirevich E, Naot Y (2000) Cloning of a glucose phosphate isomerase/neuroleukin-like sperm antigen involved in sperm agglutination. Biol Reprod 62:1016 1023
5. Feng HL, Sandlow JI, Zheng LJ (2005) C-kit receptor and its possible function in human spermatozoa. Mol Reprod Dev 70(1):103–110
6. Norton EJ, Diekman AB, Westbrook VA, Flickinger CJ, Herr JC (2001) RASA, a recombinant single-chain variable fragment (scFv) antibody directed against the human sperm surface: implications for novel contraceptives. Hum Reprod 16:1854–1860
7. Xu B, Copolla M, Herr JC, Timko MP (2007) Expression of a recombinant human sperm-agglutinating mini-antibody in tobacco (*Nicotiana tabacum* L.). Soc Reprod Fertil Suppl 63:465–477
8. Bandivdekar AH, Vernekar VJ, Moodbidri SB, Koide SS (2001) Characterization of 80kDa human sperm antigen responsible for immunoinfertility. Am J Reprod Immunol 45:28–34
9. Paasch U, Grunewald S, Glander HJ (2002) Presence of up- and downstream caspases in relation to impairment of human spermatogenesis. Andrologia 34:279–280; abstract
10. Castro A, Parodi D, Morales I, Madariaga M, Rios R, Smith R (2004) Absence of Fas protein detection by flow cytometry in human spermatozoa. Fertil Steril 81(4):1019–1025
11. Martin G, Sabido O, Durand P, Levy R (2004) Cryopreservation induces an apoptosis-like mechanism in bull sperm. Biol Reprod 71(1):28–37
12. Paasch U, Grunewald S, Wuendrich K, Jope T, Glander HJ (2005) Immunomagnetic removal of cryo-damaged human spermatozoa. Asian J Androl 7(1):61–69
13. Wündrich K, Paasch U, Leicht M, Glander HJ (2006) Activation of caspases in human spermatozoa during cryopreservation – an immunoblot study. Cell Tissue Bank 7(2):81–90

14. Hakimi H, Geary I, Pacey A, Eley A (2006) Spermicidal activity of bacterial lipopolysaccharide is only partly due to lipid A. J Androl 27(6):774–779

15. Bohring C, Krause E, Habermann B, Krause W (2001) Isolation and identification of sperm membrane antigens recognized by antisperm antibodies, and their possible role in immunological infertility disease. Mol Hum Reprod 7:113–118

16. Tsuji Y, Mitsuo M, Yasunami R, Sakata K, Shibahara H, Koyama K (2000) HLA-DR and HLA-DQ gene typing of infertile women possessing sperm-immobilizing antibody. J Reprod Immunol 46(1):31–38

17. Tasdemir I, Tasdemir M, Fukuda J, Kodama H, Matsui T, Tanaka T (1996) Sperm immobilization antibodies in infertile male sera decrease the acrosome reaction: a possible mechanism for immunologic infertility. J Assist Reprod Genet 13(5):413–416

18. Isojima S (1989) Characterization of epitopes of seminal plasma antigen stimulating human monoclonal sperm-immobilizing antibodies: a personal review. Reprod Fertil Dev 1(3):193–201

19. Koyama K, Ito K, Hasegawa A (2007) Role of male reproductive tract CD52 (mrt-CD52) in reproduction. Soc Reprod Fertil Suppl 63:103–110

20. Hasegawa A, Koyama K (2005) Antigenic epitope for sperm-immobilizing antibody detected in infertile women. J Reprod Immunol 67(1–2):77–86

21. Neilson LI, Schneider PA, Van Deerlin PG, Kiriakidou M, Driscoll DA, Pellegrini MC, Millinder S, Yamamoto KK, French CK, Strauss JF III (1999) cDNA cloning and characterization of a human sperm antigen (SPAG6) with homology to the product of the Chlamydomonas PF16 locus. Genomics 60:272–280

22. Inaba K, Morisawa S, Morisawa M (1998) Proteasomes regulate the motility of salmonid fish sperm through modulation of cAMP-dependent phosphorylation of an outer arm dynein light chain. J Cell Sci 111:1105–1115

23. Jiang H, Pillai S (1998) Complement regulatory proteins on the sperm surface: relevance to sperm motility. Am J Reprod Immunol 39:243–248

24. Kamieniczna M, Domagała A, Kurpisz M (2003) The frequency of antisperm antibodies in infertile couples–a Polish pilot study. Med Sci Monit 9(4):CR142–CR149

25. Shibahara H, Shiraishi Y, Hirano Y, Kasumi H, Koyama K, Suzuki M (2007) Relationship between level of serum sperm immobilizing antibody and its inhibitory effect on sperm migration through cervical mucus in immunologically infertile women. Am J Reprod Immunol 57(2):142–146

26. Haas GG Jr (1987) Immunologic infertility. Obstet Gynecol Clin North Am 14:1069–1085

27. Clarke GN (1985) Induction of the shaking phenomenon by IgA class antispermatozoal antibodies from serum. Am J Reprod Immunol Microbiol 9:12–14

28. Wang C, Baker HW, Jennings MG, Burger HG, Lutjen P (1985) Interaction between human cervical mucus and sperm surface antibodies. Fertil Steril 44:484–488

29. Bronson RA, Cooper GW, Rosenfeld DL, Gilbert JV, Plaut AG (1987) the effect of an IgA1 protease on immunoglobulins bound to the sperm surface and sperm cervical mucus penetrating ability. Fertil Steril 47:985–991

30. Bohring C, Skrzypek J, Krause W (2001) Influence of antisperm antibodies on the acrosome reaction as determined by flow cytometry. Fertil Steril 76(2):275–280

31. Menge AC, Christman GM, Ohl DA, Naz RK (1999) Fertilization antigen-1 removes antisperm autoantibodies from spermatozoa of infertile men and results in increased rates of acrosome reaction. Fertil Steril 71:256–260

32. Mizuno M, Harris CL, Morgan BP (2007) Immunization with autologous CD46 generates a strong autoantibody response in rats that targets spermatozoa. J Reprod Immunol 73(2):135–147

33. Auer J, Camoin L, Courtot AM, Hotellier F, De Almeida M (2004) Evidence that P36, a human sperm acrosomal antigen involved in the fertilization process is triosephosphate isomerase. Mol Reprod Dev 68(4):515–523

34. Cheng GY, Shi JL, Wang M, Hu YQ, Liu CM, Wang YF, Xu C (2007) Inhibition of mouse acrosome reaction and sperm-zona pellucida binding by anti-human sperm membrane protein 1 antibody. Asian J Androl 9(1):23–29

35. Rossato M, Galeazzi C, Ferigo M, Foresta C (2004) Antisperm antibodies modify plasma membrane functional integrity and inhibit osmosensitive calcium influx in human sperm. Hum Reprod 19(8):1816–1820

36. Feng HL, Han YB, Sparks AE, Sandlow JI (2008) Characterization of human sperm antigens reacting with anti-sperm antibodies from an infertile female patient's serum. J Androl 29(4): 440–448

37. Triphan X, Menzel VA, Petrunkina AM, Cassará MC, Wemheuer W, Hinsch KD, Hinsch E (2008) Localisation and function of voltage-dependent anion channels (VDAC) in bovine spermatozoa. Pflugers Arch 455(4):677–686

38. Wang Z, Zhang Y, Mandal A, Zhang J, Giles FJ, Herr JC, Lim SH (2004) The spermatozoa protein, SLLP1, is a novel cancer-testis antigen in hematologic malignancies. Clin Cancer Res 10(19):6544–6550

39. Chiu WW, Erikson EK, Sole CA, Shelling AN, Chamley LW (2004) SPRASA, a novel sperm protein involved in immune-mediated infertility. Hum Reprod 19(2):243–249

40. Sato Y, Son JH, Tucker RP, Meizel S (2000) The zona pellucida-initiated acrosome reaction: defect due to mutations in the sperm glycine receptor/Cl(−) channel. Dev Biol 227:211–218

41. Reddy KV, Vijayalaxmi G, Rajeev KS, Aranha C (2006) Inhibition of sperm–egg binding and fertilisation in mice by a monoclonal antibody reactive to 57-kDa human sperm surface antigen. Reprod Fertil Dev 18(8):875–884

42. Jagadish N, Rana R, Mishra D, Garg M, Chaurasiya D, Hasegawa A, Koyama K, Suri A (2005) Immunogenicity and contraceptive potential of recombinant human sperm associated antigen (SPAG9). J Reprod Immunol 67(1–2):69–76

43. Lea IA, Widgren EE, O'Rand MG (2004) Association of sperm protein 17 with A-kinase anchoring protein 3 in flagella. Reprod Biol Endocrinol 2:57

44. Lea IA, Richardson RT, Widgren EE, O'Rand MG (1996) Cloning and sequencing of cDNAs encoding the human sperm protein, Sp17. Biochim Biophys Acta 1307(3):263–266

45. Grizzi F, Chiriva-Internati M, Franceschini B, Hermonat PL, Soda G, Lim SH, Dioguardi N (2003) Immunolocalization of sperm protein 17 in human testis and ejaculated spermatozoa. J Histochem Cytochem 51(9):1245–1248

46. Kong M, Richardson RT, Widgren EE, O'Rand MG (1995) Sequence and localization of the mouse sperm autoantigenic protein, Sp17. Biol Reprod 53(3):579–590

47. Lea IA, Adoyo P, O'Rand MG (1997) Autoimmunogenicity of the human sperm protein Sp17 in vasectomized men and identification of linear B cell epitopes. Fertil Steril 67(2):355–361

48. Zhang CH, Li FQ, Yang AL, Sun W, Miao JW (2007) [Detection of anti-Sp17 antibodies in infertile patients' serum and its clinical significance]. Zhonghua Nan Ke Xue 13(1):27–29

49. Breitbart H (2002) Role and regulation of intracellular calcium in acrosomal exocytosis. J Reprod Immunol 53:151–159

50. Mahony MC, Blackmore PF, Bronson RA, Alexander NJ (1991) Inhibition of human sperm-zona pellucida tight binding in the presence of antisperm antibody positive polyclonal patient sera. J Reprod Immunol 19:287–301

51. Liu DY, Clarke GN, Baker HW (1991) Inhibition of human sperm-zona pellucida and sperm-oolemma binding by antisperm antibodies. Fertil Steril 55:440–442

52. Chan CP, Gupta S, Mark GE (1999) Identification of linear surface epitopes on the guinea pig sperm membrane protein PH-20. Life Sci 64:1989–2000

53. Mollova M, Djarkova T, Ivanova M, Stamenova M, Kyurkchiev S (1999) Isolation and biological characterization of boar sperm capacitation-related antigen. Am J Reprod Immunol 42:254–262

54. Naz RK, Zhu X, Kadam AL (2000) Identification of human sperm peptide sequence involved in egg binding for immunocontraception. Biol Reprod 62:318–324

55. Zhu X, Naz RK (1997) Fertilization antigen-1: cDNA cloning, testis-specific expression, and immunocontraceptive effects. Proc Natl Acad Sci U S A 944:704–709

56. Zayas-Pérez H, Casas E, Bonilla E, Betancourt M (2005) Inhibition of sperm-zona pellucida binding by a 55 kDa pig sperm protein in vitro. Arch Androl 51(3):195–206

57. Francavilla F, Romano R, Santucci R (1991) Effect of sperm-antibodies on acrosome reaction of human sperm used for the hamster egg penetration assay. Am J Reprod Immunol 25:77–80

58. Noor MM, Moore HD (1999) Monoclonal antibody that recognizes an epitope of the sperm equatorial region and specifically inhibits sperm–oolemma fusion but not binding. J Reprod Fertil 115:215–224

59. Focarelli R, Giuffrida A, Capparelli S, Scibona M, Fabris FM, Francavilla F, Francavilla S, Giovampaola CD, Rosati F (1998) Specific localization in the equatorial region of gp20, a 20 kDa sialylglycoprotein of the capacitated human spermatozoon acquired during epididymal transit which is necessary to penetrate zona-free hamster eggs. Mol Hum Reprod 4:119–125

60. Gabriele A, D'Andrea G, Cordeschi G, Properzi G, Giammatteo M, De Stefano C, Romano R, Francavilla F, Francavilla S (1998) Carbohydrate binding activity in human spermatozoa: localization, specificity, and involvement in sperm–egg fusion. Mol Hum Reprod 4:543–553

61. Hamatani T, Tanabe K, Kamei K, Sakai N, Yamamoto Y, Yoshimura Y (2000) A monoclonal antibody to human SP-10 inhibits in vitro the binding of human sperm to hamster oolemma but not to human zona pellucida. Biol Reprod 62(5):1201–1208

62. Nomura M, Kitamura M, Matsumiya K, Tsujimura A, Okuyama A, Matsumoto M, Toyoshima K, Seya T (2001) Genomic analysis of idiopathic infertile patients with sperm-specific depletion of CD46. Exp Clin Immunogenet 18:42–50

63. Grace KS, Bronson RA, Ghebrehiwet B (2002) Surface expression of complement receptor gC1q-R/p33 is increased on the plasma membrane of human spermatozoa after capacitation. Biol Reprod 66(3):823–829

64. Busso D, Cohen DJ, Hayashi M, Kasahara M, Cuasnicú PS (2005) Human testicular protein TPX1/CRISP-2: localization in spermatozoa, fate after capacitation and relevance for gamete interaction. Mol Hum Reprod 11(4):299–305

65. Inoue N, Ikawa M, Isotani A, Okabe M (2005) The immunoglobulin superfamily protein Izumo is required for sperm to fuse with eggs. Nature 434(7030):234–238

66. Naz RK (2008) Immunocontraceptive effect of Izumo and enhancement by combination vaccination. Mol Reprod Dev 75(2):336–344

67. Hayasaka S, Terada Y, Inoue N, Okabe M, Yaegashi N, Okamura K (2007) Positive expression of the immunoglobulin superfamily protein IZUMO on human sperm of severely infertile male patients. Fertil Steril 88(1):214–216

68. Granados-Gonzalez V, Aknin-Seifer I, Touraine RL, Chouteau J, Wolf JP, Levy R (2008) Preliminary study on the role of the human IZUMO gene in oocyte-spermatozoa fusion failure. Fertil Steril 90(4):1246–1248

69. Naz RK (1992) Effects of antisperm antibodies on early cleavage of fertilized ova. Biol Reprod 46:130–139

70. Palermo GD, Colombero LT, Rosenwaks Z (1997) The human sperm centrosome is responsible for normal syngamy and early embryonic development. Rev Reprod 2:19–27

71. Batova IN, Richardson RT, Widgren EE, O'Rand MG (2000) Analysis of the autoimmune epitopes on human testicular NASP using recombinant and synthetic peptides. Clin Exp Immunol 121:201–209

72. Cai Y, Gao Y, Sheng Q, Miao S, Cui X, Wang L, Zong S, Koide SS (2002) Characterization and potential function of a novel testis-specific nucleoporin BS-63. Mol Reprod Dev 61:126–134

73. Jager S, Kremer J, Kuiken J, Mulder I. The significance of the Fc part of antispermatozoal antibodies for the shaking phenomenon in the sperm-cervical mucus contact test. Fertil Steril. 1981 Dec;36(6):792–7

74. Li HG, Ding XF, Liao AH et al, Expression of CatSper family transcripts in the mouse testis during post-natal development and human ejaculated spermatozoa: relationship to sperm motility. Mol Hum Reprod 2007;13(5): 299–306

Section II

Antisperm Antibodies (ASA)

The Immune Privilege of the Testis

2.1

Monika Fijak, Sudhanshu Bhushan and Andreas Meinhardt

2.1.1
Introduction

Male germ cells (GC) enter meiosis beginning their complex transition into highly specialized spermatozoa at the time of puberty, after the establishment of immune competence. During the process, a myriad of surface and intracellular proteins are expressed, yet these new autoantigens are tolerated by the testis. The immunogenicity of the proteins is not diminished, as shown by their ability to induce strong autoimmune reactions when injected elsewhere in the body [1, 2]; rather it is the testis itself that confers protection. Initial suggestions that the testis was an immune privileged site were substantiated experimentally when histoincompatible allo- and xenografts placed into the interstitial space of the rat testis survived and prospered for an indefinite period of time [3]. Similarly, ectopically transplanted allogenic Sertoli cells (SC) not only survive, but when co-transplanted with allogenic pancreatic islets, also resist rejection without additional systemic immunosuppression in animals [4]. More recently, the transplantation of spermatogonia in germ cell depleted testis could restore spermatogenesis even across species borders in some instances [5]. There is general agreement that immune privilege is an evolutionary adaptation to protect vulnerable tissues with limited capacity for regeneration, thereby avoiding loss of function [6, 7]. For the testis this means safeguarding reproductive capability. Notwithstanding its immune privileged status, the testis is clearly capable of mounting normal inflammatory responses, as proven by its effective response to viral and bacterial infection. In pathological circumstances, the misbalance between the tolerogenic and the efferent limbs of the testicular immune response can lead to the formation of autosperm antibodies and in rare instances, autoimmune epididymo-orchitis in humans. Immune infertility is now estimated to be a considerable cause of sterility in couples seeking medical assistance [8–12].

The most commonly used model for the investigation of autoimmune-based inflammatory testicular impairment is experimental autoimmune orchitis (EAO), a rodent model

M. Fijak (✉)
Department of Anatomy and Cell Biology, Justus-Liebig-University of Giessen, Giessen, 35385, Germany
e-mail: monika.fijak@anatomie.med.uni-giessen.de

W. K. H. Krause and R. K. Naz (eds.), *Immune Infertility*,
DOI: 10.1007/978-3-642-01379-9_2.1, © Springer Verlag Berlin Heidelberg 2009

based on active immunization with testicular homogenate and adjuvants [13]. The clinical term "orchitis" is particularly attributed to acute, symptomatic disease due to local or systemic infection, whereas subacute or chronic, asymptomatic inflammation of the testis including noninfectious disease is difficult to diagnose and therefore likely to be ignored [14]. Orchitis may also occur in conjunction with infections of the genitourinary tract and as manifestation of sexually-transmitted diseases such as gonorrhea or *Chlamydia trachomatis* [15]. Urethral pathogens, i.e., *Escherichia coli* cause bacterial epididymo-orchitis [16]. The most common cause of viral orchitis is mumps. On balance, these data clearly indicate that the mechanism underlying immune privilege in the testis and its disruption by pathological alterations are matters of clinical importance and hence continued scientific interest. The following sections highlight some of the mechanisms that are associated with the establishment or maintenance of immune privilege.

2.1.2
Blood Testis Barrier

The blood testis barrier (BTB) is comprised of various integral membrane proteins, which in turn contain a number of interesting components such as junctional adhesion molecules (JAMs) and claudins 1 and 11 along with claudins 3–5, claudins 7–8 (also identified in the testis), and occludin [17]. The BTB divides the seminiferous epithelium into two distinct compartments: the basal carrying the spermatogonia, leptotene, and zygotene spermatocytes; and the adluminal with meiotic pachytene and secondary spermatocytes, haploid spermatids, and spermatozoa, which are all completely engulfed by cytoplasm protrusions of the Sertoli cells. The main task of the BTB is to protect the developing GC from the immune system. Meiotic and postmeiotic GC, including spermatozoa (daily production: 150×10^6 spermatozoa in rat [18]), express a large array of neo-antigens that first appear during puberty, long after the establishment of self-tolerance. With the instigation of spermatogenesis, the BTB is concurrently established and immediately sequests postpubertal GC from the immune system (Fig. 2.1.1).

Impairment of BTB integrity has been observed during inflammation, infection, and trauma which ultimately result in germ cell loss [19–21]. Mechanistically, elevated levels of tumor-necrosis factor (TNF)-α and transforming growth factor (TGF)-β, found in systemic and local testicular inflammation [22–25], have been shown to perturb the assembly of the tight junctions in cultured SC probably by downregulating occludin expression [26, 27]. Despite the junction's ability to isolate meiotic and postmeiotic GC from circulating antibodies and leukocytes, it is now accepted that the BTB alone does not account for all the manifestations of the testicular immune privilege. A proposition supported by the findings is that germ cell autoantigens are present in the basal compartment in spermatogonia and early spermatocytes which are not protected by the BTB [28, 29]. Moreover, the BTB is incomplete in the rete testis, a location where immense numbers of spermatozoa with newly adapted surface molecules traverse towards the epididymis, making it a particularly susceptible region for the development of autoimmune orchitis. Furthermore,

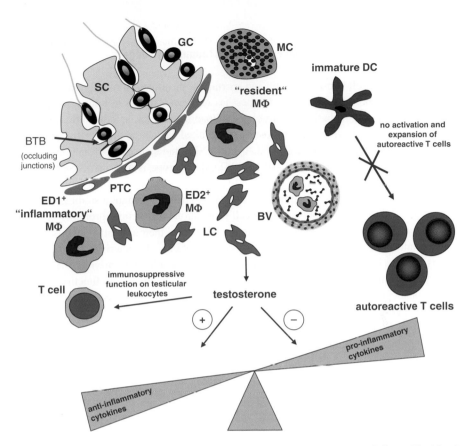

Fig. 2.1.1 Hypothetical model of factors maintaining the testicular immune privilege. The blood testis barrier (BTB) connects neighboring Sertoli cells (SC) and segregates the majority of neo-antigen expressing meiotic and postmeiotic germ cells (GC) from the testicular immune system. In the interstitial space, the ED2+-resident type of macrophages (MΦ) with their immunoregulatory and trophic functions constitute the largest subpopulation of leukocytes, whereas the ED1+ "inflammatory" macrophage cohort is much smaller in number. Most likely the phenotype of testicular dendritic cells (DC) in normal testis inhibits an activation and expansion of autoreactive T lymphocyte clones. The concentration of testosterone in the testicular interstitial fluid synthesized by the Leydig cells (LC) is about 8–10 times higher than that in serum. Recent data point to an increasingly important immunosuppressive role of androgens in inhibiting leukocyte function and reducing proinflammatory cytokine expression. *BV* blood vessels; *PTC* peritubular cells; *MC* mast cells

Head and Billingham [30] showed extended survival (i.e., no immune response/attack) of allografts that were placed under the organ capsule in the testicular interstitium. Therefore, some other mechanism, besides physical separation, must exist to maintain testicular immune privilege, which requires more robust protection of the tolerogenic environment of the testis.

2.1.3
Endocrine Regulation of Testicular Function and Immune Privilege

In addition to the well known anabolic and spermatogenic effects, a role for androgens in down regulating proinflammatory cytokines has now been shown in both experimental and clinical studies. Incubation of stimulated human monocytes, macrophages, and several nonimmune cell types with testosterone, resulted in the suppression of adhesion molecules and cytokines such as IL-1, IL-6, and TNFα and increased production of anti-inflammatory cytokines such as IL-10 [31–34]. Testosterone is also involved in T cell apoptosis [35]. A direct connection between sex steroid levels and testicular immune privilege was shown by Head and Billingham [36], when in transplantation studies, rats pretreated with estrogen to suppress Leydig cell testosterone production, promptly rejected intratesticular allografts in direct contrast to the reaction of their untreated cohorts. These studies indicate that high local testosterone concentrations, characteristic for the testis, seem to play an important role in the maintenance of testicular immune privilege. However, the precise manner in which testosterone mediates its anti-inflammatory functions on testicular leukocytes is as yet unknown. What can be surmised from the available data is that it appears likely that androgens exert their immunosuppressive function on testicular leukocytes either via nongenomic pathways [37] or indirectly by regulating the balance between pro and anti-inflammatory cytokine expressions in the Sertoli, Leydig, and peritubular cells (PTC).

2.1.4
Mechanism of Maintenance and Disturbance of Testicular Immune Privilege

2.1.4.1
Macrophages

Under normal conditions macrophages and all other leukocytes are exclusively found in the interstitial space; in humans they are also found in the tubular wall, but never within the seminiferous epithelium. There is little doubt that macrophages play a central role in the establishment and maintenance of the immune privilege of the testis. This supposition was first substantiated by in vitro studies where testicular macrophages displayed a reduced capacity to synthesize IL-1β and TNFα compared with macrophages from other tissues [38–40], and exhibited immunosuppressive characteristics [39, 41]. In the rat testis, at least two subsets of macrophages can be discerned. This heterogeneity has functional implications as in the testis the ED1+ "inflammatory" subsets, but only few ED2+ resident macrophages, express MCP-1 and iNOS in untreated and LPS challenged rats [42, 43]. The ED2+ resident population of testicular macrophages does not participate in promoting inflammatory processes; it is thought to have an immunoregulatory role in maintaining immune privilege and tropic functions, particularly on Leydig cells. Clear evidence points out that the ED1+ED2- monocytes/macrophages are involved in the testicular inflammatory response and it is the influx of ED1+ monocytes during acute and chronic inflammation that drastically alters the composition of the macrophage population and shifts the cytokine balance in favor of an inflammatory response with the potential to overcome the immune privilege [42–44].

2.1.4.2
Dendritic Cells (DC)

DC are a heterogeneous population that belongs to the most important antigen presenting cells (APC) and play a major role in the initiation and orchestration of primary immune responses of both helper and cytotoxic T and B lymphocytes – the effector cells of the adaptive immune system. DC not only activate lymphocytes, but also tolerize T cells to antigens, thereby minimizing autoaggressive immune responses [45]. DC migrate as immature or precursor cells from the bone marrow into peripheral tissue where, upon receiving an activatory signal associated with pathogens or inflammation, they migrate to the local lymph nodes, mature, and present the antigens to T cells captured in the periphery [45]. Immature DC have the highest capacity to internalize antigens, but have low T cell stimulatory activity, whereas mature DC downregulate their endocytic activity and are excellent T lymphocyte stimulators [46]. Mature DC are characterized by the upregulation of surface T cell co-stimulatory (CD40, CD80 and CD86) and MHC class II molecules, the production of bioactive IL-12 and TNFα, and changes in migratory behavior [47]. Both MHC class I and II expressions occur within the interstitial tissue of the testis including the macrophages and Leydig cells. Our own results show that also testicular DC express MHC II molecules. In contrast, on the developing GC MHC antigens are reduced in number or absent. These data indicate that spermatogenic cells are able to avoid direct recognition by CD4+ and CD8+ T cells, which may be important for reducing the potential for antigen specific immune response elicited by DC or macrophages in the seminiferous epithelium [48–53]. In spite of their potential importance in maintaining the balance of the testicular immune status between tolerance (immune privilege) and (auto-)immunogenic reply, DC in the male gonad have received little attention in the past. The presence of DC in normal (approximately 1×10^5 cells) and chronically inflamed testes from Wistar and Sprague-Dawley rats was determined and quantified for the first time using DC specific markers (Ox62 and CD11c) [54]. In experimentally induced autoimmune orchitis (EAO), DC were found in the interstitial space of the testis and, in large numbers, in the granulomas. Although increases of between 5.5- (CD11c) and 8-fold (Ox62) were seen compared to controls, these quantities are still significantly lower than the number of macrophages found in similar circumstances [54–57]. Testicular DC isolated from EAO animals significantly enhanced naïve T cell proliferation compared with control DC from untreated animals suggesting a more tolerogenic phenotype for DC in normal testis function, thereby maintaining immune privilege [58].

In light of the "danger model," the recent characterization of numerous heat shock proteins (e.g., Hsp60 and Hsp70 among others) as testicular autoantigens could provide a mechanism of how DC in the testis participate in the activation of autoreactive lymphocytes and in the subsequent damage of testicular tissue, thereby overcoming the immune privilege [59]. Millar et al. [60] provided evidence that Hsp70, when released by necrotic cells, acts like a danger signal by enhancing the maturation of DC, which then trigger autoimmunity. It is important to note that the release of endogenous inflammatory signals (e.g., Hsp70) requires necrotic cell death such as that resulting from infection or injury. On the basis of our own data and that of other autoimmune disease models, we hypothesize that immature DC, normally involved in maintaining immune privilege, under inflammatory pathological conditions sense self antigens like Hsp70 as danger signals and after maturation may overcome immune privilege/immune tolerance by local activation and expansion of autoreactive T cells.

2.1.5
Conclusions

There is now widespread agreement that the immune system, spermatogenesis, and steroidogenesis, the intrinsic testicular functions, are intricately linked by a network of complex interactions. The importance of the delicate balance needed, between the suppression of the immune response to protect the GC from autoattack on the one hand and the ability to have an active immune response to prevent damage from infection, trauma, and cancer on the other, is reflected by the fact that in the human male about 12–13%, in some studies even more, of all diagnosed infertility is related to an immunological reason, while its contribution to idiopathic infertility (31% of all cases) remains unknown [8, 10–12]. The mechanisms responsible for the testes' immune privilege are still far from being understood, but it is apparent that the identified factors involved are multiple and probably redundant. Overall, long regarded as a peculiar side issue of testis function, immune privilege is now established as part of the general scheme of male gamete formation and successful reproduction. Further research in the area will not only help to improve diagnosis and treatment of immunological male infertility, but will also open new avenues in contraceptive development and transplantation medicine.

References

1. Suescun MO, Calandra RS, Lustig L (1994) Alterations of testicular function after induced autoimmune orchitis in rats. J Androl 15:442–448
2. Tung KS, Unanue ER, Dixon FJ (1971) Immunological events associated with immunization by sperm in incomplete Freund's adjuvant. Int Arch Allergy Appl Immunol 41:565–574
3. Setchell BP (1990) The testis and tissue transplantation: historical aspects. J Reprod Immunol 18:1–8
4. Selawry HP, Cameron DF (1993) Sertoli cell-enriched fractions in successful islet cell transplantation. Cell Transplant 2:123–129
5. Brinster RL (2002) Germline stem cell transplantation and transgenesis. Science 296:2174–2176
6. Filippini A, Riccioli A, Padula F et al (2001) Control and impairment of immune privilege in the testis and in semen. Hum Reprod Update 7:444–449

7. Setchell BP, Uksila J, Maddocks S, Pollanen P (1990) Testis physiology relevant to immunoregulation. J Reprod Immunol 18:19–32
8. Mahmoud A, Comhaire FH (2006) Immunological causes. In: Schill W-B, Comhaire FH, Hargreave TB (eds) Andrology for the clinician. Springer, Berlin, pp 47–52
9. McLachlan RI (2002) Basis, diagnosis and treatment of immunological infertility in men. J Reprod Immunol 57:35–45
10. Naz RK (2004) Modalities for treatment of antisperm antibody mediated infertility: novel perspectives. Am J Reprod Immunol 51:390–397
11. Nieschlag E, Behre HM (2000) Andrology: male reproductive health and dysfunction, 2nd edn. Springer, Berlin
12. WHO (1987) Towards more objectivity in diagnosis and management of male infertility. Int J Androl (Suppl 7):1–53
13. Tung KS, Teuscher C (1995) Mechanisms of autoimmune disease in the testis and ovary. Hum Reprod Update 1:35–50
14. Schuppe HC, Meinhardt A (2005) Immune privilege and inflammation of the testis. Chem Immunol Allergy 88:1–14
15. Weidner W, Krause W, Ludwig M (1999) Relevance of male accessory gland infection for subsequent fertility with special focus on prostatitis. Hum Reprod Update 5:421–432
16. Jenkin GA, Choo M, Hosking P, Johnson PD (1998) Candidal epididymo-orchitis: case report and review. Clin Infect Dis 26:942–945
17. Wong EW, Mruk DD, Cheng CY (2008) Biology and regulation of ectoplasmic specialization, an atypical adherens junction type, in the testis. Biochim Biophys Acta 1778:692–708
18. de Kretser DM, Kerr JB (1994) The cytology of the testis. In: Knobil E, Neill J (eds) Physiology of reproduction, 2nd edn. Raven, New York, pp 1177–1300
19. Comhaire FH, Mahmoud AM, Depuydt CE, Zalata AA, Christophe AB (1999) Mechanisms and effects of male genital tract infection on sperm quality and fertilizing potential: the andrologist's viewpoint. Hum Reprod Update 5:393–398
20. Johnson MH (1970) Changes in the blood-testis barrier of the guinea-pig in relation to histological damage following iso-immunization with testis. J Reprod Fertil 22:119–127
21. Lewis-Jones DI, Richards RC, Lynch RV, Joughin EC (1987) Immunocytochemical localisation of the antibody which breaches the blood-testis barrier in sympathetic orchiopathia. Br J Urol 59:452–457
22. Hales DB, Diemer T, Hales KH (1999) Role of cytokines in testicular function. Endocrine 10:201–217
23. Hedger MP, Meinhardt A (2003) Cytokines and the immune-testicular axis. J Reprod Immunol 58:1–26
24. Huleihel M, Lunenfeld E (2004) Regulation of spermatogenesis by paracrine/autocrine testicular factors. Asian J Androl 6:259–268
25. Iosub R, Klug J, Fijak M et al (2006) Development of testicular inflammation in the rat involves activation of proteinase-activated receptor-2. J Pathol 208:686–698
26. Mankertz J, Tavalali S, Schmitz H et al (2000) Expression from the human occludin promoter is affected by tumor necrosis factor alpha and interferon gamma. J Cell Sci 113(Pt 11): 2085–2090
27. Siu MK, Lee WM, Cheng CY (2003) The interplay of collagen IV, tumor necrosis factor-alpha, gelatinase B (matrix metalloprotease-9), and tissue inhibitor of metalloproteases-1 in the basal lamina regulates Sertoli cell-tight junction dynamics in the rat testis. Endocrinology 144: 371–387
28. Saari T, Jahnukainen K, Pollanen P (1996) Autoantigenicity of the basal compartment of seminiferous tubules in the rat. J Reprod Immunol 31:65–79
29. Yule TD, Montoya GD, Russell LD, Williams TM, Tung KS (1988) Autoantigenic germ cells exist outside the blood testis barrier. J Immunol 141:1161–1167

30. Head JR, Billingham RE (1985) Immunologically privileged sites in transplantation immunology and oncology. Perspect Biol Med 29:115–131
31. Gornstein RA, Lapp CA, Bustos-Valdes SM, Zamorano P (1999) Androgens modulate interleukin-6 production by gingival fibroblasts in vitro. J Periodontol 70:604–609
32. Hatakeyama H, Nishizawa M, Nakagawa A, Nakano S, Kigoshi T, Uchida K (2002) Testosterone inhibits tumor necrosis factor-alpha-induced vascular cell adhesion molecule-1 expression in human aortic endothelial cells. FEBS Lett 530:129–132
33. Li ZG, Danis VA, Brooks PM (1993) Effect of gonadal steroids on the production of IL-1 and IL-6 by blood mononuclear cells in vitro. Clin Exp Rheumatol 11:157–162
34. Liva SM, Voskuhl RR (2001) Testosterone acts directly on CD4+ T lymphocytes to increase IL-10 production. J Immunol 167:2060–2067
35. McMurray RW, Suwannaroj S, Ndebele K, Jenkins JK (2001) Differential effects of sex steroids on T and B cells: modulation of cell cycle phase distribution, apoptosis and bcl-2 protein levels. Pathobiology 69:44–58
36. Head JR, Billingham RE (1985) Immune privilege in the testis. II. Evaluation of potential local factors. Transplantation 40:269–275
37. Benten WP, Lieberherr M, Stamm O, Wrehlke C, Guo Z, Wunderlich F (1999) Testosterone signaling through internalizable surface receptors in androgen receptor-free macrophages. Mol Biol Cell 10:3113–3123
38. Hayes R, Chalmers SA, Nikolic-Paterson DJ, Atkins RC, Hedger MP (1996) Secretion of bioactive interleukin 1 by rat testicular macrophages in vitro. J Androl 17:41–49
39. Kern S, Maddocks S (1995) Indomethacin blocks the immunosuppressive activity of rat testicular macrophages cultured in vitro. J Reprod Immunol 28:189–201
40. Kern S, Robertson SA, Mau VJ, Maddocks S (1995) Cytokine secretion by macrophages in the rat testis. Biol Reprod 53:1407–1416
41. Bryniarski K, Szczepanik M, Maresz K, Ptak M, Ptak W (2004) Subpopulations of mouse testicular macrophages and their immunoregulatory function. Am J Reprod Immunol 52:27–35
42. Gerdprasert O, O'Bryan MK, Muir JA et al (2002) The response of testicular leukocytes to lipopolysaccharide-induced inflammation: further evidence for heterogeneity of the testicular macrophage population. Cell Tissue Res 308:277–285
43. Gerdprasert O, O'Bryan MK, Nikolic-Paterson DJ, Sebire K, de Kretser DM, Hedger MP (2002) Expression of monocyte chemoattractant protein-1 and macrophage colony-stimulating factor in normal and inflamed rat testis. Mol Hum Reprod 8:518–524
44. Suescun MO, Rival C, Theas MS, Calandra RS, Lustig L (2003) Involvement of tumor necrosis factor-alpha in the pathogenesis of autoimmune orchitis in rats. Biol Reprod 68:2114–2121
45. Banchereau J, Steinman RM (1998) Dendritic cells and the control of immunity. Nature 392:245–252
46. Banchereau J, Briere F, Caux C et al (2000) Immunobiology of dendritic cells. Annu Rev Immunol 18:767–811
47. Hackstein H, Thomson AW (2004) Dendritic cells: emerging pharmacological targets of immunosuppressive drugs. Nat Rev Immunol 4:24–34
48. Haas GG Jr, D'Cruz OJ, De Bault LE (1988) Distribution of human leukocyte antigen-ABC and -D/DR antigens in the unfixed human testis. Am J Reprod Immunol Microbiol 18:47–51
49. Lustig L, Lourtau L, Perez R, Doncel GF (1993) Phenotypic characterization of lymphocytic cell infiltrates into the testes of rats undergoing autoimmune orchitis. Int J Androl 16:279–284
50. Pollanen P, Jahnukainen K, Punnonen J, Sainio-Pollanen S (1992) Ontogeny of immunosuppressive activity, MHC antigens and leukocytes in the rat testis. J Reprod Immunol 21:257–274
51. Pollanen P, Maddocks S (1988) Macrophages, lymphocytes and MHC II antigen in the ram and the rat testis. J Reprod Fertil 82:437–445
52. Pollanen P, Niemi M (1987) Immunohistochemical identification of macrophages, lymphoid cells and HLA antigens in the human testis. Int J Androl 10:37–42

53. Tung KS, Yule TD, Mahi-Brown CA, Listrom MB (1987) Distribution of histopathology and Ia positive cells in actively induced and passively transferred experimental autoimmune orchitis. J Immunol 138:752–759
54. Rival C, Lustig L, Iosub R et al (2006) Identification of a dendritic cell population in normal testis and in chronically inflamed testis of rats with autoimmune orchitis. Cell Tissue Res 324(2):311–318
55. Meinhardt A, Bacher M, Metz C et al (1998) Local regulation of macrophage subsets in the adult rat testis: examination of the roles of the seminiferous tubules, testosterone, and macrophage-migration inhibitory factor. Biol Reprod 59:371–378
56. Rival C, Theas MS, Suescun MO et al (2008) Functional and phenotypic characteristics of testicular macrophages in experimental autoimmune orchitis. J Pathol 215:108–117
57. Wang J, Wreford NG, Lan HY, Atkins R, Hedger MP (1994) Leukocyte populations of the adult rat testis following removal of the Leydig cells by treatment with ethane dimethane sulfonate and subcutaneous testosterone implants. Biol Reprod 51:551–561
58. Rival C, Guazzone VA, von Wulffen W et al (2007) Expression of co-stimulatory molecules, chemokine receptors and proinflammatory cytokines in dendritic cells from normal and chronically inflamed rat testis. Mol Hum Reprod 13:853–861
59. Fijak M, Iosub R, Schneider E et al (2005) Identification of immunodominant autoantigens in rat autoimmune orchitis. J Pathol 207:127–138
60. Millar DG, Garza KM, Odermatt B et al (2003) Hsp70 promotes antigen-presenting cell function and converts T-cell tolerance to autoimmunity in vivo. Nat Med 9:1469–1476

Immune Chemistry of ASA

2.2

Maciej Kurpisz and Marzena Kamieniczna

2.2.1
Introduction

Antisperm antibody (ASA) can be recognized as a strange immunological phenomenon. First of all, the immune response to spermatozoa is rarely sperm-specific; on the other hand, it cannot also be considered as a part of polyorgan type of reaction since such cross-reactivity was rarely found. In the older literature, ASA were occasionally linked to react with kidney (rabbit) or thyroid (beagle dog); however, such cross-reactions were not generally confirmed in mammals as long as sperm antigens were not enhanced during vaccinations in female immunocontraceptive trials when the molecular similarity of sperm PH20 protein to kidney antigens [1] was observed. Furthermore, ASA reaction is different in ontogenesis since only during puberty sperm antigens seem to appear. ASA can then be considered as the enhancement of the existing "natural" antibodies. Since the onset of puberty, we may treat ASA as the mature response to gametes of adult individuals which may interfere with infertility. Discrepancy of ASA reactions, however, still exists between female and male subjects as well as regarding its prepubertal phenomenon. This brings us to the serious questions on the nature of ASA: are they unique or too common (from immunological point of view)?, why are they so rarely sperm-specific?, and are they mostly mediated through the carbohydrate moicties? The first subdivision in their chemistry of reaction (antigenic epitopes) would be therefore ontogenically based on a) circulating "natural" autoantibodies, b) ASA developed prepuberty, c) ASA developed in females, d) ASA developed in males, and e) carbohydrate-mediated ASA antibodies with different degree of molecular identity (including "molecular mimicry").

M. Kurpisz (✉)
Department of Reproductive Biology and Stem Cells, Institute of Human Genetics, Polish Academy of Sciences, Strzeszynska 32, 60-479 Poznan, Poland
e-mail: kurpimac@man.poznan.pl

W. K. H. Krause and R. K. Naz (eds.), *Immune Infertility*,
DOI: 10.1007/978-3-642-01379-9_2.2, © Springer Verlag Berlin Heidelberg 2009

2.2.2
Natural Autoantibodies

Investigating both the female sera and their genital secretions, the presence of the antibodies with broad specificity to the so-called "public" antigenic determinants was found. These were often consisted of carbohydrates that have properties to induce IgM, pentameric antibodies reactive to the range of cells carrying common epitopes (carbohydrates). It has then been discovered through the technique of monoclonal antibodies that very often the antibodies of IgM class were the most prominent ones in detecting common sugar structures although affinity of such antibodies was not of a very high magnitude. Thus spermatozoa with a richly developed glycocalyx were one of the cells commonly reactive with such antibodies. One of the hypotheses of female genital tract formulated by Hancock regarded such "natural" broadly cross-reactive antibodies as one of the elements of female isotolerance to sperm [2]. Although a definition of "natural" autoantibodies was questioned in existing literature several times, they were subsequently rediscovered by Paradisi et al. [3, 4]. At the opportunity to detect novel sperm entities by Western immunoblotting, they found at least two strange phenomena: (1) intensity of reactions from fertile and infertile (but not infertility-mediated) polyclonal human sera were different with fertile vs. infertile sperm and (2) fertile sera represented certain fraction of positive reactions with sperm originating from in vivo fertile males. Such phenomena were then frequently reported by various other groups which reported positive reactions both by Western immunoblotting and 2D electrophoresis when using polyclonal human sera from some of the ASA-negative donors that precipitated distinct spots [5–8]. In our observations with Western immunoblotting technique [9, 10], we have found the quite broad phenomena of positive reactions presented by ASA-negative human sera while at the same time identifying the activities both to sperm as well as to human lymphocytes or erythrocytes, proving once again the character of previously formulated reactions by "natural" antibodies. Although the development of such antibodies would have most probably taken place through "molecular mimicry," it is clear that these "public" determinants may mask the more specific immune autoantibody response when sperm would appear around puberty. According to Paradisi et al. [11], some of these specificities represented by "natural" antibodies may be enhanced through the breakdown of physiological tolerance which may augment such reactions to the pathological level. So he formulated some of these "public" specificities as the ones belonging to both the groups ("natural" and the "pathological" ones), thus formulating three categories of sperm antigens: (1) "natural" ones (appearing in fertile individuals), (2) the infertile ones (assigning immune pathological reactions), and (3) enhanced reactivities derived from the first category. This could be particularly true (category 3) while looking at the antibodies reacting with sperm, which at the same time recognize antigens on lymphocytes and erythrocytes. They can be molecularly differentiated based on antigenic (carbohydrate) isoforms, which may then dissociate into antisperm and anti-lymphocytic reactions (CD52 antigen). It is unquestionable that both types of CD52 may have completely different functional meanings [12].

Another proof for "natural" antibodies originated from the studies on ASAs developed prepuberty. Although, it became recently evident that even at prepuberty we may find testicular specific antigens responsible for immunological reactions initiated by testicular pathology (cryptorchidism, torsion, mobile testis(es)), it was previously found in mammals that puberty (sperm appearance) induces physiological reactions which all of sudden become enhanced just at prepuberty. Brilliant documentation of this phenomenon was done in rodents model [13] (most of it in rats) where it was indicated that serum ASAs increased only after sexual maturation which may suggest that some differentiation antigens on sperm are processed and presented to the immune system under the normal circumstances (at least in some strains). Interestingly, it may be added that in our studies we indicated enhanced (as comparing to adults) ASA reactions prepuberty (in normal boys) while Tung et al. [14] reported it in both sexes (surely through "molecular mimicry" mechanism to microorganisms expressing similar carbohydrate groups). Physiological, sperm antigenic "leak" documented in variety of rodents (guinea pig, rats, rabbits, dark mink) could be an important mechanism reassuring immune tolerance to the newly appearing cells (sperm).

Finally, coming back to the original statement, it has to be emphasized that the level of "natural" ASAs is ontogenically driven and independent on the level of auto- and isoimmune reactions to sperm in adults. It begins from the relatively high values (until puberty), declines thereafter in order to reach another peak post 40 years and finally declines with very advanced age (>88 years) which illustrates the general immunity phenomenon and its regulatory feedback (possibly through Treg population) [15].

2.2.3
ASA Antibodies Developed Prepuberty

In the scientific literature, we may find only few reports (often contradictory) on the existence of ASA in prepubertal boys with testicular failures [16–18]. Since, until now there are undefined objective "markers" allowing prognosis of future fertility status in these boys, it is postulated to carry on surgical procedures (orchidopexy) in cryptorchidism, undescendent testis or mobile testis at the earliest opportunity as well as to suppress (possible with steroids *or* anti-globulin therapy) the immune response to eliminate a risk of high levels of circulating ASA that may persist until puberty. Urry et al. [19] have observed circulating ASA in infertile males suffering at childhood on one or both undescendent testis(es). ASA were present in 66% of such infertile males when comparing to 2.6 or 2.8% in groups consisting of infertile individuals without testicular failures or in vivo fertile men. In the patients with cryptorchidism in the past, low sperm quality (low sperm count, low sperms with progressive motility) was also observed. It could be therefore suggested that developed prepuberty antibodies may mature during different episodes of ontogenesis (including somatic mutations) and then may react with antigens of mature spermatozoa, being a reason for low sperm quality connected with infertility [20].

Undescendent testis(es) are located in the conditions of elevated temperature [21] comparing to scrotum, so it might induce the development of degenerative changes in spermatogenesis or may lead to unique exposure of membrane (integral) antigens in germ cells (spermatogonial stem cells) already present in the gonads. It can be also considered that the change in Leydig cells functioning at elevated temperature may alter the local synthesis and secretion of sex hormones (testosterone) [22]. Altogether, this may induce destructive immune response that could be initiated in favoring conditions of the lack of appropriate populations of T regulatory cells that are not triggered due to the absence of spermatozoa. It is also well known that location of the testis in abdomen may cause enhanced activity of proto-oncogenes which may result in increased frequency of testicular cancer [23].

As we know, the blood–testis barrier is not formed until the signaling from the initiated spermatogenesis; thus, circulating ASA antibodies induced through the elements of testis may freely traverse the prepubertal gonad and such phenomenon seems to be dose-dependent when testicular failure has been observed [24]. Interestingly, very often after the removal of the one gonad (involved in pathological process) significant decrease of the circulating ASA titre in comparison to preoperative stage is observed. It could be speculated that gonads are both inducive as well as the sorbent elements of the ongoing immune response. It could be also reasonable to speculate that persisting ASA may be enhanced at the time of puberty (appearance of sperm) while being on the wrong side of the barrier. At the same time, the "molecular mimicry" due to the past experience of infections ("mumps") may be still an active component. It is quite reasonable therefore to warn against the using of bacterial wall nonspecific lysates as the form of vaccination in boys around puberty [25].

It has to be pointed out that "natural antibodies" can be enhanced and/or their background may be the significant obstacle in the proper detection of the patognomic levels of ASA during that period of time. There is no established, reliable "cut off" value that would argue for suppression of immune response in such "threatened" boys, specifically the widely accepted immunobead test (IBT) does not serve the purpose. Conversely, new assays are required that would bring positive predictive value for the later observed decrease in sperm quality. In our studies on ASA developed prepuberty, we have used at least five assays (IBT, MAR test, immunosorbent assay, flow cytometry, Western immuno-blotting) to conclude on the nature of the observed ASA [16] due to visible and significant inter-individual variability in ASA levels. The sperm epitopic changes must be taken under consideration because of the subtle mechanisms of low sperm immunogenicity and possibly low affinity at the initial stages of immune response development. Sperm partial denaturation (fixation reagents), as well as assays sensitivity and specificity, should be carefully defined in each of the applied tests. Western immunoblotting vs. flow cytometry on live sperm could be interesting to be reciprocally validated.

The fact that deserves the very careful attention is that apart from the possibility raised toward the "natural antibodies" enhancement in prepuberty cases one has to admit that mass spectrometry made out of some of the spots reactive with polyclonal sera (from prepubertal boys) indicated several sperm-specific entities [5]. This may argue against no biological meaning of low affinity circulating ASA antibodies and its putative limited interference with reproductive events.

2.2.4
ASA Antibodies in Females

Immunological tolerance has also been an important factor in females. The mechanisms of quick elimination of deposited spermatoza belong to the arm of the innate immunity. The occurrence of the so-called "natural antibodies" (see, above) is one of them. Influx of leukocytes after semen deposition (clearing mechanism), opsonization of sperm, and engagement of local lymph nodes (in favor of tolerance rather than immunization) should be mentioned here [26]. However, we have to realize that both in males and females, the reproductive system is in close contact with exogenous antigens (microorganisms, antigens of natural and artificial nature, and also haptens and allergens), so both arms of immunity, the innate and adaptive ones, have to be incredibly precise in order to differentiate between the pathogenic antigens and the sperm which periodically (but in big numbers) enter the reproductive tract. No wonder that all the stimuli reaching cervix and cervical canal may affect the labile environment of selective immune tolerance. Yet, local disorder such as cervical infection, its erosion, neoplasma, and hysterectomy provide conditions of the immediate danger to initiate the response toward spermatozoa.

The chemistry of female isoimmune response is absolutely intriguing and is distinctly different from autoimmune response in males. First of all, whatever we would like to say about the common carbohydrate structures on sperm and other cells, the female isoimmune response does not follow the normal pattern of reaction. Such a difference is reflected, first of all, with some readiness to differentiate among the partners [27] but at the same time not being sperm-specific. In our earlier work, we aimed to analyze ASA-positive infertile individuals of both sexes, finding numerous false-positive reactions in female sera (but at the same time not being able to trace the polyclonal ASA in cervix) and not being able to core immune-reactive spots present in 2D to the mass spectrometry (the rate of success was far more less than for male sera). At the same time, we have to be careful about the effective local immune response, as the frequency of ASA in cervical mucus (>10%) is greater than in serum (5–8%) when analyzing the same Caucasoid populations [28]. Speaking of the ability of female local immune response to differentiate among the individual protein isoforms, at the same time not being so much sperm-specific, creates a space for the statement that most of this immune response in females interferes with sperm on the basis of "molecular mimicry." Yet, we may find a lot of differences between subtypes of female immune response regarding carbohydrate-mediated reactions as sperm agglutination and immobilization. As it was reported in a relatively old literature, the lectin-mediated sperm agglutination was mostly induced through terminally positioned common sugar residues while sperm-immobilization test [29] appears as the far more selective one and therefore not being considered as a good ASA screening assay. Yet, sperm-immobilizing antibodies also react to sperm carbohydrates.

The most representative cycle of experiments of female ASA isoimmune response originates from the work of Isojima and Koyama groups dissecting the molecular epitope of one of the glycoprotein, coded as CD52, present on both sperm and somatic cells (lymphocytes). Three classes of highly specific antibodies were developed to this epitope (first originated from woman with circulating sperm-immobilizing antibodies) [30]. Originally obtained MAb of heterohybridoma cell line was coded as H6 3C4. (This epitope can be removed by N-deglycosylation). Next two antibodies, 1G12 (IgM mouse monoclonal antibody with sperm-immobilizing activity) and Campath-1 (IgM monoclonal antibody) were then obtained, both recognized CD52 molecule, albeit with different specificity. The first one (1G12) reacted with structure formed by the GPI anchor and/or peptide portion while Campath 1 epitope included COOH-terminal three amino acid sequence on the core peptide. It was then provided (by 2D electrophoresis) different pattern of reaction, including (in case of 1G12) most possibly the reaction with three spots of O-linked carbohydrates; in the case of Campath-1, carbohydrates were not involved and they were completely absent on the lymphocytes carrying CD52 molecule. It is extremely interesting that when antiserum has been produced by immunization with CD52 core protein, it reacted to sperm causing sperm agglutination and complement-dependent sperm immobilization as well. Thus, different portions of CD52 molecule including carbohydrate moieties, core peptide and GPI anchor may induce ASA which interfere with sperm motility. So, when the studies showed that glycosylation pattern included both N-linked and O-linked carbohydrates on mrtCD52 (mrt – male reproductive tract) and they both contributed to the heterogenous negative charge of CD52 – such a structure may prevent the cells from autoagglutination and nonspecific adherence to adjacent tissues. Consequently, as the female genital tract is often subjected to frequent infections with various pathogens (bacteria, viruses, protozoa) such protection from autoagglutination seems to be a quite helpful evolutionary mechanism for sperm transport. However, the mechanism by which mrtCD52 induces ASA in female genital tract is unknown. Furthermore, it seems that N-linked carbohydrate structures are not well-recognized immunogens (similar studies on N-linked moieties were performed on autoantibodies in males), therefore sperm-immobilizing antibodies are not the most often encountered type of ASA antibodies. However, as we have said before, a plethora of factors may enhance immunological responses in the female reproductive tract and although they can be led by "natural" antibodies at first, they may fall easily (through any type of "molecular mimicry" enhancement) to the "category 3 antigens" proposed by Paradisi et al. [11].

2.2.5
ASA Antibodies in Males

Although ASAs may start to develop together with the other autoantibodies as the often quoted example of beagle dogs and associated autoimmune thyroiditis, it could be also a misleading phenomenon. This has been, however, repeated in females, in whom ASAs are mostly appearing among the other reactivities, mostly associated with thyroid, and then with the other organs as it can be encountered in women approaching IVF or those with polycystic ovary syndrome (PCOS) or premature ovarian failure (POF). These type of reactions did not become, however, a rule in respect to autoantibodies in males. It could follow well in line with lack of specificity of ASA reactions in women but it is not the essence of autoreactions in men [5]. Indeed, it is somehow a mystery that despite of the abundantly glycosylated sperm surface we can observe the formation of specific ASA (among the autoantibodies). It became very fortunate in man that, unlike in the other species (guinea pig, rabbits, monkey), we may notice a certain type of protection against the ASA autoreactivities initiated by vasectomy procedure that has never became the inducer of the polyorgan type of autoimmunity. This observation did not exclude, however, the epidemiology of ASA along the other pathologies including infectious microbial agents. Interestingly, in some reports the opposite type of reactions concerning males and females in respect to *Listeria monocytogenes* (mouse model), which was then associated with differential interleukin-10 production [31], was found. It was also more often noticed in females than in males that the ASAs appear together with chlamydial infections (often associated with infertility) [32]. It may favor the previously presented suggestion that females tend to react more readily with "common" (public) epitopes than the males who tend to be rather sperm-specific; this can be logical taking into account the presence of sperm in males (and its absence in females). Males may drive humoral response into more mature antibodies (somatic mutations) with better affinity to sperm antigens although the affinity process of ASA formation has never been directly observed (even more, this would be an urgent issue when concerning the sex differences). Another finding was the cross-reactivity of ASAs with filarial nematode (*Litomosoides sigmodontis)* [33] as well as the development of ASA circulating antibodies in diarrhoeal diseases (shigellosis, salomonellosis) [34] or their coexistence with *Helicobacter pylori* [35] and in patients with ulcerative colitis [36]. Several questions or hypotheses might be then raised concerning the initial point of ASA formation in males. First, the interesting pattern of elevated cytokines (innate immunity) associated with general inflammatory reactions that occurred in case of lethal filariosis which became associated with interferon (IFN) gamma, tumor necrosis factor (TNF) alpha, and interleukin 12 and 6 was indicated. The negative effect of these cytokines per se on sperm quality (IFN gamma), as well as the appearance of most of them in male reproductive tract inflammations (TNF, IL-12, and 6) associated with oxidative stress [37, 38] or with sperm apoptosis [39] have to be immediately noticed. The hypothesis, that apart from the blood-testis breaking down together with insufficient immunosuppressive mechanisms of active tolerance to sperm, the chemistry of ASA antibodies in males must also have its origin (at least in some cases) in acute, chronic, or latent infections of male reproductive tract together with involvement of oxidative stress, could therefore be easily formulated. This could be a basis for autoimmune reactions that could be driven either to integral sperm antigens or "coated" antigens or more specifically to prostasomes in case of autoimmune prostatitis [40].

As far as the cross-reactivity of ASA antibodies is concerned, our earlier detailed work indicated that plethora of mouse monoclonal ASAs showed specificities to "common" carbohydrates which mediated the observed reactivities both to sperm and microbial agents as: *Staphylococcus aureus, Streptococcus viridans, Escherichia coli, Salmonella typhi* [41]. This early work suggested already "molecular mimicry" as the important "trigger" point for ASA autoantibodies development. The mentioned bacteria were next analyzed in terms of in situ frequency and occurred to be (with the exception of *Salomonella*) one of the most common strains responsible for male reproductive tract infections in our cohorts as well as the potent inducers of oxidative stress reactions [42].

Apart of the fact that terminal common sugar moieties were often encountered in sperm epitopes studied (galactose, *N*-acetylgalactosamine, terminal acetylglucosamine, alpha-L-fucose, and alpha-D-mannose) [25], it has to be again emphasized that enhancement of immune response and affinity maturation process may convert initially developing low-affinity antibodies into sperm-specific response severely affecting sperm structures [5].

It is also interesting to note that the recently obtained (through human–human hybridoma technique using lymphocytes from infertile ASA-positive males) ASAs revealed interesting specificities. First, Fab homology indicated antibodies similar to those reactive with HIV gp 41/120 (fusion proteins) as well as anti-CD55 (complement relevant functions) and with anti-beta galactosidase activities (the last one may be one of the sperm–oocyte receptor mediators) [43].

2.2.6
Carbohydrate-Mediated ASA Antibodies

The chemical organization of ASA antibodies has become a complex matter. After pioneering work of molecular mapping of the sperm epitope reacting with female immobilizing antibody [44], we have also found common carbohydrates both linked with protein and lipid carriers on human sperm [41]. An interesting conclusion coming up from these studies was a bimodal curve received with virtually all antisperm monoclonal antibodies after sperm periodate oxidation, while more gentle N-deglycosylation carried out with cocktail of enzymes seemed to open sperm glycocalyx allowing to penetrate antibodies uncovering the previously seen cryptic sperm determinants [41]. Unlike, however, in Koyama et al. paper [45] where by using chemical deglycosylation (trifluoromethyl acid with sodium periodate) they abrogated all ASA reactivity, in our hands, high amounts of periodate did not remove the reactivity completely; so we could speculate that some antigenic portions were hidden beneath the cell membrane or alternatively there was retained a binding mediated through the protein (lipid) carrier. While Tsuji [46] has managed to strip off (by strong oxidation) all the carbohydrates, the conclusion was that immobilizing properties strongly depend on carbohydrates while the remaining activity of antibodies recognized the portion that was digested off by proteolytic enzymes.

The intriguing observation on sperm N- and O-deglycosylations led us to explore the partial carbohydrate digestion, although the revealed pattern by Western blotting and immunoprecipitation (reaction of antibody with denatured or "native" antigenic conformations) was quite confusing; see Fig. 2.2.1 and Table 2.2.1).

After immunoprecipitations were obtained with various families of ASAs (from infertile individuals), three types of reactions can be seen (Fig. 2.2.1). For example, O-deglycosylation procedure in same cases did not change the pattern of reaction when comparing to N-deglycosylation or the "native" sperm extract (lanes 1 vs. 2 vs. 3). In some variants, O-deglycosylation procedure (lanes 4 vs. 5 vs. 6) produced more bands with ASA polyclonal sera than after N-deglycosylation, and in some cases (lanes 16, 17, 18) O-deglycosylation abolished the antibody reaction when comparing to the other applied sperm extracts (N-deglycosylated or "native" ones).

In the next series of experiments, reactions were performed when the sperm antigens were selectively or simultaneously deglycosylated and ASAs reacted both in Western immunoblotting and immunoprecipitation techniques (Table 2.2.1).

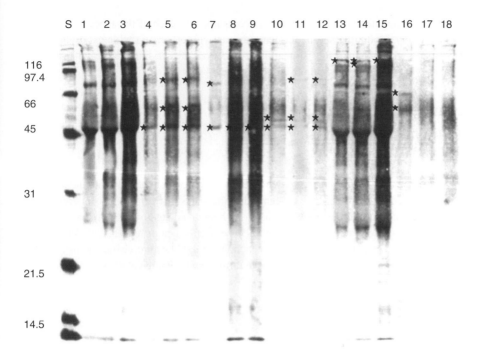

Fig. 2.2.1 Immunoprecipitation of glycosylated and deglycosylated sperm surface antigens by ASA contained in sera samples after in situ sensitisation. *S* molecular weight standards (kDa × 10⁻³). *Lanes* 1–3 control (ASA-negative) sera. *Lanes* 4–18 ASA-positive samples. *Lanes* 1, 4, 7, 10, 13, 16 sera obtained by using N-deglycosylated sperm antigens. *Lanes* 2, 5, 8, 11, 14, 17 sera obtained by using O-deglycosylated sperm antigens. *Lanes* 3, 6, 9, 12, 15, 18 sera obtained by using glycosylated sperm antigens. *Asterisk* – specific immunoprecipitated antigens

Table 2.2.1 Sera samples and ASA-reactive sperm antigens

Technique	Sperm antigens containing sugar moieties inducing antisperm antibodies		Non-glycosylated antigenic epitopes
	O-linked	N-linked	
Western immunoblotting	82, 70, 68–65, 63–61, 59–56, 53, 52, 33–30, 27–29	64, 59, 56, 53	76, 74, 68
Immunoprecipitation	160, 119, 77, 23, 19	160, 119, 108, 38, 23	111, 101, 45, 38

Molecular weights (kDa) were obtained from two independent methods: Western immunoblotting and immunoprecipitation techniques

It could be then concluded (from the Western immunoblotting) that there are more (sensitive) O-deglycosylated sites on human sperm than *N*-deglycosylated ones which could indirectly confirm our earlier reports on enhancement of ASA antibodies binding due to limited N-deglycosylation [41]. It can be clearly concluded, however, that N- and O-deglycosylation procedures applied simultaneously significantly diminished the number of bands precipitated or immunoblotted in comparison to each of the applied procedures alone. Finally, modifying sperm antigenic extract with enzymatic N-deglycosylation we have managed to obtain novel sperm antibody reactions after in situ sensitization of human lymphocytes in immunocompromised SCID mice [47].

2.2.7
Conclusions

We may again emphasize the diversity of ASA reactions which recognize abundantly gly-cosylated human sperm entities. It seems that there is sufficient data to underline once more the complex nature of ASA reactions: (1) being mediated by carbohydrate epitopes (with background of "natural" antibodies); (2) sex-dependent differences in sperm recog-nition expressed by auto- and isoimmune reactions; and (3) genuine characteristics of ASA reactions developed prepuberty that deserve further epidemiological interest.

References

1. Hardy CM, Clydesdale G, Mobbs KJ, Pekin J, Lloyd ML, Sweet C, Shellam GR, Lawson MA (2004) Assessment of contraceptive vaccines based on recombinant mouse sperm protein PH20. Reproduction 127:325–334
2. Hancock RJ (1979) Complement fixing activities of normal mammalian sera for homologous and heterologous sperm. J Reprod Immunol 1:89–96
3. Paradisi R, Pession A, Bellavia E, Focacci M, Flamigni C (1995) Characterization of human sperm antigens reacting with antisperm antibodies from autologous sera and seminal plasma in a fertile population. J Reprod Immunol 28:61–73
4. Paradisi R, Bellavia E, Pession AL, Venturoli S, Bach V, Flamigni C (1996) Characterization of human sperm antigens reacting with antisperm antibodies from autologous sera and semi-nal plasma: comparison among infertile subpopulations. Int J Androl 19:345–352
5. Domagala A, Pulido S, Kurpisz M, Herr JC (2007) Application of proteomic methods for identification of sperm immunogenic antigens. Mol Hum Reprod 13:437–444
6. Naaby-Hansen S, Flickinger CJ, Herr JC (1997) Two-dimensional gel electrophoretic analysis of vectorially labeled surface proteins of human spermatozoa. Biol Reprod 56:771–787
7. Shetty J, Naaby-Hansen S, Shibahara H, Bronson R, Flickinger CJ, Herr JC (1999) Human sperm proteome: immunodominant sperm surface antigens identified with sera from infertile men and women. Biol Reprod 61:61–69
8. Shibahara H, Sato I, Shetty J, Naaby-Hansen S, Herr JC, Wakimoto E, Koyama K (2002) Two-dimensional electrophoretic analysis of sperm antigens recognized by sperm immobiliz-ing antibodies detected in infertile women. J Reprod Immunol 53:1–12
9. Domagala A, Kamieniczna M, Kurpisz M (2000) Sperm antigens recognized by antisperm antibodies contained in sera of infertile adults and prepubertal boys with testicular failures. Int J Androl 23:150–155
10. Domagala A, Kurpisz M (2004) Immunoprecipitation of sperm and somatic antigens with antibodies from sera of sperm-sensitized and anti-sperm antibody-free individuals. Am J Reprod Immunol 51:226–234

11. Paradisi R, Bellavia E, Pession A, Venturoli S, Flamigni C (1996) Characterization of human sperm antigens reacting with sperm antibodies from autologous serum and seminal plasma in an infertile population. Biol Reprod 55:54–61

12. Domagała A, Kurpisz M (2001) CD52 antigen – a review. Med Sci Monit 7:325–331

13. Flickinger CJ, Howards SS, Baran ML, Pessoa N, Herr JC (1997) Appearance of 'natural' antisperm autoantibodies after sexual maturation of normal Lewis rats. J Reprod Immunol 33:127–145

14. Tung KS, Cooke WD Jr, McCarty TA, Robitaille P (1976) Human sperm antigens and antisperm antibodies. II. Age-related incidence of antisperm antibodies. Clin Exp Immunol 25:73–79

15. Kalaydjiev SK, Dimitrova DK, Trifonova NL, Fichorova RN, Masharova NG, Raicheva YN, Simeonova MN, Todorova EI, Todorov VI, Nakov LS (2002) The age-related changes in the incidence of 'natural' anti-sperm antibodies suggest they are not auto-/isoantibodies. Am J Reprod Immunol 47:65–71

16. Domagala A, Kamieniczna M, Kowalczyk D, Kurpisz M (1998) Antisperm antibodies in prepubertal boys and their reactivity with antigenic determinants on differentiated spermatozoa. Am J Reprod Immunol 40:223–229

17. Mirilas P, De Almeida M (1999) Absence of antisperm surface antibodies in prepubertal boys with cryptorchidism and other anomalies of the inguinoscrotal region befor and after surgery. J Urol 162:177–181

18. Sinisi AA, D'Apuzzo A, Pasquali D, Venditto T, Esposito D, Pisano G, De Bellis A, Ventre I, Papparella A, Perrone L, Bellastella A (1997) Antisperm antibodies in prepubertal boys treated with chemotherapy for malignant or non-malignant diseases and in boys with genital tract abnormalities. Int J Androl 20:23–28

19. Urry RL, Carrell DT, Starr NT, Snow BW, Middleton RG (1994) The incidence of antisperm antobodies in infertility patients with a history of cryptorchidism. J Urol 151:381–384

20. Bronson RA, O'Connor WJ, Wilson TA, Bronson SK, Chasalow FI, Droesh K (1992) Correlation between puberty and the development of the autoimmunity to spermatozoa in men with cystic fibrosis. Fertil Steril 58:1199–1204

21. Mieusset R, Fouda PJ, Vaysse P, Guitard J, Moscovici J, Juskiewenski S (1993) Increase in testicular temperature in case of cryotorchidism in boys. Fertil Steril 59:1319–1321

22. Lenzi A, Gandini L, Lombardo F, Dondero F, Culasso F, Ferro F, Cambiaso P, Caione P, Cappa M (1997) Unilateral cryptorchidism corrected in prepubertal age: evaluation of sperm parameters, hormones and antisperm antibodies in adult age. Fertil Steril 67:943–948

23. Szymkiewicz C, Baka-Jakubiak M (1998) Niezstąpione jądro – wnętrostwo. In: Semczuk M, Kurpisz M (eds) Andrologia. PZWL, Warszawa

24. Kasprzak M, Tabor J, Mazurkiewicz I, Kurpisz M (1996) Antisperm antibodies in prepubertal boys with cryptorchidism. Cent Eur J Immunol 21:101–105

25. Kurpisz M, Alexander NJ (1995) Carbohydrate moieties on sperm surface: physiological relevance. Fertil Steril 63:158–165

26. Hancock RJ, Poplham AM, Faruki S, Dresser DW (1985) Increase in the numbers of immunoglobulin-secreting cells in lymph nodes responding to sperm and other stimuli: possible relationship to immunosuppression. Immunology 55:233–239

27. Witkin SS, Vogel-Roccuzzo R, David SS, Berkeley A, Goldstein M, Graf M (1988) Heterogeneity of antigenic determinants on human spermatozoa: relevance to antisperm antibody testing in infertile couples. Am J Obstet Gynecol 159:1228–1231

28. Clarke GN, Stojanoff A, Cauchi MN, McBain JC, Speirs AL, Johnston WI (1984) Detection of antispermatozoal antibodies of IgA class in cervical mucus. Am J Reprod Immunol 5:61–65

29. Hasegawa A, Koyama K (2005) Antigenic epitope for sperm-immobilizing antibody detected in infertile women. J Reprod Immunol 67:77–86

30. Hasegawa A, Fu Y, Tsubamoto H, Tsuji Y, Sawai H, Komori S, Koyama K (2003) Epitope analysis for human sperm-immobilizing monoclonal antibodies, MAb H6–3C4, 1G12 and campath-1. Mol Hum Reprod 9:337–343

31. Pasche B, Kalaydjiev S, Franz TJ, Kremmer E, Gailus-Durner V, Fuchs H, Hrabé de Angelis M, Lengeling A, Busch DH (2005) Sex-dependent susceptibility to Listeria monocytogenes infection is mediated by differential interleukin-10 production. Infect Immun 73:5952–5960

32. Dimitrova D, Kalaydjiev S, Hristov L, Nikolov K, Boyadjiev T, Nakov L (2004) Antichlamydial and antisperm antibodies in patients with chlamydial infections. Am J Reprod Immunol 52:330–336

33. Hübner MP, Pasche B, Kalaydjiev S, Soboslay PT, Lengeling A, Schulz-Key H, Mitre E, Hoffmann WH (2008) Microfilariae of the filarial nematode *Litomosoides sigmodontis* exacerbate the course of lipopolysaccharide-induced sepsis in mice. Infect Immun 76:1668–1677

34. Kalaydjiev S, Dimitrova D, Mitov I, Dikov I, Nakov L (2007) Serum sperm antibodies after diarrhoeal diseases. Andrologia 39:101–108

35. Figura N, Piomboni P, Ponzetto A, Gambera L, Lenzi C, Vaira D, Peris C, Lotano MR, Gennari L, Bianciardi L, Renieri T, Valensin PE, Capitani S, Moretti E, Colapinto R, Baccetti B, Gennari C (2002) *Helicobacter pylori* infection and infertility. Eur J Gastroenterol Hepatol 14:663–669

36. Dimitrova D, Kalaydjiev S, Mendizova A, Piryova E, Nakov L (2005) Circulating antibodies to human spermatozoa in patients with ulcerative colitis. Fertil Steril 84:1533–1535

37. Fraczek M, Sanocka D, Kamieniczna M, Kurpisz M (2008) Proinflammatory cytokines as an intermediate factor enhancing lipid sperm membrane peroxidation in in vitro conditions. J Androl 29:85–92

38. Sanocka D, Fraczek M, Jedrzejczak P, Szumała-Kakol A, Kurpisz M (2004) Male genital tract infection: an influence of leukocytes and bacteria on semen. J Reprod Immunol 62:111–124

39. Allam JP, Fronhoffis F, Fathy A, Novak N, Oltermann I, Bieber T, Schuppe HC, Haidl G (2008) High percentage of apoptotic spermatozoa in ejaculates from men with chronic genital tract inflammation, Andrologia 40:329–334

40. Shindel AW, Naughton CK (2004) Prostatitis and male factor infertility: a review of the literature. Curr Prostate Rep 2:189–195

41. Kurpisz M, Clark GF, Mahony M, Anderson TL, Alexander NJ (1989) Mouse monoclonal antibodies against human sperm: evidence for immunodominant glycosylated antigenic sites. Clin Exp Immunol 78:250–255

42. Fraczek M, Szumala-Kakol A, Jedrzejczak P, Kamieniczna M, Kurpisz M (2007) Bacteria trigger oxygen radical release and sperm lipid peroxidation in in vitro model of semen inflammation. Fertil Steril 88(suppl 2):1076–1085

43. Fiszer D, Pupecka M, Schmidt K, Rozwadowska N, Kamieniczna M, Grygielska B, Kurpisz M (2008) Specific Fab fragments recovered by phage display technique recognizing human spermatozoa. Int J Androl [Epub ahead of print]

44. Tsuji Y, Clausen H, Nudelman E, Kaizu T, Hakomori S, Isojima S (1988) Human sperm carbohydrate antigens defined by an antisperm human monoclonal antibody derived from an infertile woman bearing antisperm antibodies in her serum. J Exp Med 168:343–356

45. Koyama K, Kameda K, Nakamura N, Kubota K, Shigeta M, Isojima S (1991) Recognition of carbohydrate antigen epitopes by sperm-immobilizing antibodies in sera of infertile women. Fertil Steril 56:954–959

46. Tsuji Y (1995) Carbohydrate antigens recognized by anti-sperm antibodies. In: Kurpisz M, Fernandez N (eds) Immunology of Human Reproduction. BIOS Scientific, Oxford, UK

47. Grygielska B, Kamieniczna M, Wiland E, Kurpisz M (2009) In situ reconstruction of humoral immune response against sperm; comparison of SCID and NOD/SCID mouse model. Am J Reprod Immunol 61(2):147–157

Sperm-Specific T Lymphocytes

2.3

Walter K. H. Krause and Michael Hertl

2.3.1
General Characteristics of T Lymphocytes (from Janeway's Immunobiology, 2007)

Sperm antigens, which can induce antibodies (the effector molecules of humoral immunity), may also be able to induce antigen-specific T cells (the effectors of cellular immunity). Specific T cells arise from the interaction of naïve T cells with antigen-presenting cells in the peripheral lymphoid organs. The migration of naïve T cells into the lymphoid organs is guided by the chemokine receptor CCR7, and L-selectin expressed by naïve T cells attracts T cells to the specialized surfaces of high endothelial venules. Facilitated by the expression of ICAM-1, the diapedesis and migration of T cells into the T cell zone is achieved, where the naïve T cells meet antigen-presenting dendritic cells. Toll-like receptors lead to maturation of dendritic cells and thereby promote antigen processing. In addition, B cells, which are able to bind and internalize soluble protein antigens and then process the peptides as peptide:MHC complexes are critical activators of T cells.

The crucial step is the priming of naïve T cells in the lymphoid organs. Naive T cells will respond to antigen only when the antigen-presenting cell presents a specific antigen in association with costimulatory molecules such as B7 (which interacts with CD28 on T cells). The activation of naive T cells leads to their proliferation and differentiation which is promoted by the production of IL-2. When antigens are presented without costimulatory molecules, effector T cells become anergic or die. Antigen-stimulated T cells develop into effector T cells, which require continous antigen recognition in association with MHC class I or II molecules for continuous activation.

T cell effector functions are elicited only when peptide:MHC complexes on the surface of the target cell are recognized. Upon antigen recognition, T cells secrete distinct cytokines , i.e., Th1 cells secrete cytokines that activate macrophages and induce cell-mediated immune response while Th2 cells secrete cytokines, such as IL-4, IL-5 and IL-13, which induce B-cell activation. Cytotoxic T cells, which are commonly CD8 positive, kill their

W. Krause (✉)
Klinik für Dermatologie und Allergologie, Philipps-Universität, Marburg, Germany
e-mail: krause@med.uni-marburg.de

W. K. H. Krause and R. K. Naz (eds.), *Immune Infertility*,
DOI: 10.1007/978-3-642-01379-9_2.3, © Springer Verlag Berlin Heidelberg 2009

target cells via different mechanisms, including secretion of granzymes, perforin and granulysin as well as by Fas-Fasl-mediated cytotoxicity.

2.3.2
What is Known About Antigen-Specific T Cells in Immune Infertility?

The knowledge on antigen-specific T lymphocytes in immune infertility is scarce, but the involvement of T cellular immune reactions to sperm antigens is likely. T lymphocytes in close association with spermatozoa were first observed in men after vasectomy within the so-called sperm granulomas. Sperm granuloma represents a dynamic structure and a site of spermatozoal phagocytosis. Intraluminal macrophages ("spermatophages") absorb degradation products, rather than whole sperm. Besides the well-known formation of antibodies, a modest T lymphocyte activity is also observed. However, the contribution of T lymphocytes and antisperm antibodies (ASA) to testicular damage after vasectomy is far from clear [1].

Following experimental vasectomy in the ram, Saravanamuthu et al. [2] identified T and B cells infiltrating the resulting sperm granulomas. They found MHC-II-restricted lymphocytes in the early granulomas, and MHC-I-restricted lymphocytes in the late granulomas. They assumed that the lymphocytes represented sperm-specific T and B cells. Mathur et al. [3] also suggested the existence of sperm-specific T lymphocytes since lymphocytes of men with ASA showed enhanced reaction to lectin-triggered stimulation by sperm antigens compared to men without ASA.

Observations of Munoz et al. [4] indicated that a proloferative response of γ/δ-T cells accompanies the development of ASA. Men with ASA fixed to the sperm surface had higher numbers of γ/δ T cells and α/β T cells in the semen than men without ASA. The number of peripheral blood T cells was not different among men with and without ASA. After incubation of blood lymphocytes of men with and those without ASA with spermatozoa, the number of γ/δ T cells increased only in men with ASA, while the T cells of men without ASA showed no proliferative response.

Yule and Tung [5] generated specific T cell clones by the incubation of peripheral lymphocytes with extracts from the testis and of spermatozoa. These T clones induced an autoimmune orchitis in syngeneic mice. This experiment demonstrated unequivocally the existence of T cells specific for sperm antigens. The absence of an immune reaction to testicular antigens in the healthy testis is obviously because of immunological tolerance by yet unknown mechanisms, but it is not due to the separation of the testicular tissue from the immune system. Evidence for suppressor mechanisms comes from the observation that the immune rejection of foreign tissues upon transplantation into the testis is delayed compared to other organs. The observation that orchitogenic T cell clones are able to induce autoimmune orchitis strongly suggests that regulatory immune mechanisms rather suppress the afferent phase and the effector phase of an immune response.

In the experiments of Qu et al. [6], immunization of syngeneic mice with testicular germ cells induced an immune response against antigens of spermatids, resulting in autoimmune orchitis. This inflammatory response was characterized by a lymphocytic infiltrate of the tests.

Subsequent vasectomy blunted the inflammation in the testis, but provoked epididymitis in the caput involving CD4+ T cells, CD8+ T cells, B cells, and macrophages. Surprisingly, although the sperm antibodies in mice without vasectomy were reactive to round and elongated spermatids, those in mice undergoing vasectomy were reactive with the acrosomes of mature spermatozoa. Thus, the site of activity of autoreactive lymphocytes determines the nature of the target antigens.

The situation is complicated by the fact that presentation of antigens to T cells by antigen-presenting cells appears to be divergent in the testis as compared to other tissues. Some costimulatory molecules, such as CD80 and CD86, are lacking in the testis. The immune privilege of the testis may thus be, in part, due to an anergy of T cells in this environment, although antigen-presenting macrophages are active in the testis [7].

Experimental results questioning the existence of sperm-specific T cells were published by O'Rand et al. [8]. These authors sequenced and cloned a sperm antigen in the rabbit, designated as Sp17. Mice which were immunized with this antigen developed antibodies, but did not show a proliferative response of T lymphocytes.

The only report on specific T cells reactive to sperm antigens is provided by a previous study of Chiriva-Internati et al. [9] relating to sperm protein 17 (Sp17). Sp17 is a specific protein of spermatozoa, which is also expressed as a cancer-testis antigen by about 30% of patients with multiple myeloma. Sp17-specific human leucocyte antigen (HLA)-A1 and B27-restricted cytotoxic T lymphocytes (CTLs) were successfully generated from peripheral blood mononuclear cells of a healthy donor. Effects on spermatogenesis are not reported since the focus of the study was on treatment of multiple myeloma.

The interaction of autoaggressive T helper cells and B cells in the course of immune infertility remains to be clearified. Autoaggressive T cell clones should be isolated and expanded ex vivo and the immunodominant T cell epitopes need to be characterized. Moreover, the T cell-dependent activation of autoaggressive B cells remains to be demonstrated. In immune infertility, it is unknown whether autoaggressive T cells of a given epitope specificity interact with autoaggressive B cells leading to T cell help for the induction and perpetuation of antibody production. Epitope-specific T cells may be identified in vitro upon coculture with synthetic peptides of a known cognate antigen of ASA (e.g., HSP70). The influence of epitope-specific T helper cells on antibody production remains to be studied.

2.3.3
T Cells in Semen

Among the normal population of leukocytes in semen at a range up to $1 \times 10^6/mL$, granulocytes are the most prevalent type with 50–60%, followed by macrophages (20–30%) and lymphocytes (2–5%). The lymphocytes were further divided into CD4-positive T cells (2.4%) and CD8-positive T cells (1.3%). B-lymphocytes were not present in healthy men, but present only in men with seminal inflammation [10]. The percentage of T lymphocytes is enhanced in men with spinal cord injury [11]. Little is known about autoreactive T cells in semen. Some studies provided evidence that their occurrence may be the consequence of immune reactions to prostatic antigens (autoimmune prostatitis) [12–14]. Witkin and Goldstein [15] performed lymphocyte and monocyte counts in the semen of 14 men with intact vas deferens and 13 men who had undergone vasovasostotomy. In both groups, the number of lymphocytes and monocytes cells was identical with 10^3/mL. However, in men with intact vasa, T suppressor/cytotoxic cells predominated. In contrast, in the vasovasostomized men the levels of CD8+ T cells were significantly reduced and CD4+ T cells predominated in their semen. The authors thus speculated that damage to the excurrent ducts was responsible for the alteration in T cell regulation leading to a decrease of CD8+ T cells and loss of tolerance permissive for the formation of ASA.

Seminal plasma possesses immunosuppressive activity. In vitro, large molecules of the seminal plasma were able to suppress the B-cell proliferative response induced by the Nocardia mitogen, while small molecules suppressed the T cell proliferatived response to phytohemagglutinin. Purification of the B-cell suppressor identified a protein with a molecular weight of 180 kDa. This molecule might be able to suppress ASA formation in females, as well as autoantibodies in men [16,17].

Munoz et al. [4] determined the number of α/β and γ/δ T cells in serum and semen of 23 men. In a cohort of seven men with ASA, the mean numbers of γ/δ and α/β T cells were 3,560 and 3,230 cells/mL semen, respectively. In contrast, a group of 16 men with no evidence of auto-immunity to sperm showed a mean number of 350 γ/δ T cells and 610 α/β T cells/mL semen. The numbers of γ/δ and α/β T cells in the peripheral blood of the identical men were unrelated to their antisperm antibody status. Thus, γ/δ T cells in human semen comprise a larger proportion of the total T cell population than of the T cells in blood. The number of γ/δ T cells appeared to be elevated in the semen of men with evidence of localized auto-immunity to their own sperm. These results suggest that the proliferative response of T cells with a γ/δ TCR accompanies an autoimmune response to sperm. The higher proportion of lymphocytes bearing the γ/δ antigen receptor in the testis, as compared to peripheral blood, was also confirmed by Bertotto et al. [18]. The rise of γ/δ T cells was mainly due to an overexpansion of cells expressing V delta 1 gene-encoded determinants on their surface. This finding points to a special immune milieu in the semen.

The presence of T lymphocytes in semen may be of relevance not only regarding their specificity to sperm antigens, but also because of their secretion of cytokines which may influence sperm functions. Sperm cells express IFN-α and IFN-γ receptors. IFN-α, IFN-γ and other cytokines have deleterious effect on sperm motility and fertilizing ability. An increase in T-helper cell activity thus may result in these effects [19]. This may concern also female lymphocytes within the genital tract, for Das et al. [20] observed a significant increase in CD8+ and CD4+ T cells in the utero–vaginal junction after repeated artifical insemination.

In addition, the membrane cofactor protein (MCP), also known as CD46, is a link between T cells and sperm function. CD46 is a multitasking molecule in complement regulation and as a costimulatory molecule for T cell activation. It exists as multiple isomeric forms while human spermatozoa express only an isoform comprising the four short consensus repeat (SCR) domains, the short Ser/Thr/Pro-rich domain C, and the Cyt2 variant of the cytoplasmic tail. Spermatozoal CD46 is identical to the previously described acrosome-restricted spermatozoal protein trophoblast-leukocyte common antigen. Because of its acrosome-restricted expression pattern, spermatozoal CD46 has been utilized as a specific acrosome marker in humans [21,22].

References

1. McDonald SW (2000) Cellular responses to vasectomy. Int Rev Cytol 199:295–339
2. Saravanamuthu V, Foster RA, Ladds PW, Gorrell MD (1991) T and B lymphocyte subsets in spermatic granulomas in five rams. Vet Pathol 28(6):482–491
3. Mathur S, Burdash NM, Williamson HO (1990) White cell subpopulations in autoimmune infertile men and their wives with cytotoxic sperm antibodies. Autoimmunity 6(3):183–193
4. Munoz G, Posnett DN, Witkin SS (1992) Enrichment of gamma delta T lymphocytes in human semen: relation between gamma delta T cell concentration and antisperm antibody status. J Reprod Immunol 22(1):47–57
5. Yule TD, Tung KS (1993) Experimental autoimmune orchitis induced by testis and sperm antigen-specific T cell clones: an important pathogenic cytokine is tumor necrosis factor. Endocrinology 133(3):1098–1107
6. Qu N, Terayama H, Naito M, Ogawa Y, Hirai S, Kitaoka M, Yi SQ, Itoh M (2008) Caput epididymitis but not orchitis was induced by vasectomy in a murine model of experimental autoimmune orchitis. Reproduction 135(6):859–866
7. Rival C, Theas MS, Suescun MO, Jacobo P, Guazzone V, van Rooijen N, Lustig L (2008) Functional and phenotypic characteristics of testicular macrophages in experimental autoimmune orchitis. J Pathol 215(2):108–117
8. O'Rand MG, Beavers J, Widgren EE, Tung KS (1993) Inhibition of fertility in female mice by immunization with a B-cell epitope, the synthetic sperm peptide, P10G. J Reprod Immunol 25(2):89–102
9. Chiriva-Internati M, Wang Z, Salati E, Wroblewski D, Lim SH (2002) Successful generation of sperm protein 17 (Sp17)-specific cytotoxic T lymphocytes from normal donors: implication for tumour-specific adoptive immunotherapy following allogeneic stem cell transplantation for Sp17-positive multiple myeloma. Scand J Immunol 56(4):429–433
10. Wolff H (1995) The biologic significance of white blood cells in semen. Fertil Steril 63(6):1143–1157
11. Basu S, Lynne CM, Ruiz P, Aballa TC, Ferrell SM, Brackett NL (2002) Cytofluorographic identification of activated T-cell subpopulations in the semen of men with spinal cord injuries. J Androl 3(4):551–556
12. Alexander RB, Brady F, Ponniah S (1997) Autoimmune prostatitis: evidence of T cell reactivity with normal prostatic proteins. Urology 50(6):893–899
13. Batstone GR, Doble A, Gaston JS (2002) Autoimmune T cell responses to seminal plasma in chronic pelvic pain syndrome (CPPS). Clin Exp Immunol 128(2):302–307
14. Motrich RD, Maccioni M, Ponce AA, Gatti GA, Oberti JP, Rivero VE (2006) Pathogenic consequences in semen quality of an autoimmune response against the prostate gland: from animal models to human disease. J Immunol 177(2):957–967
15. Witkin SS, Goldstein M (1988) Reduced levels of T suppressor/cytotoxic lymphocytes in semen from vasovasostomized men: relationship to sperm autoantibodies. J Reprod Immunol 14(3):283–290
16. Bouvet JP, Couderc J, Quan CP, Pirès R, D'Azambuja S, Pillot J (1988) Delineation between T- and B-suppressive molecules from human seminal plasma: I. Partial characterization of a 180-kD protein inhibiting the B response to T-independent antigens. Am J Reprod Immunol Microbiol 18(3):87–93
17. Thomas IK, Erickson KL (1984) Seminal plasma inhibits lymphocyte response to T-dependent and–independent antigens in vitro. Immunology 52(4):721–726
18. Bertotto A, Spinozzi F, Gerli R, Bassotti G, Fabietti GM, Castellucci G, Vagliasindi C, Vaccaro R (1995) Gamma delta T-cell subset distribution in human semen from fertile donors. Am J Reprod Immunol 34(3):176–178

19. Naz RK (2006) Effect of sperm DNA vaccine on fertility of female mice. Mol Reprod Dev 73(7):918–928
20. Das SC, Nagasaka N, Yoshimura Y (2005) Changes in the localization of antigen presenting cells and T cells in the utero–vaginal junction after repeated artificial insemination in laying hens. J Reprod Dev 51(5):683–687
21. Mizuno M, Harris CL, Morgan BP (2007) Immunization with autologous CD46 generates a strong autoantibody response in rats that targets spermatozoa. J Reprod Immunol 73(2): 135–147
22. Mizuno M, Harris CL, Suzuki N, Matsuo S, Morgan BP (2005) Expression of CD46 in developing rat spermatozoa: ultrastructural localization and utility as a marker of the various stages of the seminiferous tubuli. Biol Reprod 72(4):908–915

Site and Risk Factors of Antisperm Antibodies Production in the Male Population

2.4

Marcelo Marconi and Wolfgang Weidner

2.4.1
Introduction

During the last 25 years, conflicting data regarding the risk factors and site of anti-sperm antibodies (ASA) formation in men have been published. Inflammatory and/or infectious (inflammatory/infectious) diseases of the male reproductive tract (MRT), varicocele, genital trauma, testicular tumors, and testicular sperm extraction (TESE) between others have been proposed as risk factors for the generation of ASA, deteriorating the fertilizing capacity of the affected men (Table 2.4.1) [1]. However, as demonstrated in numerous clinical trials, the association between these entities and the presence of ASA is still controversial, indicating that the understanding of these conditions in the development of ASA is incomplete.

Although many questions regarding the site and risk factors of ASA production in males remain unanswered, there seems to be a consensus in the literature on three important facts: First – vasectomy followed by vasovasostomy (VV) is the only clinical condition that shows almost permanently high titers of ASA in numerous clinical series [2–5]. Second – circulating ASA do not play an important role and do not show any negative influence on the fertility prognosis of the affected men. In contrast, local ASA act negatively on the motility of spermatozoa, on their ability to pass through the female genital secretions and/or on the fusion of gametes, which is the key event of fecundation [6]. Third – the lack of a standardized method and an established cut-point for ASA detection in the ejaculate makes the comparison difficult among different clinical trials [7].

Taking into account the increased prevalence of the above mentioned diseases in an uro-andrological setting (i.e., inflammatory/infectious diseases of the MRT, varicocele, TESE, etc.) and the negative impact of ASA on fertility of these men, this chapter evaluates the existing data trying to identify the possible risk factors and sites of ASA production in the MRT.

M. Marconi (✉)
Department of Urology, University of Chile, Santos Dumont 999, Santiago, Chile
e-mail: mmarconi@med.uchile.cl

W. K. H. Krause and R. K. Naz (eds.), *Immune Infertility*,
DOI: 10.1007/978-3-642-01379-9_2.4, © Springer Verlag Berlin Heidelberg 2009

Table 2.4.1 Suggested risk factors for ASA formation

Chronic obstruction of the MRT
Congenital
    Congenital bilateral absence of the vas deferens (CBAVD)
    Müllerian prostatic cysts
Acquired
    Vasectomy
    Iatrogenic obstruction of the epididymis and/or vas deferens
Inflammation and/or infection of the male reproductive tract
Varicocele
Cryptorchidism
Testicular trauma
Testicular torsion
Testicular surgery
Testicular sperm extraction (TESE)
Testicular biopsy
Organ-sparing surgery for testicular tumors
Testicular tumors
Homosexuality

2.4.2
Risk Factors and Site of ASA Formation

2.4.2.1
Chronic Obstruction of the MRT

Surgical interventions of the epididymis and vas deferens that cause an obstruction have demonstrated to be the only widely accepted conditions [2–5], demonstrating almost permanently high titers of ASA. Several reports suggest that between 50 and 100% of men who undergo vasectomy subsequently have sera positive for ASA [4, 8] and the prevalence of ASA in the ejaculate of these men is also extremely high (70–100%) [5]. It is not that only acquired obstruction of the seminal tract may trigger the formation of ASA. Bronson et al. [9] demonstrated that ASA were detected after the onset of puberty in a cohort of men with cystic fibrosis and congenital bilateral aplasia of the vas deferens (CBAVD).

Following vasectomy, epididymal distension and sperm granuloma formation may result from raised intraluminal pressure. The sperm granuloma is a dynamic structure and a site of much spermatozoal phagocytosis by its macrophage population; however, it is not a permanent finding in patients who have undergone vasectomy [10]. In many species, spermatozoa in the obstructed ducts are destroyed by intraluminal macrophages, and degradation products, rather than the whole sperm getting absorbed by the epididymal epithelium. Humoral immunity against spermatozoal antigens following vasectomy would be secondary to the combination of a constant leak of sperm antigens that by far surmounts all known mechanisms against autoimmunity present in the epididymis and a chronic increase in intraluminal pressure.

The time-course for post-vasectomy ASA production does not seem to be triggered exclusively by acute, sudden, and massive reabsorption of spermatozoa after vasectomy but also by slow, gradual, and late sperm antigen reabsorption. Data from a rat model suggests that IgM ASA develop within 2 weeks after vasectomy, decreasing in the next 4–8 weeks followed by increasing titers of ASA IgG between 8 and 12 weeks [11].

Cellular immuno-tolerance mechanicisms are also implicated in the ASA production of VV patients, as demonstrated by Witkin ang Goldstein (12) who described reduced concentrations of T suppressor lymphocytes in their semen when compared men with undisturbed vasa.

The immunologic response to spermatozoa is polyclonal, so that the populations of ASA directed against different epitopes vary from individual to individual. As far as the antigenic structure of spermatozoa is concerned, several groups of specific substances have been studied: the ABO groups antigens (Ags), acrosin, HLA Ags, hyaluronidase, protamines, and DNA polymerase [13].

The strength of the ASA formation after vasectomy is variable but there are some patients who have a genetic predisposition to develop ASA [14]. It can be postulated that a breakdown of sperm immune tolerance depends on an individual's immune responsiveness, the nature of the precipitating event, and the length of exposure of inoculum. The genetic predisposition for the development of an autoimmune sperm reaction as has been demonstrated in monozygotic twins were the antisperm immune reaction is triggered by genetic predisposition rather than by the amount of the inoculum (spermatozoa concentration) [15].

Still under debate is the location in the genital tract where ASA transuded from serum and locally produced antibodies, respectively, become attached to the surface of the spermatozoa. In spermatozoa retrieved directly from the distal end of the vas in patients undergoing VV, IgG and IgA ASA determined by the Immunobead test were present in 78.6 to 32.1% of the patients [16], respectively, indicating that in these patients, the epididymis would be the primary site of ASA local production and transudation from serum. The question whether the rest of the MRT contributes to ASA deposition in the ejaculate of these patients was addressed by Meinertz et al. [17], who performed the mixed antiglobulin reaction (MAR) for IgG and IgA in the whole ejaculate and the fractions of the split ejaculate of 11 men with history of vasectomy and successful VV. The MAR test revealed almost identical concentrations of ASA in the first and second fractions of the ejaculate. The results suggest that ASA in the ejaculate from VV patients are transuded from serum not only at the epididymal but also at the prostatic and seminal vesicle levels.

In conclusion, chronic obstruction at the level of the vas deferens constitutes a clear risk factor for ASA formation (Table 2.4.2). In these patients, the most probable site of ASA production is the epididymis; however, once autoimmunization happens transudation of ASA seems to occur also at other levels of the MRT (i.e., seminal vesicles and prostate). The pathophysiology of ASA formation in these patients would involve, among others, an increased intraductal pressure associated with chronic absorption of spermatozoa or sperm fragments and a decrease in the cellular immunomodulatory factors present in the seminal plasma, namely reduced concentrations of T suppressor lymphocytes. It seems logical that any pathologic condition that causes chronic obstruction of the MRT can constitute a risk factor for ASA formation through the same mechanisms.

2.4.2.2
Infection and/or Inflammation of the MRT as Cause of ASA Formation

Infection/inflammation of the MRT would be a risk factor for ASA formation through four main mechanisms:

- Obstruction of the MRT because of inflammatory and postinflammatory changes
- Tearing of the blood–testis barrier (BTB) because of local inflammation
- Decrease of the immunomodulatory factors (cellular and humoral) present in seminal plasma that normally prevent sperm autoimmunization
- Cross-reactivity between antigens of the microorganisms responsible for MRT infections (i.e., *Chlamydia Trachomatis*) and sperm antigens

Controversial data exist on the association between inflammation/infection of the MRT and ASA [7]. In a recently presented series of 79 infertile patients with inflammatory/ infectious diseases of the MRT [5], the comparative results of the two tests for ASA detection in seminal plasma, the MAR and Immunobead test, demonstrated no clear role of this association for male infertility. In a second series of 365 patients with documented inflammation/infection of the MRT, such as chronic bacterial prostatitis (CBP), inflammatory Chronic Prostatitis / Chronic Pelvic Pain Syndrome (CP/CPPS), noninflammatory CPPS, chronic urethritis, and chronic epididymitis, again we found no association between ASA formation and these diseases [7]. Controversially, Witkin and Toth [18], using an ELISA, reported a 48% incidence of ASA in seminal plasma of men with a history of urethritis and CBP. Jarow et al. [19] also found a positive association between CP/CPPS and ASA using the gel agglutination assay in serum.

The number of clinical series dealing with the detection of "significant" ASA levels in seminal plasma of men with inflammation/infection of the MRT is small; the tests used for ASA detection and the positive cut-points for the different methods vary between the different studies. All these factors may explain the fact that the relationship between these two conditions is still debatable.

From a pathophysiological point of view, the absence of a confirmed clinical association between infectious/inflammatory diseases of the MRT and ASA formation would rely on the fact that the four previously mentioned mechanisms, by which these diseases would constitute a risk factor for ASA formation, are not regular findings in patients with these conditions.

Even though both acute and chronic infection/inflammation of the MRT have been claimed as risk factors for partial and total obstruction of the MRT, further reports have demonstrated that the link between these two conditions, with the exception of epididymal tuberculosis, is weak [20]. Especially, for CP/CPPS obstructive findings seem to be rare, either not evident or evaluable in less than 10% [21]. Apparently, inflammatory/infectious related obstructions of the MRT do not seem to be as important as usually considered [22].

Inflammatory-induced tears of the distal segments of the epididymal duct or efferent duct epithelium may occur in inflammatory/infectious diseases of the MRT breaching the blood–epithelial barriers [12]. This would activate the immunological defense and induce the production of ASA [23, 24]. As there are no sensitive markers for the disruption of the

BTB and blood epididymal barrier (BEB), it is not possible to evaluate if this event really occurs in patients with inflammation/infection of the MRT or up to what degree it may be present. Questionable the presence of leukocytes in seminal fluid could indicate some degree of disruption; however, it is a known fact that the levels of seminal leukocytes in patients with inflammation/infection of the MRT are extremely variable and their exact role and meaning are not clear. Moreover, if this would be the case we [7] and other authors [25–29] have found no association between the presence of ASA and elevation of inflammatory parameters in seminal fluid, such as leukocytes and elastase. Associated with the fact that the disruption of the blood–epithelial barriers is a questionable event in the mentioned diseases, there is also the important fact that a breach of the barrier alone is not enough in many patients to trigger the formation of ASA. This finding was clarified by the studies of Komori et al. [30] and Leonhartsberger et al. [31], in which patients undergoing TESE and organ-sparing surgery for testicular tumors, where certainly a disruption of the BTB occurs, no increased risk of ASA formation has been reported.

Even though the significance of white blood cells in the ejaculate remains a matter of debate, several authors have suggested that such cells are important in the modulation of an ASA response, in the sense that the role of the suppressor lymphocyte predominance over helper lymphocytes prevents the formation of ASA. Some reports support the idea that inflammatory/infectious diseases of the MRT would not only not promote granulocyte migration into the MRT but also the activation of B- and T-helper lymphocytes [32], modulating the physiological predominance T suppressor lymphocytes over helper T lymphocytes [12]. Local production of cytokines at the epididymal epithelium would be an important factor for recruiting lymphocytes into the semina fluid [33].

In agreement with this theory, Munoz and Witkin [24] postulated that an asymptomatic, undetected *Chlamydia Trachomatis* infection of the MRT may induce the local activation of $\gamma\delta$ T lymphocytes that are believed to comprise the first line of immunological defense against infection at mucosal surfaces. Once activated, these would react with those sperm antigens that do not require presentation by MHC class I or class II molecules, resulting in further amplification and activation of $\gamma\delta$ T lymphocytes and increase cytokine expression. This in turn would activate $\gamma\delta$ T lymphocytes in the genital tract and lead to the induction of an autoimmune response to spermatozoa.

However, as previously mentioned several authors [25–28, 34] have reported no relation between the presence of ASA and the number of leukocytes in the ejaculate, suggesting that despite the fact that both abnormalities are manifestations of an immunological response they are not interrelated. Moreover, Barratt et al. [35] reported that in men with ASA the predominance of T helper lymphocytes over T suppressor lymphocytes is very rare.

Owing to their similarity, immunological cross-reactivity between antigens of the sperm membrane and *Chlamydia Trachomatis* has also been proposed as a theory to explain the questionable association between infections of the MRT and ASA formation [7]. Immune response against stress proteins (i.e., heat shock proteins, HSP – essential mammalian and bacterial stress proteins) can be highly cross-reactive. It has been suggested that the antibodies against conserved epitopes on *Chlamydial* HSP 60 may cross-react with those on human HSP 60 and initiate an autoimmune response [36]. However, once again, clinical data fail to detect an association between chlamydial infections and the presence of ASA in seminal plasma [7, 37].

In the hypothetical scenario that inflammatory/infectious diseases of the MRT are associated with ASA formation, for anatomical reasons previously discussed the epididymis would be the most probable site of ASA formation (Table 2.4.2). However, the prostate gland is another site where a localized immune response can be induced, since prostatic fluids have been identified to contain specific IgA antibody against Escherichia Coli and spermatozoa [18]. Some authors suggest that inflammation/infection of the MRT in some men may interfere with the complete closure of prostatic ducts during ejaculation, resulting in leakage of sperm into the prostate gland inducing an immune response [38].

Patients with inflammatory/infectious diseases of the MRT seem to bring together many favorable conditions for ASA formation; however, evidence in clinical studies indicates that the association between these two conditions is extremely weak. A probable explanation for this contradiction would be that all the favorable conditions for ASA formation, supposed to be present in these patients, do not seem to be as important or prevalent as usually considered.

2.4.2.3
Varicocele as Cause of ASA Formation

In 1959, Rümke and Hellinka [39] first suggested a probable association between varicocele and ASA; since then, the association between these two entities is a matter of debate. Clinical studies supporting an association have been based in the detection of ASA in serum and in the ejaculate of patients with varicocele. Using enzyme-linked immunoabsorbant assay (ELISA), Golomb et al. [40] and Gilbert et al. [41] found significantly higher levels of ASA in the serum of patients with varicocele vs. controls (90 vs. 41% and 32 vs. 14%, respectively). Both concluded that varicocele was a risk factor for ASA formation. During the 1990s, other authors [42, 43], testing ASA in the ejaculate by means of Immunobead and MAR test, came to the same conclusion. Djadalat et al. [44] using the MAR test found a weak association between varicocele and ASA; moreover, he concluded that even though surgical treatment for varicocele may reduce the ASA level in some patients, it may increase it in others.

Contradicting the previous evidence, Oshinsky et al. [45] and Heidenreich et al. [46] reported in two different series of patients that varicocele is not a risk factor for ASA production. This finding was confirmed by Veräjänkorva et al. [47] who, using the MAR test, analyzed the predisposing factors for male immunological infertility in 508 patients that had been treated for infertility. Patients with a history of varicocele had statistically significant lower level ASA than patients without.

Basic research evidence is also controversial: Shook et al. [48] demonstrated in an animal model that a surgically induced varicocele triggers ASA formation. However, Turner et al. [49], working also with surgically induced varicocele model in rats, demonstrated that the BTB was not damaged in these animals, suggesting that the impairment of spermatogenesis in this disease is not immunologically mediated. Interestingly, in patients with varicocele and ASA in the ejaculate these immunoglobulins are also present in testicular biopsies, more specifically inside the seminiferous tubule, suggesting that if in fact there is an association between these two conditions, the most probable site of formation would be the testis [42] (Table 2.4.2).

2.4.2.4
Cryptorchidism as a Cause of ASA Formation

Cryptorchidism is defined as a condition in which one or both testis fail to descend to the scrotal position. The incidence of this condition varies from 1.4 to 2.7% in male births and is increased in premature birth [50]. Several studies have reported an increased incidence of ASA (up to 28%) in patients with history of cryptorchidism either treated or untreated by orchidopexy [51, 52]. However, as most of the studies include prepuberal population they have tested ASA only in serum, not addressing the important issue of the presence of ASA in the ejaculate. Moreover, there is a high probability that an undefined percentage of the patients who have undergone orchidopexy develop, as a complication of surgery, some degree of obstruction at the epididymal or ductal level. Those patients have a high probability of ASA formation, but the etiology would be falsely classified to cryptorchidism and not to chronic obstruction.

These later studies oppose to the findings of others [53, 54], who evaluated ASA in the serum and ejaculate of patients with history of cryptorchidism, orchidopexy, and testicular biopsy not finding any association between the mentioned conditions and the presence of ASA. Clinical evidence in agreement with this last fact was published by Mirilas et al. [55, 56] who found no evidence of ASA in prepuberal boys with history of cryptorchidism.

In prepuberal population, the clinical evidence is even more conflicting, since before puberty, the absence of mature spermatozoa with its antigenic material should exclude any possible immune reaction against sperm antigens; however, several studies report the presence of ASA in the serum of prepuberal boys with cryptorchidism [51, 57, 58]. Sinisi et al. [59] suggested that in these patients the sperm surface antigens are already present before meiosis and the BTB is either immature or impaired by heat due to the abnormal position. However, evidence in experimental rat models of cryptorchidism demonstrates that the BTB remains competent under this situation [60, 61].

As with other previous conditions, the association between cryptorchidism and ASA remains controversial (Table 2.4.2). If the association is real and the bias from surgical treatment complications, namely iatrogenic obstruction of the vas deferens is excluded, the most probable site of ASA production in these patients would be the testis.

2.4.2.5
Testicular Trauma, Surgery, and Torsion as Cause of ASA Formation

It seems logical that every condition where the BTB is breached should constitute a clear risk factor for ASA production, since the immune system establishes a direct contact with the antigens present in the sperm surface. Surprisingly, the data are not clear. Kukadia et al. [62] evaluated the presence of ASA in the ejaculate, using the direct Immunobead test, in eight patients with history of severe testicular trauma who underwent surgical exploration. Only one patient had detectable levels of ASA, all other patients were negative for ASA. He concluded that there is no association between these factors. Surgical procedures to the testis have also proved not to be a risk factor for ASA formation; successful TESE

[5], open and needle testicular biopsy [63], and organ-sparing surgery for testicular tumor do not constitute a risk factor for ASA production [31].

Testicular torsion is a surgical emergency, which requires prompt diagnosis and immediate treatment. One of the consequences that patients may face in the follow-up is a compromise of the exocrine testicular function (spermatogenesis) [64]. The generation of ASA because of the rupture of the BTB is claimed to be one of the possible causes of this exocrine impairment. Arap et al. [65] evaluated ASA formation in the ejaculate of 24 patients with history of testicular torsion; 15 were treated with orchiectomy and 9 were treated with orchidopexy. He used 20 proven fertile men as controls and found no significant differences in the ASA levels between patients and controls, regardless of the treatment applied. These results agree with the findings of Anderson et al. [66] who studied a similar population and were unable to find an increased rate of ASA detection in these patients. Identifying the risk factors for ASA production in a population of 226 male patients, Heidenreich et al. [46] also concluded that testicular torsion is not associated with this condition.

Even though clinical evidences seem to be conclusive, studies in animal models generally confirm the presence of ASA [67]. However, animal models for testicular torsion may not exactly reproduce the conditions found in humans, so care should be taken in extrapolating these data [65].

With the available evidence, trauma, surgery, and torsion of the testis do not seem to constitute a risk factor for ASA formation; however, larger studies are needed (Table 2.4.2). Nevertheless, the BTB is clearly disturbed in all these cases; ASA formation is not regularly triggered, this fact demonstrates that the pathophysiology of ASA formation is still unclear.

2.4.2.6
Testicular Tumors as Cause of ASA Formation

Testicular tumors have been reported to be a risk factor for ASA formation. The incidence of ASA in these patients ranges from 18 to 73%; however, all the studies were biased because only serum ASA were evaluated, and most important did not include a control group to evaluate if the detection rates were significantly higher [68–70]. With the available evidence, the link between testicular tumors and ASA remains questionable (Table 2.4.2); larger studies including healthy fertile controls are needed.

2.4.2.7
Homosexuality as Cause of ASA Formation

During the 1980s, experimental studies in rabbits demonstrated that nontraumatic weekly deposition of sperm in the rectum led to the formation of ASA [71, 72]. Taking into account this evidence, it seems logical that unprotected anal intercourse in homosexual men could constitute a risk factor for ASA formation. Wolff and Schill [1] evaluated the incidence of ASA in the serum of different groups of men. Four percent of dermatologic patients ($n=223$), 9.6% of andrologic patients ($n=178$), and 28.6% of homosexual men ($n=42$) were positive for IgG and/or IgM antibodies. They concluded that there was a high inci-

Table 2.4.2 Suggested risk factors and sites of ASA production in the MRT

Risk factor	Status	Most probable site of first immunization and ASA production
Chronic obstruction of the MRT	Confirmed risk factor	Epididymis
Inflammation/infection of the MRT	Not confirmed	Epididymis/Prostate
Varicocele	Not confirmed	Testis
Cryptorchidism	Not confirmed	Testis
Testicular trauma	No risk factor (more evidence is needed)	–
Testicular torsion	No risk factor (more evidence is needed)	–
Testicular surgery	No risk factor (more evidence is needed)	–
Testicular tumors	Not confirmed	Testis
Homosexuality	Not confirmed	Gastrointestinal mucosa

dence of ASA among homosexual men, probably because of contact of spermatozoa with the immune system by passive anal intercourse.

Five years later, Mulhall et al. [73] reported a 10% prevalence of ASA in homosexual men and 17% in those who had practiced unprotected anal receptive intercourse in the previous 6 months. They found no correlation between the presence of ASA and human immunodeficiency virus (HIV) infection. They speculated that rectal intercourse may be a risk factor for ASA formation, even though a comparison with a healthy fertile population was not performed. Contradicting the previous results, Sands et al. [74] found no significant difference in the serum ASA titers between sexually active heterosexual men and homosexual men with or without HIV infection, concluding that ASA levels are not higher in homosexual men.

In conclusion, there is not enough evidence to support homosexuality as a risk factor for ASA formation; however, taking into account clinical evidence and basic research studies, it seems highly probable that, if this association exists, the primary site of ASA production would be the distal gastrointestinal mucosa (Table 2.4.2).

2.4.3
Conclusions

The pathophysiology of ASA formation is still unclear; the old concept that a simple tear or breach in the BTB is enough to trigger ASA formation has been pulled down by clinical evidence. As the exact mechanisms operating in ASA formation remain to be elucidated, it is not surprising that many clinical conditions still have a questionable association with ASA formation. The only condition that is a confirmed risk factor for ASA formation is chronic obstruction of the MRT, especially after vasectomy. With the available evidence, testicular trauma, surgery, and torsion should not be considered as risk factors for ASA production; in all other conditions, the association is still questionable. In patients with chronic obstruction of the MRT, the most probable site of ASA production is the epididymis; however, once the immune reaction is triggered and the systemic production of ASA starts, immunoglobulins may enter the MRT at other levels (i.e., seminal vesicles and prostate).

References

1. WHO (2000) World Health Organization manual for the standardized investigation and diagnosis of the infertile couple, 2nd edn. Cambridge University Press, Cambridge
2. Gubin DA, Dmochowski R, Kutteh WH (1998) Multivariant analysis of men from infertile couples with and without antisperm antibodies. Am J Reprod Immunol 39:157–160
3. Jarow JP, Sanzone JJ (1992) Risk factors for male partners antisperm antibodies. J Urol 148:1805–1807
4. Lee R, Goldstein M, Ullery B, Ehrlich J, Soares M, Razzano R, Herman M, Callahan M, Li P, Schlegel P, Witkin S (2009) Value of serum antisperm antibodies in diagnosing obstructive azoospermia. J Urol 181:264–269
5. Marconi M, Nowotny A, Pantke P, Diemer T, Weidner W (2008) Antisperm antibodies detected by MAR and immunobead test are not associated with inflammation and infection of the seminal tract. Andrologia 40:227–234
6. Eggert-Kruse W, Rohr G, Böckem-Hellwig S, Huber K, Christmann-Edoga M, Runnebaum B (1995) Immunological aspects of subfertility. Int J Androl 18:43–52
7. Marconi M, Pilatz A, Wagenlehner F, Diemer T, Weidner W (2009) Are really antisperm antibodies associated with inflammatory/infectious diseases of the male reproductive tract. Eur Urol (in press)
8. Mazumdar S, Levine A (1998) Antisperm antibodies: etiology, pathogenesis, diagnosis, and treatment. Fertil Steril 70:799–810
9. Bronson RA, O'Connor WJ, Wilson TA, Bronson SK, Chasalow FI, Droesch K (1992) Correlation between puberty and the development of autoimmunity to spermatozoa in men with cystic fibrosis. Fertil Steril 58:1199–1204
10. Boorjian S, Lipkin M, Goldstein M (2004) The impact of obstructive interval and sperm granuloma on outcome of vasectomy reversal. J Urol 171:304–306
11. Flickinger CJ, Howards SS, Bush LA, Baker LA, Herr JC (1994) Temporal recognition of sperm autoantigens by IgM and IgG autoantibodies after vasectomy and vasovasostomy. J Reprod Immunol 27:135–150
12. Witkin SS, Goldstein M (1988) Reduced levels of T suppressor/cytotoxic lymphocytes in semen from vasovasostomized men: relationship to sperm autoantibodies. J Reprod Immunol 14:283–290
13. Dondero F, Lenzi A, Gandini L, Lombardo F (1993) Immunological infertility in humans. Exp Clin Immunogenet 10:65–72
14. Choi YJ, Reiner L (1983) Autoimmune response following vasectomy. N Y State J Med 83: 819–822
15. Lenzi A, Gandini L, Claroni F, Dondero F (1987) Post-vasectomy antisperm immune reaction after testosterone-induced azoospermia. Br J Urol 59:277–279
16. Wen RQ, Li SQ, Wang CX, Wang QH, Li QK, Feng HM, Jiang YJ, Huang JC (1994) Analysis of spermatozoa from the proximal vas deferens of vasectomized men. Int J Androl 17(4):181–185
17. Meinertz H (1991) Antisperm antibodies in split ejaculates. Am J Reprod Immunol 26(3): 110–113

18. Witkin SS, Toth A (1983) Relationship between genital tract infections, sperm antibodies in seminal fluid and infertility. Fertil Steril 40:805–808
19. Jarow JP, Kirkland JA, Assimos DG (1990) Association antisperm antibodies with chronic non bacterial prostatitis. Urology 36:154–156
20. Dohle GR (2003) Inflammatory-associated obstructions of the male reproductive tract. Andrologia 35:321–324
21. Engeler DS, Hauri D, John H (2003) Impact of prostatitis NIH IIIB (prostatodynia) on ejaculate parameters. Eur Urol 44:546–548
22. Weidner W, Anderson RU (2008) Evaluation of acute and chronic bacterial prostatitis and diagnostic management of chronic prostatitis/chronic pelvic pain syndrome (CP/CPPS) with special reference to infection/inflammation. Int J Antimicrob Agents 31:S91–S95
23. Dondero F, Radicioni A, Gandini L, Lenzi A (1984) Immunoglobulins in human seminal plasma. Andrologia 16:228–236
24. Muñoz MG, Witkin SS (1995) Autoimmunity to spermatozoa, asymptomatic *Chlamydia trachomatis* genital tract infection and gamma delta T lymphocytes in seminal fluid from the male partners of couples with unexplained infertility. Hum Reprod 10:1070–1074
25. Eggert-Kruse W, Buhlinger-Gopfarth N, Rohr G, Probst S, Aufenanger J, Naher H, Runnebaum B (1996) Antibodies to chlamydia trachomatis in semen and relationship with parameters of male fertility. Hum Reprod 11:1408–1417
26. Gil T, Castilla JA, Hortas ML, Redondo M, Samaniego F, Garrido F, Vergara F, Herruzo AJ (1998) Increase of large granular lymphocytes in human ejaculate containing antisperm antibodies. Hum Reprod 13:296–301
27. Gonzales GF, Kortebani G, Mazzolli AB (1992) Leukocytospermia and function of the seminal vesicles on seminal quality. Fertil Steril 57:1058–1065
28. Kortebani G, Gonzales GF, Barrera C, Mazzolli AB (1992) Leucocyte populations in semen and male accessory gland function: relationship with antisperm antibodies and seminal quality. Andrologia 24:197–204
29. Wolff H, Politch JA, Martinez A, Haimovici F, Hill JA, Anderson DJ (1990) Leukocytospermia is associated with poor semen quality. Fertil Steril 53:528–536
30. Komori K, Tsujimura A, Miura H, Shin M, Takada T, Honda M, Matsumiya K, Fujioka H (2004) Serial follow-up study of serum testosterone and antisperm antibodies in patients with non-obstructive azoospermia after conventional or microdissection testicular sperm extraction. Int J Androl 27:32–37
31. Leonhartsberger N, Gozzi C, Akkad T, Springer-Stoehr B, Bartsch G, Steiner H (2007) Organ-sparing surgery does not lead to greater antisperm antibody levels than orchidectomy. BJU Int 100:371–374
32. Abbas AK, Burstein HJ, Bogen SA (1993) Determinants of helper T cell-dependent antibody production. Semin Immunol 5:441–447
33. Seiler P, Cooper TG, Nieschlag E (2000) Sperm number and condition affect the number of basal cells and their expression of macrophage antigen in the murine epididymis. Int J Androl 23(2):65–76
34. Wolff H, Schill WB (1985) Antisperm antibodies in infertile and homosexual men: relationship to serologic and clinical findings. Fertil Steril 44:673–677
35. Barratt CL, Harrison PE, Robinson A, Cooke ID (1990) Antisperm antibodies and lymphocyte subsets in semen–not a simple relationship. Int J Androl 13:50–58
36. Dimitrova D, Kalaydjiev S, Hristov L, Nikolov K, Boyadjiev T, Nakov L (2004) Antichlamydial and antisperm antibodies in patients with chlamydial infections. Am J Reprod Immunol 52:330–336
37. Eggert-Kruse W, Rohr G, Demirakca T, Rusu R, Näher H, Petzoldt D, Runnebaum B (1997) Chlamydial serology in 1303 asymptomatic subfertile couples. Hum Reprod 12:1464–1475
38. Blacklock NJ (1974) Anatomical factors in prostatitis. Br J Urol 46:47–54

39. Rumke P, Hellinga G (1959) Autoantibodies against spermatozoa in sterile men. Am J Clin Pathol 32:357–363

40. Golomb J, Vardinon N, Homonnai ZT, Braf Z, Yust I (1986) Demonstration of antispermatozoal antibodies in varicocele-related infertility with an enzyme-linked immunosorbent assay (ELISA). Fertil Steril 45:397–402

41. Gilbert BR, Witkin SS, Goldstein M (1989) Correlation of sperm-bound immunoglobulins with impaired semen analysis in infertile men with varicoceles. Fertil Steril 52:469–473

42. Isitmangil G, Yildirim S, Orhan I, Kadioglu A, Akinci M (1999) A comparison of the sperm mixed-agglutination reaction test with the peroxidase-labelled protein A test for detecting antisperm antibodies in infertile men with varicocele. BJU Int 84:835–838

43. Knudson G, Ross L, Stuhldreher D, Houlihan D, Bruns E, Prins G (1994) Prevalence of sperm bound antibodies in infertile men with varicocele: the effect of varicocele ligation on antibody levels and semen response. J Urol 151:1260–1262

44. Djaladat H, Mehrsai A, Rezazade M, Djaladat Y, Pourmand G (2006) Varicocele and antisperm antibody: fact or fiction? South Med J 99:44–47

45. Oshinsky GS, Rodriguez MV, Mellinger BC (1993) Varicocele-related infertility is not associated with increased sperm-bound antibody. J Urol 150:871–873

46. Heidenreich A, Bonfig R, Wilbert DM, Strohmaier WL, Engelmann UH (1994) Risk factors for antisperm antibodies in infertile men. Am J Reprod Immunol 31:69–76

47. Veräjänkorva E, Laato M, Pöllänen P (2003) Analysis of 508 infertile male patients in southwestern Finland in 1980–2000: hormonal status and factors predisposing to immunological infertility. Eur J Obstet Gynecol Reprod Biol 10:173–178

48. Shook TE, Nyberg LM, Collins BS, Mathur S (1988) Pathological and immunological effects of surgically induced varicocele in juvenile and adult rats. Am J Reprod Immunol Microbiol 17:141–144

49. Turner TT, Jones CE, Roddy MS (1987) Experimental varicocele does not affect the blood–testis barrier, epididymal electrolyte concentrations, or testicular blood gas concentrations. Biol Reprod 36:926–931

50. Trussell JC, Lee PA (2004) The relationship of cryptorchidism to fertility. Curr Urol Rep 5:142–148

51. Sinisi AA, Pasquali D, Papparella A, Valente A, Orio F, Esposito D, Cobellis G, Cuomo A, Angelone G, Martone A, Fioretti GP, Bellastella A (1998) Antisperm antibodies in cryptorchidism before and after surgery. J Urol 160:1834–1837

52. Urry RL, Carrell DT, Starr NT, Snow BW, Middleton RG (1994) The incidence of antisperm antibodies in infertility patients with a history of cryptorchidism. J Urol 151:381–383

53. Cortes D, Brandt B, Thorup J (1990) Direct mixed antiglobulin reaction (MAR) test in semen at follow-up after testicular biopsy of maldescended testes operated in puberty. Z Kinderchir 45:227–228

54. Patel RP, Kolon TF, Huff DS, Carr MC, Zderic SA, Canning DA, Snyder HM 3rd (2005) Testicular microlithiasis and antisperm antibodies following testicular biopsy in boys with cryptorchidism. J Urol 174:2008–2010

55. Mirilas P, Mamoulakis C, De Almeida M (2003) Puberty does not induce serum antisperm surface antibodies in patients with previously operated cryptorchidism. J Urol 170: 2432–2435

56. Mirilas P, De Almeida M (1999) Absence of antisperm surface antibodies in prepubertal boys with cryptorchidism and other anomalies of the inguinoscrotal region before and after surgery. J Urol 162:177–181

57. Lenzi A, Gandini L, Lombardo F, Cappa M, Nardini P, Ferro F, Borrelli P, Dondero F (1991) Antisperm antibodies in young boys. Andrologia 23:233–235

58. Mininberg DT, Chen ME, Witkin SS (1993) Antisperm antibodies in cryptorchid boys. Eur J Pediatr 152(Suppl 2):S23–S24

59. Sinisi AA, D'Apuzzo A, Pasquali D, Venditto T, Esposito D, Pisano G, De Bellis A, Ventre I, Papparella A, Perrone L, Bellastella A (1997) Antisperm antibodies in prepubertal boys treated with chemotherapy for malignant or non-malignant diseases and in boys with genital tract abnormalities. Int J Androl 20:23–28

60. Hagenäs L, Plöen L, Ritzen EM, Ekwall H (1977) Blood-testis barrier: maintained function of inter-Sertoli cell junctions in experimental cryptorchidism in the rat, as judged by a simple lanthanum-immersion technique. Andrologia 9:250–254

61. Stewart RJ, Boyd S, Brown S, Toner PG (1990) The blood–testis barrier in experimental unilateral cryptorchidism. J Pathol 160:51–55

62. Kukadia AN, Ercole CJ, Gleich P, Hensleigh H, Pryor JL (1996) Testicular trauma: potential impact on reproductive function. J Urol 156:1643–1646

63. Harrington TG, Schauer D, Gilbert BR (1996) Percutaneous testis biopsy: an alternative to open testicular biopsy in the evaluation of the subfertile man. J Urol 156:1647–1651

64. Lievano G, Nguyen L, Radhakrishnan J, Fornell L, John E (1999) New animal model to evaluate testicular blood flow during testicular torsion. J Pediatr Surg 34:1004–1006

65. Arap MA, Vicentini FC, Cocuzza M, Hallak J, Athayde K, Lucon AM, Arap S, Srougi M (2007) Late hormonal levels, semen parameters, and presence of antisperm antibodies in patients treated for testicular torsion. J Androl 28:528–532

66. Anderson MJ, Dunn JK, Lipshultz LI, Coburn M (1992) Semen quality and endocrine parameters after acute testicular torsion. J Urol 147:1545–1550

67. Koşar A, Küpeli B, Alçigir G, Ataoglu H, Sarica K, Küpeli S (1999) Immunologic aspect of testicular torsion: detection of antisperm antibodies in contralateral testicle. Eur Urol 36:640–644

68. Foster RS, Rubin LR, McNulty A, Bihrle R, Donohue JP (1991) Detection of antisperm-antibodies in patients with primary testicular cancer. Int J Androl 14:179–185

69. Guazzieri S, Lembo A, Ferro G, Artibani W, Merlo F, Zanchetta R, Pagano F (1985) Sperm antibodies and infertility in patients with testicular cancer. Urology 26:139–142

70. Höbarth K, Klingler HC, Maier U, Kollaritsch H (1994) Incidence of antisperm antibodies in patients with carcinoma of the testis and in subfertile men with normogonadotropic oligoasthenoteratozoospermia. Urol Int 52:162–165

71. Richards JM, Bedford JM, Witkin SS (1984) Rectal insemination modifies immune responses in rabbits. Science 27:390–392

72. Witkin SS, Sonnabend J, Richards JM, Purtilo DT (1983) Induction of antibody to asialo GM1 by spermatozoa and its occurrence in the sera of homosexual men with the acquired immune deficiency syndrome (AIDS). Clin Exp Immunol 54:346–350

73. Mulhall BP, Fieldhouse S, Clark S, Carter L, Harrison L, Donovan B, Short RV (1990) Antisperm antibodies in homosexual men: prevalence and correlation with sexual behaviour. Genitourin Med 66:5–7

74. Sands M, Phair JP, Hyprikar J, Hansen C, Brown RB (1985) A study on antisperm antibody in homosexual men. J Med 16:483–491

Walter K. H. Krause

2.5.1
ASA Are Immunoglobulins

There are five main types of these proteins distributed in a specific manner and with a specific activity (see Table 2.5.1). IgM antibodies are the first immunoglobulins to be synthesized in the course of immune response. They form pentramers, which exhibit ten antigen binding sites. Because of the large size, IgM concentrations in the extravascular space including seminal fluid are low. The immunoglobulins of glandular secretions and in the extraepithelial spaces are IgG and IgA. IgA is secreted in dimers, in which two molecules are connected by the secretory piece, a fragment of the IgA receptor of the epithclial cell.

Antibodies are secreted from plasma cells, which are derived from activated B lymphocytes. The activation of B cells requires both antigen binding and the support by antigen-specific T helper cells. The B cells internalize the antigens which are bound to surface immunoglobulins and present it as peptide bound to MHC class II molecules to the helper T cells. Subsequently, T helper cells stimulate the B lymphocytes through binding different mechanisms including CD40 and tumor-necrosis factor (TNF) and finally induce differentiation of the clonally B cells into plasma cells. The antibody-producing plasma cells may be systemically active, but also topical activity is possible. This may explain different antigen specifities of antibodies present in the different compartments.

A study of the B-cell activation process producing antisperm antibodies (ASA) has been published by Dimitrova et al. [1]. They were able to produce three stable cell populations derived from transformed B-lymphocytes from infertile patients with ASA. The cDNA of the heavy chain of this immunoglobulin showed high homology to the DNA of immunoglobulins in general. Thus the authors concluded that it was more likely that the ASA were natural antibodies (iso-antibodies) as they were induced by stimulation of a specific sperm antigen.

ASA may be present in the human biological fluids – blood serum of both sexes, seminal fluid and fluid of male accessory glands, cervix mucus, tubal, and follicular fluid. They are

W. Krause
Klinik für Dermatologie und Allergologie, Philipps-Universität, Marburg, 35033, Germany
e-mail: krause@med.uni-marburg.de

W. K. H. Krause and R. K. Naz (eds.), *Immune Infertility*,
DOI: 10.1007/978-3-642-01379-9_2.5, © Springer Verlag Berlin Heidelberg 2009

Table 2.5.1 Activity and distribution of immunoglobulins (from Janeway et al. 2001 [45])

	IgM	IgD	IgG	IgA	IgE
Neutralizing antibody	+	−	+	+	−
Sensibilization of mast cells	−	−	+	−	++
Activation of complement	+	−	+	+	−
Transepithelial transport	+	−	−	++	−
Diffusion into extravascular spce	−	−	+	+	+
Mean serum concentration (mg/mL)	1.5	0.04	13	2.1	30.000

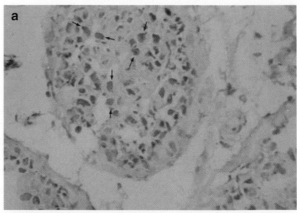

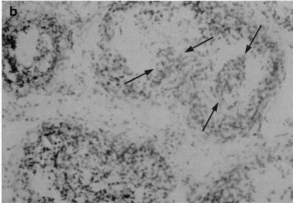

Fig. 2.5.1 (**a**) Direct immunofluorescence on seminiferous tubules. Mature spermatocytes (*arrows*) in the lumen from a patient with varicocele show the binding of ASA by the brown staining from the POPA method. (**b**) A slide from the control group without ASA binding (no brown staining arrows) (from Isitmangi et al. [2], with permission)

also demonstrable after binding to spermatozoa or even to testicular progenitor cells [2; Fig. 2.5.1]. These ASA are predominantly IgG and IgA. Various tests used for the demonstration of ASA are able to differentiate between these immunoglobulins (see Chap. 3.2).

ASA will influence sperm function only when they are bound to spermatozoa [43]. In general, antibodies may influence the function of a cell in different manners:

1. The most relevant mechanisms are inhibition of function provided by that protein, which includes the cognate antigen (epitope). The proteins influenced by ASA binding will be outlined in the appropriate chapter.

2. The complement activation is of minor importance. Complement activating ASA are not effective in the seminal plasma because it contains complement inhibitors. However, during their residence in the cervical mucus, spermatozoa are exposed to complement activity, which is approximately 12% of that of serum [3]. But also here the spermatozoa themselves are protected against complement attacks mainly by CD46, the main complement-regulation protein [4; Fig. 2.5.2]. Human spermatozoa express CD46 on the inner acrosomal membrane after the acrosome reaction.

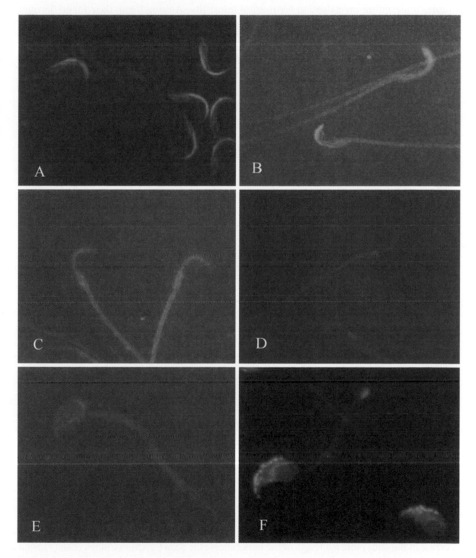

Fig. 2.5.2 Distribution of membrane CReg on rodent spermatozoa. CD46 expression in the rat is restricted to the acrosome (**a**), whereas CD55 is also found on the tail (**b**). CD59 in the rat is broadly distributed (**c**). CD59a in the mouse is broadly distributed (**e**) whereas CD59b is restricted to the head (**f**). (**d**) Negative control. Original magnification is 1,000×, magnified a further three times electronically in (**e**) and (**f**) (from Harris et al. [4], with permission)

3. Antibodies may activate accessory effector cells (phagocytes) or natural killer cells after binding of the Fc fragment of the immunoglobulin. Sperm-destructing phagocytes (spermiophages) are normal constituents of seminal cells. They are, however less, the consequence of the destruction of spermatozoa bearing ASA [5] than the elimination sperm undergoing apoptosis [6].

An important question is whether ASA influence the conception rate in general and ASA of which compartments are of greatest significance. Collins et al. [7] investigated 471 couples undergoing investigation for marital infertility. Among them, they found 38 men and six women being positive for ASA in serum. In 23.7% of the couples with male ASA in serum a pregnancy occurred, in 27% of the couples without ASA, the difference being not significant. Men with ASA, however, had a significantly longer time-to-pregnancy (TTP) and a significantly lower sperm concentration. The authors hypothezised that not ASA themselves might be the cause of subfertility, but the ASA were a consequence of errors in the spermatogenesis, which in turn decreased fertility. With proportional hazards analysis, however, antibody status in either partner was not a significant independent predictor of time to pregnancy (Fig. 2.5.3). Also Vujisic et al. [8] could not observe any correlations of ASA concentrations in semen, serum, and follicular fluid with the fertilization rate in vitro fertilization (IVF) outcome in 52 couples.

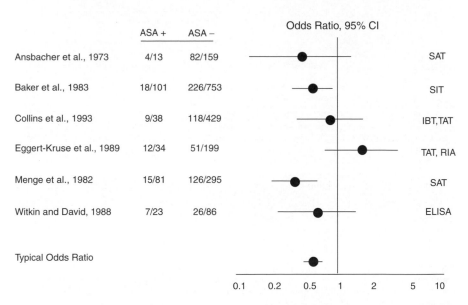

Fig. 2.5.3 The association of the presence of ASA in infertile men and the pregnancy rate in their partners as calculated on the basis of different studies. The vertical line in the middle indicates an odds ratio of 1, i.e., no association. The bars including this line indicate no significant increase or decrease of the odds ratio, the length of the bars indicate the 95% CI. (from Collins et al. [7], with permission). *SAT* serum agglutination test; *SIT* serum immobilization test; *IBT* immunobead binding test; *TAT* tray agglutination test; *RIA* radioimmunoassay; *ELISA* enzyme linked immunosorbent assay

2.5.2
ASA in Serum

ASA may occur in the blood serum of male and female patients. With increasing knowledge on the cognate antigens of ASA and their biological relevance it has become evident that some of the ASA in serum are not a consequence of the contact to sperm antigens, but they are indenpendently existing isoantibodies. This concerns mainly antibodies in female serum, such as the sperm-immobilizing antibodies [9], antibodies to the proacrosin/acrosin system [10], and antibodies to the fertilization antigen-1 or YLP12 [11]. Also the antibodies detected in cryptorchid boys may represent isoantibodies [12–14].

Another hypothesis for the induction of ASA is based on the crossreactivity between antigens of spermatozoa and exogenous antigens. Common antigenicity has been established between spermatozoa and *Escherichia coli, streptococcal antigens, Trichomonas vaginalis, Mycoplasma hominis*, and *Ureaplasma urealyticum* [15]. Also a correlation of ASA testing and the presence of antibodies against chlamydia trachomatis has been described [16]. Since the antibodies have been detected only in the serum of patients with genital chlamydial infection, but not in those with ocular infection, it appeared likely that the ASA formation is a result of the chlamydial inflammatory process with genital localization, but not of cross-reactivity between sperm and C. trachomatis antigens. Also the ASA observed in patients with colitis-ulcerosa might be provoked by the systemic inflammatory responses or by a polyclonal activation of B-cells [15].

2.5.3
ASA in Seminal Fluid

The main determinant for the concentration of immunoglobulins in seminal fluid is inflammation, whereupon acute inflammation increases the concentrations to a much higher extent than chronic inflammation [17; Table 2.5.2]. Similar results were described also by Marconi et al. [18], who have included also the results of ASA determination in seminal fluid and have found no difference of this value between healthy men and men with inflammations.

Table 2.5.2   Concentration of different proteins in seminal fluid [4]

	Healthy men [26]	Acute prostatitis [26]	Chronic prostatitis [38]
Albumin	0.59	4.7	1.6
Haptoglobulin	0	0.14	0.001
Transferrin	0.04	0.28	0.11
α-1 Antitrypsin	0.08	0.22	0.12
α-2 Macroglobulin	0	0.12	0.007
IgG	0.21	2.4	0.49
IgA	0.02	0.35	0.13

Usually, men expressing ASA in the seminal fluid also have ASA in blood serum. Andreou et al. [19] have described a close correlation between the concentration of ASA fixed to spermatozoa (direct mixed antiglobulin reaction (MAR) test) and that of ASA solubilized in serum and serminal plasma (indirect MAR test). For IgG, a correlation was found between ASA in seminal plasma and in serum. Vujisic et al. [8], on the other hand, could not find a correlation between ASA concentrations in the different biological fluids.

The studies indicate that ASA in semen predominantly are the product of locally active B lymphocytes. This is less pronounced in IgG, since IgG in semen is mainly derived from the serum IgG. ASA of the IgA fraction, however, clearly originate from a local production [19]. The conditions are complicated by the fact that human semen contains antibody-binding proteins with IgG-Fc affinity, which is not present in other compartments. The function of these proteins is unclear [20].

As a consequence of different B cell populations present in the different compartments it appears that ASA must not recognize identical antigens. Domagala et al. [21] have demonstrated that local antibodies in seminal plasma may bind to other cognate antigens than those in blood serum.

2.5.4
ASA in Cervix Mucus

The cervical fluid has no unique origin. It is a mixture of secretions from cervical vestibular glands, plasma transudate, endometrial, and oviductal fluids. As cellular components leukocytes are present, the molecular components include inorganic salts, urea, amino acids, proteins, and a number of fatty acids. Among the proteins albumin, transferrin, and immunoglobulins are demonstrable. The characteristic mucins are high-molecular, which are heavily glycosylated glycoproteins products of the different mucin genes. They are similar to the mucins of other origin such as saliva, respiratory tract, and the gastrointestinal tract [22, 47].

Immunoglobulin concentrations in the cervix mucus vary with hormonal conditions and with inflammation [23, 24]. During menstrual cycle, they are highest at the day of ovulation, while the levels outside this period are far lower (see Table 2.5.3). Eighty percent of the IgA occur in the polymeric forms [25]. The concentrations also vary in the course of pregnancy. Immunoglobulin A remained stable during each trimester of pregnancy (26 mg/dL). Cervical mucus immunoglobulin G decreased from a first-trimester high of 44.4 mg/dL to lower levels in the second and third trimesters [26]. At term of pregnancy, levels of IgG [median 3,270 µg/mL] and IgA [540 µg/mL], but not IgM [30.5 µg/mL], were

Table 2.5.3 Immunoglobulin amount in cervix mucus (concentration multiplicated by volume of mucus) at midcycle [30]

	IgA	IgG	IgM	Total Ig
Ovulation day 1	11.9±9.2	29.2±26.7	5.9±3.3	47.0
Ovulation day 4	2.0±1.5	4.8±3.9	2.5±1.4	9.3

significantly elevated compared to cervical mucus from nonpregnant women [27]. IgG and IgM originate mainly from serum, whereas a local synthesis provided total-IgA and secretory IgA [28].

The occurrence of ASA in cervical mucus is generally quoted to be rare. Stern et al. [29] compared retrospectively the concentration of ASA in serum and mucus by means of the indirect immunobead binding test (IBT) in patients undergoing evaluation for infertility. They found that ASA levels in serum did not correlate with the ASA levels in mucus, which is not in line with the changing levels of immunoglobulins as described by Kutteh et al. [25]. They also could not demonstrate an alteration with the menstrual cycle. In those couples, in which ASA were demonstrable as a possible cause of infertility, ASA were found in serum in 58% of patients, but in cervix mucus only in 25% of patients [30].

Eggert-Kruse et al. [31] found among 192 infertile patients, in only 2% of cervical mucus samples significant ASA levels by means of the indirect MAR test. All ASA positive women had a negative outcome of the postcoital test, but a greater number of negative post-coital tests was independent of ASA. Among 48 patients of Domagala et al. [32] were only two CM samples (4.6%), which yielded positive results in the indirect IBT. Among 155 infertile women, Kamieniczna et al. [33] demonstrated ASA in 3.2% of cervix mucus samples by means of the IBT.

Menge and Naz [34] used a special enzyme linked immunosorbent assay (ELISA) for the detection of ASA directed to the fertilization antigen-1 (FA-1). In 32 infertile women, 10 sera were negative and 22 positive. Of the 22 CM samples from ASA-positive women, 9 were positive for IgG antibodies, 9 for IgA, 7 for IgA1, and 6 for IgA2.

An interesting question is whether insemination may induce local ASA. Friedman et al. [35] observed 51 women, which underwent 1–9 cycles of intrauterine insemination (IUI). In these women, mucus or serum ASA titres did not increase. The observation indicated that the local immune response is not activated by intrauterine insemination. Consequently, this question was not resumed in later studies.

2.5.5
ASA in Follicular Fluid

Serum proteins and immunoglobulins in follicular fluid are of lower or equal concentration as in blood serum (Table 2.5.4), the interrelationship between the protein fractions, however, is similar to that in serum [36]. Only few proteins present in the follicular fluid showed an association to the follicule maturation [37]. Additionally, also other cofactors of the immune system such as various cytokines such as SCF, IL-2 and IL-11 are present in the follucular fluid, IL-6, IL-8, TNF-α, MIP-1α, and IFN-γ were detected in oviductal fluid [38]. The proteomics of follicular fluid has been analyzed by Anahory et al. [39]. A 2D-electrophoresis revealed up to 600 protein spots.

Kohl et al. [40] tested follicular fluid for ASA in 38 women by means of an ELISA. Positive results were found only in women with antibodies circulating in serum ($r > 0.88$, $p < 0.001$). There was no correlation between ASA in serum with sperm agglutination and the post-coital test. Neither was there any correlation between antibodies in follicular fluid

Table 2.5.4 Follicular fluid and serum concentration of proteins (g/L) in relation to ovarian stimulation (from Suchanek et al. [42])

	n	Clomiphene-hMG-hCG	n	hMG-hCG	Serum range
Total proteins	40	46.33±7.26	20	43.66±7.36	65–80
Fibrinogen	38	0.24±0.17	17	0.23±+0.15	2.0–4.5
α-2 Macroglobulin	40	0.20±0.11	20	0.17±0.09	1.75–4.20
α-1 Antitrypsin	40	4.29±1.66	20	4.22±1.09	1.9–3.5
IgG	40	7.56±1.87	20	8.02±1.88	8–18
IgA	39	1.03±0.52	19	0.73±0.30	0.8–4.5
IgM	7	0.44±0.12	3	0.28±0.03	0.7–2.8

and the post-coital test, the pregnancy rate or successful IVF [44]. Nip et al. [41] described a higher prevalence of ASA in infertile women, and a relation between the concentration found in serum and follicular fluid. Marín-Briggiler et al. [46] demonstrated the presence of ASA in the follicular fluid which were able to induce the AR in capacitated human donor spermatozoa. It has, however, to be taken in consideration that also normal follicular fluid is able to induce acrosome reaction, depending on the amount of progesterone present.

Vujisic et al. [8] found no associotion of ASA concentrations in the follicular fluid have with those of the blood serum. In their study, the authors also have described no association of ASA concentrations in the different biological fluids and with the fertilization rate.

References

1. Dimitrova-Dikanarova DK, Tsuji Y, Nakata Y, Shibahara H, Mitsuo M, Hashimoto T, Furuyama J, Koyama K (1996) Characterization of anti-sperm antibodies and their coding cDNA sequences by Epstein-Barr virus transformed B cell lines from lymphocytes of infertile women possessing anti-sperm antibodies. J Reprod Immunol 32(2):171–191
2. Isitmangi G, Yildirim S, Orhan K, Kadiog A, Akinci M (1999) A comparison of the sperm mixed-agglutination reaction test with the peroxidase-labelled protein A test for detecting antisperm antibodies in infertile men with varicocele. BJU Int 84:835–838
3. Haas GG Jr (1987) Immunologic infertility. Obstet Gynecol Clin North Am 14:1069–1085
4. Harris CL, Mizuno M, Morgan BP (2006) Complement and complement regulators in the male reproductive system. Mol Immunol 43:57–67
5. Pelliccione F, D'Angeli A, Cordeschi G, Mihalca R, Ciociola F, Necozione S, Francavilla F, Francavilla S (2008) Seminal macrophages in ejaculates from men with couple infertility. Int J Androl epub ahead of print Sept. 2008
6. Said TM, Paasch U, Glander HJ, Agarwal A (2004) Role of caspases in male infertility. Hum Reprod Update 10(1):39–51
7. Collins JA, Burrows EA, Yeo J, YoungLai EV (1993) Frequency and predictive value of anti-sperm antibodies among infertile couples. Hum Reprod 8(4):592–598
8. Vujisić S, Lepej SZ, Jerković L, Emedi I, Sokolić B (2005) Antisperm antibodies in semen, sera and follicular fluids of infertile patients: relation to reproductive outcome after in vitro fertilization. Am J Reprod Immunol 54(1):13–20
9. Isojima S (1989) Human sperm antigens corresponding to sperm-immobilizing antibodies in the sera of women with infertility of unknown cause: personal review of our recent studies. Hum Reprod 4(6):605–612

10. Veaute C, Furlong LI, Bronson R, Harris JD, Vazquez-Levin MH (2008) Acrosin antibodies and infertility. I. Detection of antibodies towards proacrosin/acrosin in women consulting for infertility and evaluation of their effects upon the sperm protease activities. Fertil Steril 2009; 91(4): 1245–1255

11. Williams J, Samuel A, Naz RK (2008) Presence of antisperm antibodies reactive with peptide epitopes of FA-1 and YLP12 in sera of immunoinfertile women. Am J Reprod Immunol 59(6):518–524

12. Domagala A, Havryluk A, Nakonechnyj A, Kamieniczna M, Chopyak V, Kurpisz M (2006) Antisperm antibodies in prepubertal boys with cryptorchidism. Arch Androl 52(6):411–416

13. Mirilas P, Mamoulakis C, De Almeida M (2003) Puberty does not induce serum antisperm surface antibodies in patients with previously operated cryptorchidism. J Urol 170(6 Pt 1):2432–2435

14. Sinisi AA, Pasquali D, Papparella A, Valente A, Orio F, Esposito D, Cobellis G, Cuomo A, Angelone G, Martone A, Fioretti GP, Bellastella A (1998) Antisperm antibodies in cryptorchidism before and after surgery. J Urol 160(5):1834–1837

15. Dimitrova D, Kalaydjiev S, Mendizova A, Piryova E, Nakov L (2005) Circulating antibodies to human spermatozoa in patients with ulcerative colitis. Fertil Steril 84(5):1533–1535

16. Dimitrova D, Kalaydjiev S, Hristov L, Nikolov K, Boyadjiev T, Nakov L (2004) Antichlamydial and antisperm antibodies in patients with chlamydial infections. Am J Reprod Immunol 52(5):330–336

17. Blenk H, Hofstetter A (1985) The behaviour of complement C3 and other serum proteins in the ejaculate in chronic prostatitis and their diagnostic importance. In: Brunner H, Krause W, Rothauge CF, Weidner W (eds) Chronic prostatitis. Schattauer, Stuttgart-New York

18. Marconi M, Nowotny A, Pantke P, Diemer T, Weidner W (2008) Antisperm antibodies detected by mixed agglutination reaction and immunobead test are not associated with chronic inflammation and infection of the seminal tract. Andrologia 40(4):227–234

19. Andreou E, Mahmoud A, Vermeulen L, Schoonjans F, Comhaire F (1995) Comparison of different methods for the investigation of antisperm antibodies on spermatozoa, in seminal plasma and in serum. Hum Reprod 10(1):125–131

20. Chiu WW, Chamley LW (2002) Antibody-binding proteins in human seminal plasma. Am J Reprod Immunol 48(4):269–274

21. Domagała A, Pulido S, Kurpisz M, Herr JC (2007) Application of proteomic methods for identification of sperm immunogenic antigens. Mol Hum Reprod 13(7):437–444

22. Thornton DJ, Howard M, Devine PL, Sheehan JK (1995) Methods for separation and deglycosylation of mucin subunits. Anal Biochem 227(1):162–167

23. Shaw JL, Smith CR, Diamandis EP (2007) Proteomic analysis of human cervico-vaginal fluid. J Proteome Res 6(7):2859–2865

24. Tang LJ, De Seta F, Odreman F, Venge P, Piva C, Guaschino S, Garcia RC (2007) Proteomic analysis of human cervical-vaginal fluids. J Proteome Res 6(7):2874–2883

25. Kutteh WH, Prince SJ, Hammond KR, Kutteh CC, Mestecky J (1996) Variations in immunoglobulins and IgA subclasses of human uterine cervical secretions around the time of ovulation. Clin Exp Immunol 104(3):538–542

26. Kutteh WH, Franklin RD (2001) Quantification of immunoglobulins and cytokines in human cervical mucus during each trimester of pregnancy. Am J Obstet Gynecol 184(5):865–872

27. Hein M, Petersen AC, Helmig RB, Uldbjerg N, Reinholdt J (2005) Immunoglobulin levels and phagocytes in the cervical mucus plug at term of pregnancy. Acta Obstet Gynecol Scand 84(8):734–742

28. Bard E, Riethmuller D, Biichlé S, Meillet D, Prétet JL, Mougin C, Seillès E (2002) Validation of a high sensitive immunoenzymatic assay to establish the origin of immunoglobulins in female genital secretions. J Immunoassay Immunochem 23(2):145–162

29. Stern JE, Dixon PM, Manganiello PD, Brinck-Johnsen T (1992) Antisperm antibodies in women: variability in antibody levels in serum, mucus, and peritoneal fluid. Fertil Steril 58(5): 950–958

30. Kapoor A, Talib VH, Verma SK (1999) Immunological assessment of infertility by estimation of antisperm antibodies in infertile couples. Indian J Pathol Microbiol 42(1):37–43
31. Eggert-Kruse W, Böckem-Hellwig S, Doll A, Rohr G, Tilgen W, Runnebaum B (1993) Antisperm antibodies in cervical mucus in an unselected subfertile population. Hum Reprod 8(7):1025–1031
32. Domagala A, Kasprzak M, Kurpisz M (1997) Immunological characteristics of cervical mucus in infertile women. Zentralbl Gynakol 119(12):616–620
33. Kamieniczna M, Domagała A, Kurpisz M (2003) The frequency of antisperm antibodies in infertile couples–a Polish pilot study. Med Sci Monit 9(4):CR142–CR149
34. Menge AC, Naz RK (1993) Immunoglobulin (Ig) G, IgA, and IgA subclass antibodies against fertilization antigen-1 in cervical secretions and sera of women of infertile couples. Fertil Steril 60(4):658–663
35. Friedman AJ, Juneau-Norcross M, Sedensky B (1991) Antisperm antibody production following intrauterine insemination. Hum Reprod 6(8):1125–1128
36. Munuce MJ, Quintero I, Caille AM, Ghersevich S, Berta CL (2006) Comparative concentrations of steroid hormones and proteins in human peri-ovulatory peritoneal and follicular fluids. Reprod Biomed Online 13(2):202–207
37. Nagy B, Pulay T, Szarka G, Csömör S (1989) The serum protein content of human follicular fluid and its correlation with the maturity of oocytes. Acta Physiol Hung 73(1):71–75
38. Srivastava MD, Lippes J, Srivastava BI (1996) Cytokines of the human reproductive tract. Am J Reprod Immunol 36(3):157–166
39. Anahory T, Dechaud H, Bennes R, Marin P, Lamb NJ, Laoudj D (2002) Identification of new proteins in follicular fluid of mature human follicles. Electrophoresis 23(7–8):1197–1202
40. Kohl B, Kohl H, Krause W, Deichert U (1992) The clinical significance of antisperm antibodies in infertile couples. Hum Reprod 7(10):1384–1387
41. Nip MM, Taylor PV, Rutherford AJ, Hancock KW (1995) Autoantibodies and antisperm antibodies in sera and follicular fluids of infertile patients; relation to reproductive outcome after in-vitro fertilization. Hum Reprod 10(10):2564–2569
42. Suchanek E, Mujkic-Klaric A, Grizelj V, Simunic V, Kopjar B (1990) Protein concentration in pre-ovulatory follicular fluid related to ovarian stimulation. Int J Gynaecol Obstet 32(1):53–59
43. Bohring C, Krause W (2003) Immune infertility: towards a better understanding of sperm (auto)-immunity by proteomic analysis. Human Reprod 18:915–924
44. Hammadeh ME, Ertan AK, Zeppezauer M, Baltes S, Georg T, Rosenbaum P, Schmidt W (2002) Immunoglobulins and cytokines level in follicular fluid in relation to etiology of infertility and their relevance to IVF outcome. Am J Reprod Immunol 47(2):82–90
45. Charles Janeway, Kenneth Murphy, Paul Travers, Mark Walport, Mark Jeremy (eds) (2008) Janeway's immunobiology, 7th edn. Garland Science, New York
46. Marín-Briggiler CI, Vazquez-Levin MH, Gonzalez-Echeverría F, Blaquier JA, Miranda PV, Tezón JG (2003) Effect of antisperm antibodies present in human follicular fluid upon the acrosome reaction and sperm-zona pellucida interaction. Am J Reprod Immunol 50(3):209–219
47. Tang S, Garrett C, Baker HW (1999) Comparison of human cervical mucus and artificial sperm penetration media. Hum Reprod 14(11):2812–2817

ASA in the Female

2.6

Gary N. Clarke

2.6.1
Introduction

The main aim of this chapter is to review selected literature which is pertinent to understanding why some females develop sperm immunity, with primary focus on antisperm antibodies (ASA) detectable in serum, follicular fluid, or cervical mucus. Another important aim is to discuss several aspects or observations from animal models which have so far received little consideration from the clinical perspective with the objective of stimulating more research focus in these areas. Other chapters in this volume cover in detail the tests available for detecting ASA (Chap. 3.2), antigens (Chap. 1.2), impact on assisted reproduction (Chap. 3.4), and treatment of immune infertility (Chap. 3.5) and other important aspects.

2.6.2
Historical Background

During the first few decades of the twentieth century many studies in animals had indicated that homologous or heterologous immunization of females with sperm or testis preparations could induce sperm antibody activity and infertility (see [1] for review). The considerable evidence derived from animal models, combined with preliminary evaluation of patients provided stimulus for "clinical trials" involving immunization of women with their partner's semen with the aim of inducing immuno-contraception. Baskin [2] reported on a study of 20 fertile women immunized three times intramuscularly at weekly intervals, with their partner's whole ejaculate. All but one of the women showed sperm immobilizing activity in their serum by 1 week after the last injection which persisted for up to 1 year. One woman became pregnant after 12 months when the sperm immobilizing activity was

G. N. Clarke
Andrology Unit, Royal Women's Hospital, Melbourne, Australia
e-mail: gary.clarke@thewomens.org.au

W. K. H. Krause and R. K. Naz (eds.), *Immune Infertility*,
DOI: 10.1007/978-3-642-01379-9_2.6, © Springer Verlag Berlin Heidelberg 2009

no longer detectable in her serum. These trials demonstrated that women could be immunized to develop sperm immobilizing activity, and that this was associated with reduced fecundity.

Further significant evidence for female ASA association with human infertility awaited the report by Franklin and Dukes [3]. They found that 20.1% of 214 women undergoing infertility investigations had detectable sperm agglutinating activity in their serum. Women with unexplained infertility had a much higher incidence (72.1%) than women with organic causes for their infertility (8.4%) or fertile women (5.7%). It should be noted that this study found a very high incidence of ASA and the results are not supported by recent studies using immunologically specific procedures such as the immunobead test (IBT). However, this report was notable from a historical perspective in that it stimulated significant interest in the idea that female immunological responses to sperm could be involved in the development of otherwise unexplained infertility and in the concept of an antisperm contraceptive vaccine.

2.6.3
More Recent Studies on ASA in Females

Since the early reports described above, a multitude of studies have examined the effects of ASA on sperm-cervical mucus penetration, in vitro fertilization (IVF), and infertility. Many reviews have described the clinical and experimental research in this area [4–7]. It is pertinent however to review some of the background information and studies which are relevant to explaining the pathogenesis of female immuno-infertility associated with ASA.

The uterine cervix is a highly competent mucosal immune site (for review, see [8]), which contains many IgA positive plasma cells located in the sub-epithelial layers of the endocervix. Most of the IgA in cervical mucus is secretory IgA consisting of two IgA monomers linked by J-chain and secretory piece. The secretory IgA antibodies directed against potential pathogens and occasionally sperm [9] can immobilize the invaders by cross-linking them to the cervical mucus strands, effectively blocking their progress to the upper reaches of the reproductive tract [10]. There are obviously mechanisms which normally prevent such immunological reactions to sperm in women. However, in a small percentage of couples these are somehow circumvented or disrupted, resulting in local and often circulating ASA production and reduced chances of natural conception. In women with otherwise unexplained infertility, sperm antibody activity has been detected in cervical mucus in more than 10% of cases [11–13].

Investigations using zona-free hamster eggs or salt-stored human zona pellucida indicated that high level ASA might be expected to interfere with human fertilization [6], but this could not be adequately confirmed using fresh human oocytes until the availability of routine clinical IVF around 1985. Retrospective analysis of IVF results by Clarke et al. [14] provided some of the first evidence that ASA from female serum could inhibit the fertilization of viable human oocytes by human spermatozoa. They observed a fertilization rate of only 15% for patients who had significant titres of IgG and IgA class ASA in their serum which was used as a supplement in the IVF culture medium, vs. 69% for those patients where replacement serum was used during the fertilization culture. Their later experimental results confirmed that high titre ASA of IgG immunoglobulin class in female serum could effectively inhibit fertilization of fresh human oocytes [15]. Subsequent reports from other laboratories have also indicated that high level ASA can inhibit human fertilization [16–18]. In addition, more recent animal studies have also provided considerable evidence that experimentally induced sperm iso-immunity could have detrimental effects on fertility and IVF [6]. Consequently, it is now generally accepted, at least with strong sperm immunity, that ASA can block sperm functions such as cervical mucus penetration and fertilization and thereby impair fertility.

2.6.4
Clinical Evaluation of ASA

It is strongly recommended that both the female and male partners should be tested for ASA during infertility assessment. The initial investigation of the male partner of an infertile couple should include a direct IBT or mixed antiglobulin reaction (MAR) screen for sperm-bound antibodies [5]. A positive result (>50% of motile sperm being antibody coated) should be followed up with a repeat test and mucus penetration testing to make an assessment of the potential functional significance of the antibodies. High levels of circulating antibodies in the female may severely reduce the chances of successful treatment by IVF [6] or donor insemination. Assessment of in vitro sperm–mucus interaction by means of the capillary (Kremer) test and/or the semen/cervical mucus contact test (SCMCT) may suggest the likely presence of sperm antibodies in CM, even though circulating ASA may have been weak or undetectable. The presence of antibodies in CM should be confirmed by testing liquefied CM using the indirect IBT. The presence of high CM antibody levels and associated negative or low titre circulating ASA suggests a good prognosis for treatment of the couple by intrauterine artificial insemination. In contrast, the presence of high antibody concentrations or titres both locally and systemically suggests a poor prognosis. Couples with apparently intractable immunoinfertility can be effectively treated using intra-cyto-plasmic sperm injection (ICSI) [19].

2.6.5
Postfertilization Effects of ASA on Fertility

Definitive studies in various animal models have shown an association between ASA and pre- or postimplantation embryonic degeneration [20]. In one study on rabbits, reproductive tract secretions containing ASA were found to cross-react with rabbit morulae and blastocysts, resulting in embryotoxic effects during in vitro culture [21]. In a number of tightly controlled experiments, this group demonstrated that only secretory IgA (sIgA) from the uterine fluid of semen-immunized does was embryotoxic during in vitro culture. In contrast, blood sera with high levels of ASA were not embryotoxic, nor were IgG fractions isolated from the immune uterine fluid (IUF). Absorption of IUF with either sperm or anti-sIgA removed the embryotoxicity, thereby providing evidence of specificity. Other experiments indicated that the sperm antigen stimulating the sIgA embryotoxic antibody in IUF was distinct from the antigen stimulating IgG and IgA class ASA with the ability to inhibit fertilization. In unpublished observations, absorption of the IUF with paternal lymphocytes did not remove the embryotoxicity, indicating that transplantation antigens were unlikely to be involved. Additional investigations suggested that the antigen responsible for the sIgA-associated embryotoxicity was a sub-surface component. Thus, immunization with isolated sperm membrane fractions resulted in reduced fertilization, whereas immunization with sub-membrane fractions caused only the postfertilization effects on embryos.

Why should ASA react with embryos? Firstly, the sperm membrane is integrated as a mosaic into the zygote membrane during the process of fertilization, so that sperm antigens are incorporated, although at relatively low densities, into the developing embryo [22]. Secondly, embryonic gene expression commencing from the four to eight cell stage results in the synthesis of various developmental antigens which can cross-react with sperm antigens (for review, see [23]). Consequently, during embryo development and perhaps particularly around the time of blastocyst hatching, there is a chance for the ASA to bind to cross-reacting embryonic antigens and potentially cause embryo degeneration or possibly prevent implantation.

There is also some evidence for postfertilization effects associated with ASA in humans. Concerning negative effects, Warren Jones [24] reported that around 50% of pregnancies conceived in women with ASA subsequently ended in first trimester spontaneous miscarriages. Similar observations have been reported by other groups [13, 25]. In the latter study, it was found that 7/16 (44%) of women who miscarried were positive for ASA in their serum, compared with only 2/17 (12%) of women who had successful ongoing pregnancies. Examination of the immunoglobulin classes of the antibodies revealed that IgA was significantly ($p < 0.01$) more common in those women who miscarried. The IgA class antibodies in serum may be a marker for local secretory IgA in the female reproductive tract. However, despite the strong evidence in rabbits, it is not known whether sIgA class ASA in humans are embryotoxic. In another clinical study [26] it was found that of 173 women referred for a history of three or more consecutive spontaneous miscarriages, there was a significantly higher incidence of sperm immobilizing antibodies when compared with the infertile group. Interestingly, they also observed a higher incidence of ASA in the group of women shown to have an immunological basis for their recurrent miscarriages (for example, couples sharing at least three HLA determinants, or couples with the female showing a relatively low response to her partner's lymphocytes in mixed lymphocyte culture). Other groups have reported a significant association between ASA and some auto-antibodies such as antiphospholipids which may be involved in deleterious effects on the fetus. In contrast to the studies cited above which have reported an association between ASA and recurrent miscarriage, others have not seen a statistically significant association [27, 28]. Further investigations in this area would be useful, particularly focusing on the possible involvement of subsurface sperm antigens which react with IgA class ASA. It is important to note that sperm antibodies specific for subsurface antigens are unlikely to be detected by assays such as the IBT and MAR which are designed to measure reactivity with membrane antigens on motile sperm. It could be very informative to conduct a clinical investigation of IVF patients with repeated implantation failure or early spontaneous miscarriages, using a new generation of highly specific ELISA and immunofluorescence assays in conjunction with the IBT or MAR.

With respect to positive effects of sperm immunity, there is some evidence from analysis of IVF data suggesting that some ASA may be associated with increased implantation rates [29, 30]. If confirmed, this could add an interesting new dimension to our analysis and understanding of sperm immunity. It also underlines the potential importance of efforts to develop routine assays which can identify sperm antibodies reacting with defined antigens.

2.6.6
Origins of ASA in Females

It is obvious that normal fertile women do not usually mount strong immune reactions to sperm resulting in high titres of ASA capable of blocking sperm function and reducing fertility. Although it is still uncertain what exact mechanism is acting to suppress the female immune response to sperm antigen after sexual intercourse, there are several possible ways in which this could occur. Firstly, experimental evidence indicates that seminal plasma contains potent immunosuppressive factors. Some sperm antigens may carry suppressor epitopes which could inhibit an effective B-cell response and ensuing sperm antibody production. If the initial immunosuppressive mechanisms fail to prevent the initiation of sperm antibody production, then it is also possible that anti-idiotype antibodies, if produced in sufficient quantities, could inhibit production of the related idiotype (anti-idiotypes are discussed in more detail below). Despite these safeguards, a small proportion of women do develop significant levels of ASA in their blood and reproductive tract.

What information is currently available regarding the development of, or predisposing factors for sperm immunity in females? Observations of potential relevance to understanding the underlying causes of ASA in women include evidence that they are more likely to have detectable sperm antibodies if their male partner also has ASA in his semen [31]. Another important observation was that in about one third of cases women apparently react only to their partner's sperm antigens, rather than to sperm-specific antigens [32]. Several hypotheses have been proposed in order to explain the origins of female sperm immunity and the observed association between male and female sperm immunity in a proportion of couples.

The first hypothesis is based on observations that human spermatozoa have antigens which cross-react immunologically with certain microbial antigens. Thus, Sarkar [33] reported that antibodies with specificity for certain yeast mannan molecular configurations cross-reacted with sperm membrane antigens. For example, 75% of sera from men with ASA were found to react with the 1, 6 yeast mannan specificity. In addition, some patients reacted with the 1, 3 mannan specificity or with chemotype C1 from Salmonella paratyphi C. In another investigation Blum et al. [34] observed a strong association between Chlamydia antibodies and ASA in young women using oral contraceptives.

Similarly, Cunningham et al. [35] reported that 56% of women with primary pelvic inflammatory disease had ASA detectable by the indirect mixed agglutination reaction. Sera from these patients uniformly reacted with a 69 KDa band by Western blotting. Because both partners would be likely to be exposed to the same microbes during unprotected sexual intercourse, they would also be expected to have an increased chance of concurrently developing ASA. In summary, although several clinics have reported significant associations between genital tract infections and ASA [34, 35], a more recent and very thorough study did not confirm such an association [36]. More research in this fascinating area should be encouraged.

A second interesting hypothesis was based on the observation by Steven Witkin [37] that antibody coated sperm stimulated in vitro interferon gamma (IFN-γ) synthesis by lymphocytes from female donors. In contrast, antibody free sperm did not cause IFN-γ production. Given the evidence that IFN-γ induces macrophages to express Ia antigen (MHC class II marker) on the cell surface, the resulting juxtaposition of sperm antigen and Ia on the macrophage cell surface would be expected to facilitate the recruitment of T-helper cells and subsequent initiation of ASA production by B lymphocytes. These observations are consistent with the finding that women are more likely to develop sperm antibodies if their partner has sperm autoimmunity. Although supported by solid experimental data in the original publication by Steven Witkin, this hypothesis should be tested by other laboratories in the light of more recent immunological knowledge.

A third tentative hypothesis has recently been postulated [38] based on the likelihood that if a male had ASA in his semen, then during repeated acts of sexual intercourse his female partner would be expected to develop a range of anti-idiotype antibodies which could potentially facilitate an immune response to his sperm. A summary of the background to this hypothesis is presented below.

Jerne [39] proposed that antibodies should be antigenic to the individual's own immune system, resulting in the production of autoantibodies directed against the unique (idiotypic) parts of the antibody which comprise the antigen binding site. The result is a network of idiotype/anti-idiotype interactions which are involved in regulation and modulation of the immune system. The antigen binding site of the anti-idiotype often mimics the original antigenic structure which was recognized by the individuals' immune system (Fig. 2.6.1). Consequently, immunization against a particular antibody idiotype can provide an effective means of stimulating or at least facilitating an immune response directed towards the original "native" antigen. There have been numerous investigations into the application of anti-idiotypes for generating enhanced immune responses to cancer cells and infectious agents [41].

Several groups have shown that polyclonal heterologous anti-idiotype antibodies can be generated against the idiotypes on monoclonal ASA [42–44], and that the anti-idiotype could significantly inhibit the binding of the monoclonal antibody to sperm. Testing of the anti-idiotype supported the hypothesis that its' ability to inhibit the original monoclonal antibody was due to its antigen binding site forming a similar shape to the original antigenic epitope, the so-called "internal antigen image" [43].

If the male partner had ASA in his semen, how would the female immune system respond to repeated exposure to these antibodies? In light of the above information about idiotype/anti-idiotype responses, it is likely that the female would produce anti-idiotype antibodies which could ultimately potentiate an antisperm immune response. It is also

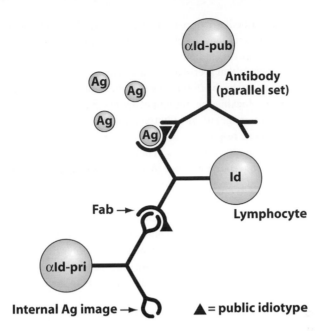

Fig. 2.6.1 The immune response to antigen (Ag) generates antibodies bearing unique idiotypic (Id) signatures comprising the antigen binding site or paratope of the antibody [40]. The individual's immune system subsequently sees the unique Id as foreign and responds by forming anti-Id (α-Id) antibodies, some of which recognize public Ids (Id-pub) present on other antibodies of different Ag specificity, whilst some recognize internal or private (Id-pri) parts of the Fab (internal Ag image). The former may recruit B lymphocytes producing antibodies of various specificities (the parallel set), whilst the latter can potentially augment the production of antibodies reacting with the original Ag

important to note that the female could potentially form anti-idiotype antibodies directed against the male partner's antibodies specific for internal sperm components, in addition to those specific for sperm membrane antigens. The associated "parallel set" of anti-anti-idiotypes could potentially react with some sperm surface epitopes. In other words, it is feasible that the idiotype hypothesis could potentially explain most of the observed range of female ASA activity.

An extremely interesting study by Naz et al. [45] demonstrated the presence of anti-idiotype antibodies in women (albeit against their own antibodies, rather than their partner's, however it provides solid evidence that women can produce anti-idiotype antibodies against sperm antibodies). These authors concluded that both fertile and infertile women form immune responses to sperm, but that sperm antibodies are usually not detected in fertile women because their reactivity in assays is blocked by high levels of anti-idiotype antibodies. They concluded that higher levels and incidence of sperm antibodies are detected in infertile women because their sera contain relatively low concentrations of the blocking anti-idiotype antibodies. However, an alternative explanation of these findings is more consistent with current knowledge about the immune response [40]. Thus, higher levels of anti-idiotype antibodies to a particular antigen lead to active suppression of the host immune response, whereas low levels can lead to a significant stimulation of production of the idiotype (i.e., sperm antibody in this case). Thus, with respect to the study by Naz et al. [45], it is probable that sperm antibodies were not detected in the fertile women because their production had been inhibited by the anti-idiotype antibodies, rather than the anti-idiotype antibodies blocking the binding of sperm antibodies during the assay. Low concentrations (nanogram range) of anti-idiotype antibodies on the other hand can lead to enhancement of the immune response to the original antigen (i.e., sperm in this case). Naz et al. [45] detected anti-idiotype antibodies in only 3/23 infertile women, but the sensitivity of their assay at this concentration range may have been a factor. Further investigation of this phenomenon is vital in order to improve our understanding of female immune reactions to sperm.

With regard to the idiotype hypothesis further research is required to try to understand the relationship between anti-male idiotype antibody which could be generated in women exposed to semen containing ASA, and anti-female anti-idiotype antibody formed when women react to their own sperm antibodies. Another consideration is whether seminal plasma contains anti-idiotype antibody in suitable amounts to have direct effects on the female immune system?

It is quite possible that the development of ASA in some women may involve one or more of the three main postulated mechanisms operating in concert. For example, the stimulation by antibody-coated sperm of IFN-γ gamma synthesis in the female partner's lymphocytes could potentially augment her immunological response to antibody idiotypes in semen. It is also feasible that some women initially respond to microbial antigens (microbes attached to the sperm surface can also stimulate IFN-γ gamma production by the female's lymphoid cells), resulting in the formation of antibodies which cross-react with sperm-this immune response could then be maintained over a longer period by her ongoing exposure and response to antisperm idiotypes in semen and/or generation of anti-idiotype antibodies against her own sperm antibodies. The relationship between the three hypothesized mechanisms requires investigation.

2.6.7
Conclusions

Unfortunately there has been relatively little research interest in female sperm immunity in recent years. Further understanding of the reactivity of the female immune system to semen antigenicity, including experimental investigation of the idiotype hypothesis, may help to explain immuno-infertility, but could also have significant implications for the development of immuno-contraceptive vaccines and for the wider understanding of normal pregnancy and its' associated pathology. Thus, the recognition of the male partner's antibody idiotype spectrum in semen by the female's immune system provides a potentially important means of cross-talk which could prove vital for the establishment of normal pregnancy. It would also be very interesting to explore the possible implications of idiotype responses within the seminal priming hypothesis proposed by Robertson et al. [46].

References

1. Katsh S (1959) Immunology, fertility, and infertility: a historical survey. Am J Obstet Gynecol 77(5):946–956
2. Baskin MJ (1932) Temporary sterilization by the injection of human spermatozoa. Am J Obstet Gynecol 24:892–897
3. Franklin RR, Dukes CD (1964) Further studies on sperm-agglutinating antibody and unexplained infertility. JAMA 190:682–683
4. Bronson RA (1999) Antisperm antibodies: a critical evaluation and clinical guidelines. J Reprod Immunol 45(2):159–183
5. Chamley LW, Clarke GN (2007) Antisperm antibodies and conception. Semin Immunopathol 29(2):169–184
6. Clarke GN (1988) Sperm antibodies and human fertilization. Am J Reprod Immunol Microbiol 17(2):65–71
7. Marshburn PB, Kutteh WH (1994) The role of antisperm antibodies in infertility. Fertil Steril 61(5):799–811
8. Anderson DJ (1996) The importance of mucosal immunology to problems in human reproduction. J Reprod Immunol 31(1-2):3–19
9. Ingerslev HJ, Moller NP, Jager S et al (1982) Immunoglobulin class of sperm antibodies in cervical mucus from infertile women. Am J Reprod Immunol 2(6):296–300
10. Kremer J, Jager S (1992) The significance of antisperm antibodies for sperm-cervical mucus interaction. Hum Reprod 7(6):781–784
11. Cantuaria AA (1977) Sperm immobilizing antibodies in the serum and cervicovaginal secretions of infertile and normal women. Br J Obstet Gynaecol 84(11):865–868
12. Clarke GN, Stojanoff A, Cauchi MN et al (1984) Detection of antispermatozoal antibodies of IgA class in cervical mucus. Am J Reprod Immunol 5(2):61–65
13. Menge AC, Medley NE, Mangione CM et al (1982) The incidence and influence of antisperm antibodies in infertile human couples on sperm-cervical mucus interactions and subsequent fertility. Fertil Steril 38(4):439–446
14. Clarke GN, Lopata A, Johnston WI (1986) Effect of sperm antibodies in females on human in vitro fertilization. Fertil Steril 46(3):435–441
15. Clarke GN, Hyne RV, du Plessis Y et al (1988) Sperm antibodies and human in vitro fertilization. Fertil Steril 49(6):1018–1025
16. de Almeida M, Gazagne I, Jeulin C et al (1989) In-vitro processing of sperm with autoantibodies and in-vitro fertilization results. Hum Reprod 4(1):49–53
17. Ford WC, Williams KM, McLaughlin EA et al (1996) The indirect immunobead test for seminal antisperm antibodies and fertilization rates at in-vitro fertilization. Hum Reprod 11(7):1418–1422
18. Yeh WR, Acosta AA, Seltman HJ et al (1995) Impact of immunoglobulin isotype and sperm surface location of antisperm antibodies on fertilization in vitro in the human. Fertil Steril 63(6):1287 1292
19. Clarke GN, Bourne H, Baker HW (1997) Intracytoplasmic sperm injection for treating infertility associated with sperm autoimmunity. Fertil Steril 68(1):112–117
20. Menge AC (1970) Immune reactions and infertility. J Reprod Fertil Suppl 10:171–186
21. Menge AC, Lieberman ME (1974) Antifertility effects of immunoglobulins from uterine fluids of semen-immunized rabbits. Biol Reprod 10(4):422–428
22. O'Rand MG, Irons GP, Porter JP (1984) Monoclonal antibodies to rabbit sperm autoantigens. I. Inhibition of in vitro fertilization and localization on the egg. Biol Reprod 30(3):721–729
23. Menge AC, Naz RK (1988) Immunologic reactions involving sperm cells and preimplantation embryos. Am J Reprod Immunol Microbiol 18(1):17–20

24. Jones WR (1981) Immunology of infertility. Clin Obstet Gynaecol 8(3):611–639
25. Witkin SS, David SS (1988) Effect of sperm antibodies on pregnancy outcome in a subfertile population. Am J Obstet Gynecol 158(1):59–62
26. Haas GG Jr, Kubota K, Quebbeman JF et al (1986) Circulating antisperm antibodies in recurrently aborting women. Fertil Steril 45(2):209–215
27. Clarke GN, Baker HW (1993) Lack of association between sperm antibodies and recurrent spontaneous abortion. Fertil Steril 59(2):463–464
28. Ingerslev HJ, Ingerslev M (1980) Clinical findings in infertile women with circulating antibodies against spermatozoa. Fertil Steril 33(5):514–520
29. Clarke GN (2006) Association between sperm autoantibodies and enhanced embryo implantation rates during in vitro fertilization. Fertil Steril 86(3):753–754
30. Daitoh T, Kamada M, Yamano S et al (1995) High implantation rate and consequently high pregnancy rate by in vitro fertilization-embryo transfer treatment in infertile women with antisperm antibody. Fertil Steril 63(1):87–91
31. Witkin SS, Chaudhry A (1989) Relationship between circulating antisperm antibodies in women and autoantibodies on the ejaculated sperm of their partners. Am J Obstet Gynecol 161(4):900–903
32. Witkin SS, Vogel-Roccuzzo R, David SS et al (1988) Heterogeneity of antigenic determinants on human spermatozoa: relevance to antisperm antibody testing in infertile couples. Am J Obstet Gynecol 159(5):1228–1231
33. Sarkar S (1974) Carbohydrate antigens of human sperm and autoimmune induction of infertility. J Reprod Med 13(3):93–99
34. Blum M, Pery J, Blum I (1989) Antisperm antibodies in young oral contraceptive users. Adv Contracept 5(1):41–46
35. Cunningham DS, Fulgham DL, Rayl DL et al (1991) Antisperm antibodies to sperm surface antigens in women with genital tract infection. Am J Obstet Gynecol 164(3):791–796
36. Eggert-Kruse W, Rohr G, Probst S et al (1998) Antisperm antibodies and microorganisms in genital secretions–a clinically significant relationship? Andrologia 30(Suppl 1):61–71
37. Witkin SS (1988) Production of interferon gamma by lymphocytes exposed to antibody-coated spermatozoa: a mechanism for sperm antibody production in females. Fertil Steril 50(3): 498–502
38. Clarke GN (2009) Etiology of sperm immunity in women. Fertil Steril 91(2):639–643
39. Jerne NK (1974) Towards a network theory of the immune system. Ann Immunol (Paris) 125C(1-2):373–389
40. Delves PJ, Martin SJ, Burton DR, Roitt IM (2006) Roitt's essential immunology. Blackwell, Oxford
41. Monroe JG, Greene MI (1986) Anti-idiotypic antibodies and disease. Immunol Invest 15(3): 263–286
42. Carron CP, Jarvis HW, Saling PM (1988) Characterization of antibodies to idiotypic determinants of monoclonal anti-sperm antibodies. Biol Reprod 38(5):1093–1103
43. Carron CP, Mathias A, Saling PM (1989) Anti-idiotype antibodies prevent antibody binding to mouse sperm and antibody-mediated inhibition of fertilization. Biol Reprod 41(1):153–162
44. Kuo CY, Sun P, Lee CY (1988) Sperm antibodies induced by anti-idiotype antibodies: a strategy in development of immunocontraceptive vaccines. J Reprod Immunol 13(3):193–209
45. Naz RK, Ahmad K, Menge AC (1993) Antiidiotypic antibodies to sperm in sera of fertile women that neutralize antisperm antibodies. J Clin Invest 92(5):2331–2338
46. Robertson SA, Bromfield JJ, Tremellen KP (2003) Seminal 'priming' for protection from preeclampsia-a unifying hypothesis. J Reprod Immunol 59(2):253–265

Sperm–Immobilizing Antibody and Its Target Antigen (CD52)

2.7

Akiko Hasegawa and Koji Koyama

2.7.1
Introduction

Antisperm antibodies detected by sperm immobilization tests are present exclusively in unexplained infertile women [1, 2]. When sperm-immobilizing antibodies (SI-Abs) are present in the serum, they are also found in the peritoneal fluid, follicular fluid, and cervical mucus. Patients with a high titer of SI-Abs are found to have difficulty to conceive a child [3, 4]. We have reported that SI-Abs impair passage of sperm in female reproductive tracts (frt) from the cervix through the fallopian tubes and also block binding of sperm to the zona pellucida [5, 6]. Although previous studies have shown that carbohydrate moieties of sperm and seminal plasma are major target antigens for SI-Abs [7, 8], the identification of antigenic epitopes has been difficult due to heterogeneity of SI-Abs in patients. Elucidation of the epitopes recognized by SI-Abs is important not only for understanding the mechanism of immunological infertility but also for developing a means of treatment for infertility resulting from SI-Abs.

2.7.2
Characterization of Sperm-Immobilizing Monoclonal Antibodies

For characterization of antigen epitopes for SI-Abs, a number of human and mouse monoclonal antibodies with complement-dependent sperm-immobilizing activity were generated in our laboratory [9–11]. A human monoclonal antibody, Mab H6–3C4, with a high titer of SI activity was established using peripheral B-lymphocytes from an infertile woman [12]. A mouse monoclonal antibody, 1G12, reactive to human sperm membrane also showed a high titer of SI activity [13]. Another mouse monoclonal antibody, S19, generated by Herr's

A. Hasegawa (✉)
Laboratory of Developmental Biology and Reproduction, Advanced Medical Sciences, Hyogo College of Medicine, Nishinomiya, Japan
e-mail: zonapel@hyo-med.ac.jp

W. K. H. Krause and R. K. Naz (eds.), *Immune Infertility*,
DOI: 10.1007/978-3-642-01379-9_2.7, © Springer Verlag Berlin Heidelberg 2009

Table 2.7.1 Characteristic properties of antibodies recognizing CD52

Name	Species	Ig class	Sperm immobilization	Sperm agglutination	Immunogen	Reactivity
MAb H6–3C4	Human	IgM	++	++	Unknown	mrt
1G12	Mouse	IgM	++	++	Sperm membrane	mrt Lymphocytes
Campath-1	Rat	IgM	++	++	Spleen cells	mrt Lymphocytes
Anti-CD52	Rabbit	Poly-clone	+	±	Synthetic peptide of CD52 core	mrt lymphocytes

mrt male reproductive tracts

group, showed strong sperm agglutinating and SI activities, and the corresponding antigen was termed as SAGA-1 (sperm agglutination antigen-1) [14]. Campath-1 is a rat monoclonal antibody defining CD52 as an antigen [15]. It was established against human spleen cells and reacted with virtually all leucocytes. Subsequent studies showed that campath-1 was cross-reactive to mature human sperm [16] with sperm agglutinating and immobilizing activities similar to monoclonal antibodies generated by sperm antigens. The characteristic properties of the monoclonal antibodies are summarized in Table 2.7.1.

Tandem mass spectrometric analysis shows that there are distinct differences in the N-linked carbohydrates between lymphocyte-CD52 and mrt-CD52 [17, 18]. Both lymphocyte- and mrt-CD52 are glycosylphosphatidylinositol (GPI) anchor glycoproteins and the molecular conformation, formed by three C-terminal amino acids and the GPI anchor, is recognized by campath-1 [19]. The observation that Mab H6–3C4 indentifies exclusively with sperm suggests that this monoclonal antibody reacts with a sperm-specific antigen present in a carbohydrate moiety [20]. Another monoclonal antibody, 1G12, reacts with sperm and also with lymphocytes [13].

Figure 2.7.1 shows indirect immunofluorescent stainings of human sperm and lymphocytes with Mab H6–3C4 and campath-1. Both monoclonal antibodies stain the whole sperm surface but lymphocytes are stained with campath-1 only. It appears that the antigens recognized by these monoclonal antibodies are similarly distributed on the sperm surface. Mab H6–3C4 did not react with lymphocytes and exclusively recognizes mrt-specific antigen while campath-1 recognizes a core structure of CD52 shared by lymphocytes and mrt.

For detailed analysis of the epitopes, sperm extracts were subjected to high-resolution two-dimensional polyacrylamide gel electrophoresis with the first dimension in a pH 2–4 range and the second dimension in molecular sieving followed by Western blot analysis [20]. As positive control, anti-CD52 antibody produced to a core peptide comprising 12 amino acids was used. For carbohydrate analysis, mrt-CD52 extracted from sperm was treated with *N*-glycosidase F to remove the N-linked carbohydrate. The presence of O-linked carbohydrates was examined by mild alkaline treatment. Figure 2.7.2 shows that anti-CD52 peptide antibody reacts with intact mrt-CD52 molecules showing a heterogeneous staining pattern of PI<2.8 and MW 15–25 K (Fig. 2.7.2a). This heterogeneity is markedly reduced by deglycosylation of N-linked carbohydrate (Fig. 2.7.2e). Additional removal of O-linked carbohydrates results in staining of a single spot (Fig. 2.7.2i), suggesting that the O-linked carbohydrate contributes to molecular polymorphism of mrt-C52.

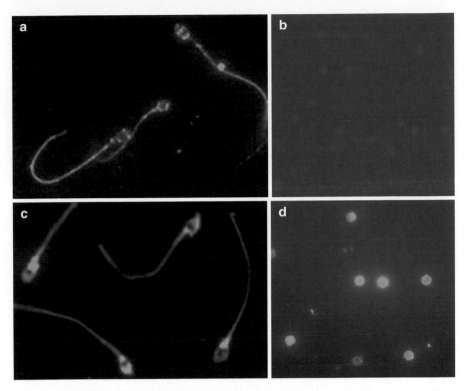

Fig. 2.7.1 Immunofluorescent stainings of formalin-fixed human sperm with monoclonal antibodies. Mab II6–3C4 reacts exclusively with sperm (**a**) but not with lymphocytes (**b**), while campath-1 recognizes the lymphocytes (**d**) as well as sperm (**c**)

Recently, the existence of the O-linked carbohydrate in mrt-CD52 has been demonstrated by lectin-binding assay [21] and MALDI-TOF mass spectrometry [22]. Monoclonal antibodies, Mab H6–3C4, 1G12, and campath-1, show similar polymorphic staining pattern in the region of PI<2.8 and MW 15–25 K (Fig. 2.7.2b–d). The patterns of staining change after removal of the N-linked carbohydrate. In the case of Mab H6–3C4, no staining is observed after the removal of the N-linked carbohydrate (Fig. 2.7.2f). In the case of 1G12 and campath-1, heterogeneity is reduced but still several spots remained. 1G12 shows with six spots at different pH, while campath-1 reacted with three spots, suggesting that the epitope for 1G12 is not identical to that for campath-1 (Fig. 2.7.2g, h). These results show that Mab H6–3C4 recognizes the N-linked carbohydrate moiety of mrt-CD52, while 1G12 and campath-1 recognize the core portion of mrt-CD52. After further removal of the O-linked carbohydrate, 1G12 and campath-1 yield single spots like the positive control (Fig. 2.7.2k, l). Collectively, these results confirm that Mab H6–3C4 and 1G12 recognize mrt-CD52 but the epitopes are different. The epitope for Mab H6–3C4 is present in the N-linked carbohydrate, while the epitope for 1G12 is present in the core portion of CD52. These results indicate that SI-Abs in some infertile women are produced against mrt-specific carbohydrate antigens in the mrt-CD52 molecule. Indeed, it has been reported that mrt-CD52 contains specific carbohydrate chains [17].

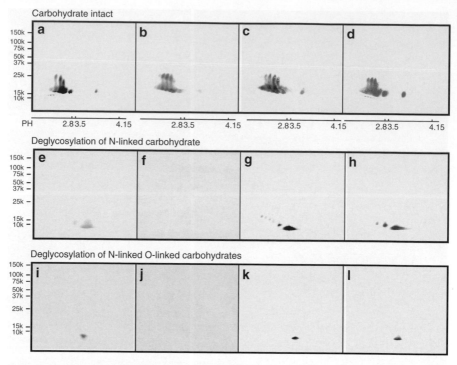

Fig. 2.7.2 Two-dimensional PAGE and Western blot analysis of sperm extracts with monoclonal antibodies before and after the treatment with deglycosylation. The sperm extracts were separated by two-dimensional PAGE, blotted onto a Polyvinylidene Fluoride membrane and probed with antibodies. (**a–d**) Intact mrt-CD52; (**e–h**) N-linked carbohydrate–deglycosylated mrt-CD52; (**i–l**) N- and O-linked carbohydrate–deglycosylated mrt-CD52. (**a, e, i**) anti-peptide antibody (positive control); (**b, f, j**) Mab H6–3C4; (**c, g, k**) 1G12; (**d, h, l**) Campath-1

2.7.3
Hypothetical Structure of CD52

On the basis of biochemical and immunological analyses, a hypothetical structure of mrt-CD52 is presented in Fig. 2.7.3. The core peptide of CD52 is composed of just 12 amino acids, common to lymphocytes and mrt. This suggests that the peptide portion is a scaffold for supporting carbohydrate moieties. The core peptide contains ^{3}Asn(N)^{4}Asp(X)^{5}Thr(T), a consensus sequence, for N-linked carbohydrate binding. It has been reported that mrt-CD52 is heavily glycosylated with heterogeneous carbohydrate chains comprising more than 50 different glycoforms which are almost completely sialylated and fucosylated in 10–15% of total mrt-CD52 [17]. In contrast, the carbohydrate moieties in lymphocyte CD52 are much smaller and only lightly sialylated but not fucosylated [18]. Another distinct structure of the mrt-CD52 carbohydrate is [GlcNAcβ1–6Man] in the N-linked carbohydrate chain. The presence of the β1–6 bond possibly allows branching of a carbohydrate

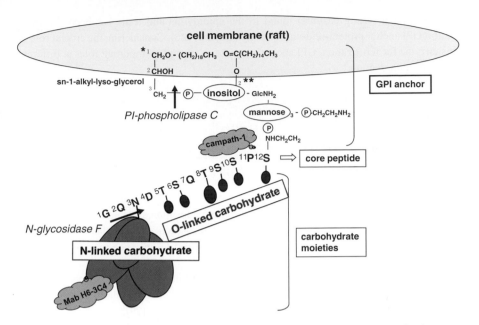

Fig. 2.7.3 Hypothetical structure of male reproductive tract CD52. The male reproductive tract CD52 molecule is composed of 12 amino acid residues, N-linked and O-linked carbohydrates, and a GPI anchor portion inserted in the plasma membrane. The amino acid sequence of core peptide is shown in capitals. Carbohydrate chains are shown by ovals

chain to the backbone. The carbohydrate branching via this bond has been reported to contribute to the metastatic potential of tumor [23].

The GPI anchor portion, consisting of glucerolipid, inositol and mannose, is bound to Ser residue at the carboxyl terminal through ethanolamine. Approximately 80% of the inositol residue are acylated (mainly palmitoylate) at the 2-position as shown by ** in Fig. 2.7.3. The low susceptibility of mrt-CD52 to phospholipase C may be due to this acyl group anchoring into the cell membrane because this anchoring is known to be refractory to phospholipase C. Another structural difference of lymphocyte CD52 is that the glycerolipid portion of mrt-CD52 is a sn-1-alkyl-lyso-glycerol type (single-footed) in which only one fatty acid chain at the 1-position is linked as shown by * in Fig. 2.7.3. The 1-alkyl structure is reported to be synthesized by sperm as a 1-alkyl-2-acetyl-sn-glycero-3-phosphocholine but monoalkyl structure has not been documented in mammalian species. Phospholipase A_2, which is detected abundantly in seminal plasma, removes the acylation at the 2-position, although inhibitory factors are also detected in the seminal plasma. The lyso- (single-footed) glycerolipid anchor may play an important role in the transportation of this molecule to sperm from the epithelium in the cauda epididymis or from seminal plasma.

mrt-CD52 has been reported to be transferred easily from epithelial cells to mature sperm in the epididymis [24]. Epididymosome, exosome from epithelial cells, may be a possible transporter of mrt-CD52 as reported by Sullivan et al. [25]. More recently, ACE (angioteisin-converting enzyme) found in the epididymis and testis has been shown to exhibit GPI anchor protein-releasing activity (GPIase) [26]. Considering the crucial role of this enzyme for fertilization, GPI anchoring proteins may play important roles at different stages of reproduction.

2.7.4
Biological Function of CD52

CD52 is a GPI anchor glycoprotein present in lymphocytes and male reproductive tissues including mature sperm and seminal plasma. It has been reported that CD52 on the lymphocyte surface induces regulatory T cells with immunosuppressive activities [27], while soluble mrt-CD52 from epididymis induces clot formation and liquefaction of human semen [28]. However, the biological significance of mrt-CD52 anchoring to the sperm membrane is not well understood.

Not only the N-linked carbohydrate, but also the O-linked carbohydrate, possibly contributes to the heterogeneous negative charge of mrt-CD52. These molecules may prevent sperm from autoagglutination and nonspecific tissue adherence [29].

Considering that the monoclonal antibodies targeted to mrt-CD52, Mab H6–3C4, campath-1, and 1G12 exhibit strong complement-dependent sperm-immobilizing activities, it is speculated that CD52 possesses a function to suppress complement activity. Campath-1 has also been shown to induce strong complement-dependent cytolysis of lymphocytes [30]. The female genital tracts are subject to frequent infection with various pathogens including sexually transmitted bacteria and viruses. However, its antibody-producing ability is not so strong compared to other mucosal tissues [31]. Innate immunological systems including complement activation are thought to play a major role in the host defense. Functionally active complement has been shown to be present in the female genital tract [32] and follicular fluid [33].

Complement-regulatory proteins such as C1-INH, CD55, CD46, and CD59 are present in spermatozoa and seminal plasma [34–36], and CD55 and CD59 have been shown to serve as GPI anchor proteins like CD52. CD55 and CD59 protect the cells expressing these molecules from complement-dependent cytotoxicity. CD55 is known to be a dacay-accelerating factor that inhibits C3/C5 convertase formation and CD59 inhibits MAC (membrane attack complex) formation in the final stage of the complement pathway. These molecules are suggested to protect sperm from complement-dependent cytotoxicity.

Recently, Kinoshita et al. have reported an interesting clinical observation that a clonally acquired disorder in PNH (paroxysmal nocturnal hemoglobinuria) leads to intravascular hemolysis due to the defect in the synthesis of GPI anchors such as CD55 and CD59 [37]. Campath-1H, humanized anti-CD52 antibody cross-reactive to CD55 and CD59 GPI anchors, has extensively been used clinically for the elimination of T-cells from bone marrow to prevent graft-versus-host disease. It has also been reported that patients treated with campath-1H develop PNH-like symptoms with hemolysis and thrombosis [38]. These patients show increased numbers of cells deficient in CD55 and CD59. The reactivity of campath-1H with GPI anchor induces a lack of CD55 and CD59 and causes PNH-like disease. These results suggest that CD52, like CD55 and CD59, has a role in complement regulation. In hemolytic assay of sensitized erythrocytes, the addition of purified mrt-CD52 significantly reduces hemolytic activity (CH50) by complement and this inhibitory effect of mrt-CD52 is neutralized by the addition of anti-CD52 antibody to the reaction mixture. These results indicate that mrt-CD52 regulates the complement system. In complement pathway analysis [39], purified mrt-CD52 interfered with the classical pathway but not with the lectin-binding and alternative pathways.

2.7.5
Animal Studies on CD52

As shown in Fig. 2.7.4, the amino acid sequence of mature peptides of CD52 in human and four animal species are quite different but signal peptide region and GPI anchoring signal are conserved in these species [29]. Mouse mrt-CD52 has Asn(N)-linked and Thr/Ser(O)-linked carbohydrates bound to the core peptide [40] but Mab H6–3C4 did not react to mouse mrt-CD52. Mouse CD52, like human CD52, is present in lymphocytes and male reproductive tissues. Immunohistochemical studies show that mouse CD52 is localized in the epididymis and vas deferens but not in testis, liver, or kidney [40]. In our study, the testis was not stained with rabbit antiserum produced to mouse CD52 core peptide

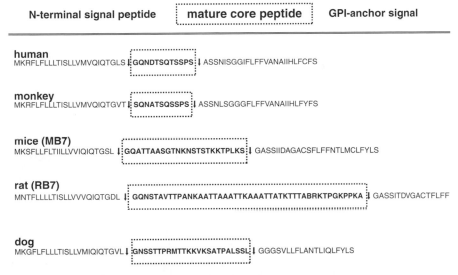

Fig. 2.7.4 Alignment of deduced amino acid sequences of CD52 of various animals. CD52 molecules are highly conserved among the five species analyzed in the signal peptide and GPI-addition signal, mature CD52 peptide sequences show low similarity except for the putative N-glycosylation site (NXT) and proline near the COOH-terminus. The potential sites of Ser/Thr (O)-linked carbohydrate moieties are conserved. Dash means no corresponding amino acid residue

but the epididymis, especially corpus and cauda, and vas deferens were strongly stained (Fig. 2.7.5c). The result of quantitative analysis of CD52 mRNA is compatible with immu-nohistochemical data shown in Fig. 2.7.5b. CD52 mRNA is not detected in the testis but detected in the epididymis and vas deferens in large amounts.

Immunization with mrt-CD52 purified from vas deferens sperm produced auto and iso-antibodies in the male and female mice, respectively. The raised antibodies showed a strong complement-dependent sperm-immobilizing activity. These results indicated that mouse CD52 has biochemical and immunological properties similar to those of human CD52. However, immunized female animals did not develop infertility, although the anti-bodies exhibited the complement-dependent sperm-immobilizing activity. This may reflect differences in physiological and reproductive systems between the two species. For instance, it has been reported that mouse mrt-CD52 is detected in only 30% of mature sperm [41], whereas human mrt-CD52 is detected in 80% of ejaculated sperm [42]. In addition, CD52-knockout male mice have been reported to show no impairment of fertility [41]. It is possible that ejaculated mouse sperm may be protected by vaginal plug that forms after coitus so that excessive expression of CD52 on the sperm unnecessary.

However, when CD52-knockout female mice were mated with CD52-knockout male mice, the number of offspring is significantly reduced. This suggests that CD52 is present in frt as well as in mrt. In fact, we found that frt-CD52 is expressed in cumulus cells in mice and humans. Mouse frt-CD52 is detected in cumulus cells and intercellular matrix, but not in oocytes, and its amount was significantly increased after ovulation [43, 44]. CD52 is also

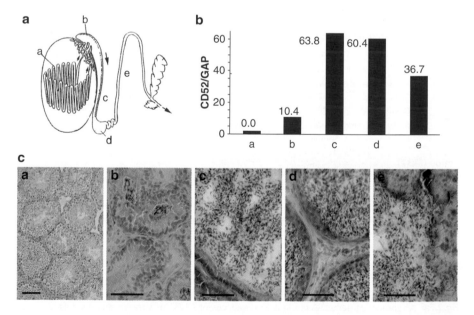

Fig. 2.7.5 Localization of CD52 in male reproductive tracts (mrt). (**a**) Schematic drawing of mrt. (**b**) Levels of CD52 mRNA in mrt analyzed by real-time Polymerase Chain Reaction. (**c**) Immunohistochemical staining of mrt with rabbit antiserum to mouse CD52 core peptide. (**a**) Testis; (**b**) caput epididymis; (**c**) corpus epididymis; (**d**) cauda epididymis; (**e**) vas deferens

detected in the endometium and significantly increased after nidation of embryos. These results suggest that frt-CD52 protects not only sperm but also embryos from cytotoxic effects of complement activation. Further studies are necessary to determine the molecular features of frt-CD52 and biological functions of mrt- and frt-CD52 in reproduction.

References

1. Isojima S, Li TS, Ashitaka Y (1968) Immunological analysis of sperm immobilizing factor found in sera of women with unexplained sterility. Am J Obstet Gynecol 101:677–683
2. Isojima S, Tsuchiya K, Koyama K et al (1972) Further studies on sperm-immobilizing antibody found in sera of unexplained cases of sterility in women. Am J Obstet Gynecol 112:199–207
3. Kobayashi S, Bessho T, Shigeta M et al (1990) Correlation between quantitative antibody titers of sperm immobilizing antibodies and pregnancy rates by treatments. Fertil Steril 54:1107–1113
4. Koyama K, Kubota K, Ikuma K et al (1988) Application of the quantitative sperm immobilization test for follow-up study of sperm-immobilizing antibody in the sera of sterile women. Int J Fertil 33:201–206
5. Menge AC, Medley NE, Mangione CM et al (1982) The incidence and influence of antisperm antibodies in infertile human couples on sperm-cervical mucus interactions and subsequent fertility. Fertil Steril 38:439–446
6. Shibahara H, Shigeta M, Toji H et al (1995) Sperm immobilizing antibodies interfere with sperm migration from the uterine cavity through the fallopian tubes. J Reprod Immunol 34:120–124
7. Koyama K, Kameda K, Nakamura N et al (1991) Recognition of carbohydrate antigen epitopes by sperm-immobilizing antibodies in sera of infertile women. Fertil Steril 56:954–959
8. Kurpisz M, Alexander NJ (1995) Carbohydrate moieties on sperm surface: physiological relevance. Fertil Steril 63:158–165
9. Kameda K, Tsuji Y, Koyama K et al (1992) Comparative studies of the antigens recognized by sperm-immobilizing monoclonal antibodies. Biol Reprod 46:349–357
10. Kyurkchiev SD, Shigeta M, Koyama K et al (1986) A human-mouse hybridoma producing monoclonal antibody against human sperm coating antigen. Immunology 57:489–492
11. Shigeta M, Watanabe T, Maruyama S et al (1980) Sperm-immobilizing monoclonal antibody to human seminal plasma antigens. Clin Exp Immunol 42:458–462
12. Isojima S, Kameda K, Tsuji Y et al (1987) Establishment and characterization of a human hybridoma secreting monoclonal antibody with high titers of sperm immobilizing and agglutinating activities against human seminal plasma. J Reprod Immunol 10:67–78
13. Komori S, Kameda K, Sakata K et al (1997) Characterization of fertilization-blocking monoclonal antibody 1G12 with human sperm-immobilizing activity. Clin Exp Immunol 109:547–554
14. Diekman AB, Norton EJ, Klotz KL et al (1999) N-linked glycan of a sperm CD52 glycoform associated with human infertility. FASEB J 13:1303–1313
15. Hale G, Xia MQ, Tighe HP et al (1990) The CAMPATH-1 antigen (CDw52). Tissue Antigens 35:118–127
16. Hale G, Rye PD, Warford A et al (1993) The glycosylphosphatidylinositol-anchored lymphocyte antigen CDw52 is associated with the maturation of human spermatozoa. J Reprod Immunol 23:189–205
17. Schröter S, Derr P, Conradt HS et al (1999) Male-specific modification of human CD52. J Biol Chem 274:29862–29873

18. Treumann A, Lifely R, Schneider P (1995) Primary structure of CD52. J Biol Chem 270: 6088–6099
19. Hale G (1995) Synthetic peptide mimotope of the CAMPATH-1 (CD52) antigen, a small glycosylphosphatidylinositol-anchored glycoprotein. Immunotechnology 1:175–187
20. Hasegawa A, Fu Y, Tsubamoto H et al (2003) Epitope analysis for human sperm-immobilizing monoclonal antibodies, MAb H6–3C4, 1G12 and campath-1. Mol Hum Reprod 9:337–343
21. Hasegawa A, Sawai H, Tsubamoto H et al (2004) Possible presence of O-linked carbohydrate in the human male reproductive tract CD52. J Reprod Immunol 62:91–100
22. Parry S, Wong NK, Easton RL et al (2007) The sperm agglutination antigen-1 (SAGA-1) glycoforms of CD52 are O-glycosylated. Glycobiology 17:1120–1126
23. Dennis J, Laferte S, Waghorne C et al (1987) Beta 1–6 branching of Asn-linked oligosaccharides is directly associated with metastasis. Science 236:582–585
24. Kirchhoff C, Hale G (1996) Cell-to-cell transfer of glycosylphosphatidylinositol-anchored membrane proteins during sperm maturation. Mol Hum Reprod 2:177–184
25. Sullivan R, Frenette G, Girouard J (2007) Epididymosomes are involved in the acquisition of new sperm proteins during epididymal transit. Asian J Androl 9:483–491
26. Kondoh G, Toji H, Nakatani Y et al (2005) Angiotensin-converting enzyme is a GPI-anchored protein releasing factor crucial for fertilization. Nat Med 11:160–166
27. Watanabe T, Masuyama J, Sohma Y et al (2006) CD52 is a novel costimulatory molecule for induction of CD4+ regulatory T cells. Clin Immunol 120:247–259
28. Flori F, Ermini L, La Sala GB et al (2008) The GPI-anchored CD52 antigen of the sperm surface interacts with semenogelin and participates in clot formation and liquefaction of human semen. Mol Reprod Dev 75:326–335
29. Kirchhoff C, Schröter S (2001) New insights into the origin, structure and role of CD52: a major component of the mammalian sperm glycocalyx. Cells Tissues Organs 168:93–104
30. Xia MQ, Hale G, Lifely MR et al (1993) Structure of the CAMPATH-1 antigen, a glycosylphosphatidylinositol-anchored glycoprotein which is an exceptionally good target for complement lysis. Biochem J 293:633–640
31. Wu HY, Abdu S, Stinson D et al (2000) Generation of female genital tract antibody responses by local or central (common) mucosal immunization. Infect Immun 68:5539–5545
32. Price RJ, Boettcher B (1979) The presence of complement in human cervical mucus and its possible relevance to infertility in women with complement-dependent sperm-immobilizing antibodies. Fertil Steril 32:61–66
33. Perricone R, Pasetto N, De Carolis C et al (1992) Functionally active complement is present in human ovarian follicular fluid and can be activated by seminal plasma. Clin Exp Immunol 89:154–157
34. Cummerson JA, Flanagan BF, Spiller DG et al (2006) The complement regulatory proteins CD55 (decay accelerating factor) and CD59 are expressed on the inner acrosomal membrane of human spermatozoa as well as CD46 (membrane cofactor protein). Immunology 118:333–342
35. Jiang H, Pillai S (1998) Complement regulatory proteins on the sperm surface: relevance to sperm motility. Am J Reprod Immunol 39:243–248
36. Rooney IA, Heuser JE, Atkinson JP (1996) GPI-anchored complement regulatory proteins in seminal plasma. An analysis of their physical condition and the mechanisms of their binding to exogenous cells. J Clin Invest 1:1675–1686
37. Kinoshita T, Inoue N, Takeda J (1995) Defective glycosyl phosphatidylinositol anchor synthesis and paroxysmal nocturnal hemoglobinuria. Adv Immunol 60:57–103
38. Ruiz P, Weppler D, Tryphonopoulos P et al (2006) CD55 and CD59 deficiency in transplant patient populations: possible association with paroxysmal nocturnal hemoglobinuria-like symptoms in Campath-treated patients. Transplant Proc 38:1750–1752
39. Walport M (2001) Complement. N Engl J Med 344(1058–1066):1140–1144

40. Ito K, Hasegawa A, Komori S et al (2007) Biochemical property and immunogenicity of mouse male reproductive tract CD52 (mrt-CD52). J Reprod Immunol 75:32–39

41. Yamaguchi R, Yamagata K, Hasuwa H et al (2008) Cd52, known as a major maturation-associated sperm membrane antigen secreted from the epididymis, is not required for fertilization in the mouse. Genes Cells 13:851–861

42. Yeung CH, Cooper TG, Nieschlag E (1997) Human epididymal secreted protein CD52 on ejaculated spermatozoa: correlations with semen characteristics and the effect of its antibody. Mol Hum Reprod 3:1045–1051

43. Hasegawa A, Takenobu T, Kasumi H et al (2008) CD52 is synthesized in cumulus cells and secreted into the cumulus matrix during ovulation. Am J Reprod Immunol 60:187–191

44. Hernandez-Gonzalez I, Gonzalez-Robayna I, Shimada M et al (2006) Gene expression profiles of cumulus cell oocyte complexes during ovulation reveal cumulus cells express neuronal and immune-related genes: does this expand their role in the ovulation process? Mol Endocrinol 20:1300–1321

Section III

The Clinical Impact of Sperm Antibodies

Male Autoimmune Infertility

3.1

Felice Francavilla and Arcangelo Barbonetti

3.1.1
Introduction: Does Antisperm-Antibodies-Related Infertility Really Exist?

An etiological link between naturally occurring ASA and male infertility has been claimed since Rumke [1] and Wilson [2] reported the presence of serum sperm-agglutinating activity (SAA) in some infertile men, in 1954. However, although the clinical significance of ASA has been extensively investigated, it is still a matter for debate. While, on one hand, any link between sperm antibody presence and impaired conception has been considered hypothetical [3] and the routine use of current ASA testing has been questioned as an essential procedure in the fertility work-up, because any treatment on the basis of such tests would not be justified [4], on the other hand, intracytoplasmatic sperm injection (ICSI) has been claimed as the primary choice of treatment in the presence of sperm autoimmunization [5].

Different approaches used for the recognition of the ASA-related infertility and the lack of prospective studies on the occurrence of spontaneous pregnancies and well-designed and controlled studies on treatment's effectiveness have strongly contributed to the confusion on the clinical significance of ASA. Furthermore, although substantial evidence has been provided that ASA can affect sperm fertilizing ability at various levels, it is still hard to establish in each individual patient, whether, or to what extent, these interfering effects occur. The major reason is the inability of current diagnostic tests in quantifying the antibody density on the sperm surface and defining the antigenic specificities of ASA, main determinants of their antifertility effect.

This chapter critically reviews current understanding of the clinical relevance of naturally occurring ASA in men.

F. Francavilla (✉)
Department of Internal Medicine, Andrologic Unit, University of L'Aquila, Coppito, 67100, L'Aquila, Italy
e-mail: francavi@cc.univaq.it

W. K. H. Krause and R. K. Naz (eds.), *Immune Infertility*,
DOI: 10.1007/978-3-642-01379-9_3.1, © Springer Verlag Berlin Heidelberg 2009

3.1.2
Prevalence of Antisperm Antibodies

A variable prevalence of ASA has been reported depending on the specificity and sensitivity of the test used for their detection and on the screened population. The first assays to be utilized were indirect tests detecting biological activities of ASA in serum and seminal plasma, i.e., sperm agglutination techniques and complement-dependent sperm-immobilization/cytotoxicity techniques. Subsequently, widespread acceptance has been gained for antiglobulins-based tests, used to detect antibodies coated to the surface of ejaculated spermatozoa, including the mixed antiglobulin reaction (MAR) test and the immunobead binding test (IBT). They reveal the percentage of antibody-coated spermatozoa, the Ig-isotype, and grossly the regional specificity of ASA. Multicentric comparative studies [6, 7] have shown that all these tests determine in large measure the same antibody specificities for surface antigens, but with different sensitivity, which is lower for complement-dependent sperm-immobilization/cytotoxicity techniques.

In epidemiologic studies, serum SAA ranged from 8.1 to 30.3% in unselected men with infertile marriages [8–11], but at low titers it was also reported up to 10% of control sera [10]. When stricter criteria were used (i.e., the occurrence of sperm-immobilizing activity in addition to high titers of SAA in the serum and/or SAA in seminal plasma, indicating an excess of free antibodies in the semen), the prevalence of ASA in men with infertile marriages ranged from 4.6 to 5.7% [9, 12]. Direct tests (MAR or IBT) gave positive results (>10 or >20%) in 7.6–12.9% of unselected infertile patients [9, 12–14], but highly positive results (≥50%) were restricted to 5–6% of patients [9, 13, 14].

Although a higher prevalence of ASA has been reported in some clinical conditions, mainly acquired genital tract obstructions and genitourinary infections, especially by Chlamydia trachomatis (see Chap. 2.4), only for vasectomy the association is well established with a prevalence of ASA ranging from 33 to 74% [15–18], and with their persistence in 38–60% following successful vasovasostomy [15, 18].

3.1.3
Prognostic Studies

Although suggested by epidemiologic studies, the proof of a causal link between ASA and fertility impairment could only be produced by prospective studies comparing the occurrence of natural pregnancies in patients with and without ASA. But the feasibility of these studies is hindered by the following: (1) the low incidence of sperm autoimmunization in unselected infertile couples requires multicentric studies including a large number of patients and a large number of observed cycles; (2) the inter-individual variability of semen parameters, not related to the presence of ASA, makes it very difficult to obtain a study- and a control-population, homogeneous for semen quality. Owing to these limitations, little information along with conflicting results has been produced by prospective studies comparing ASA-positive and ASA-negative patients [8, 19, 20].

However, what is worth noting is that in retrospective studies, when the degree of sperm autoimmunization was taken into account, it exhibited a significant inverse correlation with the incidence of spontaneous pregnancies. In an old report by Rumke et al. [21], during a 10-year follow-up of 254 infertile men with serum SAA, the titer of SAA was inversely correlated with the occurrence of spontaneous pregnancies. Notably, restricting the analysis to normozoospermic men, no pregnancy was observed with very high titer of serum SAA ($\geq$1:1,024), a low (15.8%) pregnancy rate (PR) with titers ranging from 1:32 to 1:512 and a high PR (48.4%) with titers <1:32. Ayvaliotis et al. [22] reported that in 108 infertile couples where the male exhibited a direct IBT >10%, and the female was treated for other factors leading to impaired reproduction, PR was significantly higher when IBT was <50% than when it was >50% (43.4 vs. 21.8%) during a follow-up after at least 18 months. The difference in PR was ever of greater significance in a subgroup of 35 couples, where no other cause of infertility was found (15.3 vs. 66.7%). Abshagen et al. [23] reported that in 157 infertile couples with a direct IBT >10%, cumulative spontaneous PR over 6 years was high (~50%) when IBT was <50%, low (~30%) when IBT was 50–90%, and very low (~15%) when IBT was >90%, independent from the IgG-class (IgG and/or IgA). A significant inverse correlation between the degree of sperm autoimmunization and PR was also found in a follow-up study of 216 men after vasovasostomy by Meinertz et al. [24]. While no pregnancy was observed in a median period of ~4 years in men where all spermatozoa were antibody-coated at MAR test, in association with a high titer of serum SAA, pregnancy occurred in 64.3% of couples with a less degree of spermautoimmunization. While in this study only a prevalent IgA autoimmunization was associated to a reduced fertility, a major role of IgA was not found in another study on vasovasostomized men by Matson et al. [18].

Altogether, the analysis of epidemiologic and prognostic studies indicates that ASA are a relative, rather than absolute, cause of infertility. The degree of fertility impairment appears to be related to the extent of sperm autoimmunization.

3.1.4
Mechanisms of Fertility Impairment by Antisperm Antibodies: Clinical Relevance

Only ASA directed toward surface antigens have a physiopathological and clinical significance in the male immunological infertility, because subsuperficial antigens cannot be exposed to antibodies by living cells along the male genital tract.

3.1.4.1
Effect on Semen Quality

Sperm agglutination is the only well-established semen alteration related to the presence of ASA [25]. However, sperm agglutination, which is a time-dependent phenomenon, only rarely involves a large proportion of motile spermatozoa soon after liquefaction, even when all ejaculated spermatozoa are antibody coated. Therefore, sperm agglutination, although extremely suggestive of sperm autoimmunization, does not represent an important mechanism of the antibody interference with fertility in most cases. Apart from sperm-agglutination, there is little evidence that suggests a cause/effect relationship between ASA and the abnormality of semen parameters [25]. Actually, an effect on sperm motility/vitality should involve a complement (C)-mediated sperm injury, but it is prevented by anticomplementary activity in human seminal plasma [26, 27].

3.1.4.2
Interference with Cervical Mucus Penetration

The impairment of sperm penetration through the cervical mucus represents the most established mechanism of ASA interference with fertility. Several studies have shown a significant association between a poor PCT outcome and sperm autoimmunization [28–30]. Furthermore, the degree of the impairment of sperm penetration "in vivo" through the cervical mucus was found to correlate with the proportion of antibody-covered spermatozoa [28], as well as with the titer of circulating ASA [30]. The demonstration of the actual responsibility of ASA in impairing cervical mucus penetration has been provided by matching donor sperm suspensions exposed to sera containing ASA against the same sperm suspensions exposed to control sera without ASA, using the in vitro cervical mucus penetration test [31]. Although a prominent role for IgA-ASA in impairing sperm penetration of cervical mucus has been reported [32–34], other findings indicate that an abnormal interaction between the Fc portion of both IgA and IgG bound to the sperm surface and the constituents of the cervical mucus is responsible for the impairment of mucus penetration [35]. Antibodies directed against the tail-tip do not impair sperm/cervical mucus interaction [34]; therefore, they have no role in infertility.

3.1.4.3
Complement-Mediated Cytotoxicity Through the Female Genital Tract

When spermatozoa coated with complement-fixing antibodies enter the female reproductive tract, they could undergo deleterious effects of complement activation, supposing that complement components are present in a sufficient amount in the female genital tract. In a study by Price and Boettcher [36], although the level of complement activity in cervical mucus was only 11.5% of the serum activity, it was enough to cause complement-dependent immobilization of 50% of ASA-coated spermatozoa after 1 h and of 70% after 3 h. Higher levels of complement activity were detected in human follicular fluid (one-half of that in serum), and IgG-ASA were able to activate follicular fluid complement on human spermatozoa [37]. Owing to the dilution of follicular fluid after ovulation, any sperm damage or dysfunction related "in vivo" to its complement activity is difficult to ascertain. Therefore, its clinical relevance is not proven.

3.1.4.4
Interference with Sperm/Egg Interaction

Although experimental "in vitro" studies have largely demonstrated that ASA can affect sperm functions involved in the sperm/egg interaction (see Chap. 1.4), the clinical relevance of these effects might be proven above all by the results of in vitro fertilization (IVF) as a model of study. In most reports, the overall fertilization rate was significantly lower in the presence of sperm-bound antibodies than in the case of other indications for IVF [38–44]. But, in some other reports no significant difference was found [45–48].

Indeed, the assessment of the actual interference of ASA on sperm fertilizing ability from the analysis of IFV results is hindered by the effect of concomitant nonimmunological sperm abnormalities and by the different degree of sperm autoimmunization. Nevertheless, when the extent of sperm autoimmunization was taken into account, it was inversely correlated with the overall fertilization rate [49–51]. But, notably (1) even when the percentage of fertilized oocytes was reduced in the presence of ASA, some oocytes were fertilized and (2) in some individual patients, a high fertilization rate was achieved even in the presence of a high extent of sperm autoimmunization.

This variable interfering effect emerging from the analysis of IVF results is also supported by experimental laboratory-based studies aimed to determine the level of the interference of ASA on sperm functions involved in gametes interaction [25; see also Chap. 1.3]. Particularly illustrative is a study from our group where the occurrence of the ASA interference with zona pellucida (ZP)-binding was tested in 22 patients exhibiting all ejaculated spermatozoa coated "in vivo" with antibodies against the sperm head [52]. Excluding patients with abnormal semen from the analysis, an impairment of the ZP-binding was observed in 50% of cases, by matching patients and donor spermatozoa, labeled with different fluorochromes, for their binding ability to the same ZPs. It is worth noting that (1) in no case, the inhibition of ZP-binding was complete and (2) a normal ZP-binding was observed even when all ejaculated spermatozoa were coated with both IgG- and IgA-ASA.

On the whole, human IVF results and experimental laboratory-based studies suggest that, at the level of the sperm/egg interaction, ASA exert a relative impairment, which, to some extent, is related to the degree of sperm autoimmunization. However, the degree of autoimmunization does not completely explain the variability of the antibody impairment. Apparently, at the level of gamete interaction, more than at other levels (i.e., cervical mucus penetration), the interference of ASA exhibits qualitative, apart from quantitative, differences among patients. Most likely, this interference also depends on the relevance of the specific antigens, targeted by natural ASA, to the fertilization process.

3.1.5
Clinical Implications

Given that the only ASA-related semen alteration is sperm agglutination, which, however, is not a sensitive indicator, a direct screening test (MAR or IBT) should be performed on all semen samples examined in the couple-infertility work-up. As IgA-antibodies, whenever they occur, are always found in association with IgG [12, 53, 54], only IgG-ASA have to be screened. In all positive samples for IgG, even at a low degree, IgA-ASA should be screened to determine whether and at what extent they are also bound to the sperm surface.

If ASA-direct tests are negative or with a low positive rating (<50%), an ASA-related subfertility may be excluded. On the other hand, when >50% of motile spermatozoa are coated by ASA, the degree of the interfering effect on cervical mucus penetration should be verified and quantified by a carefully performed PCT, and, if possible, confirmed "in vitro" by a poor sperm penetration into donor cervical mucus with the capillary tube test.

When this is the case (>50% ASA-covered motile spermatozoa associated with a poor PCT and a poor "in vitro" sperm penetration), an immunological male subfertility can be diagnosed.

Whether, or to what extent, an ASA-interfering effect occurs, in each individual patient, downstream from the impairment of cervical mucus penetration, when all or nearly all spermatozoa are antibody-coated, is still hard to establish. The main reason is the inability of current diagnostic tests in quantifying the antibody density on the sperm surface and in defining the antigenic specificities of ASA, main determinants of the ASA-impairment at the level of sperm/oocyte interaction, which, however seems to be less effective and certain than that at the level of cervical mucus penetration.

In any case, from a clinical point of view, to establish whether, or to what extent, an ASA-interfering effect occurs, in each individual patient, downstream from the impairment of cervical mucus penetration, is not needed to diagnose ASA-related subfertility, because such an impairment cannot occur in the absence of the more effective interference on mucus penetration. But, it would be relevant in choosing the more appropriate assisted reproductive treatment option. Although ICSI has been claimed as the primary choice of treatment for ASA-related subfertility, because it overcomes any potential interference of ASA with sperm fertilizing ability [5], it would be better to reserve it for patients for whom achieving a pregnancy with less invasive techniques would be most unlikely. In the light of preventing inappropriate aggressive intervention, the main question is whether/when intrauterine insemination (IUI) could represent an effective first-line ART treatment, as discussed elsewhere in the book.

References

1. Rumke PH (1954) The presence of sperm antibodies in the serum of two patients with oligospermia. Vox Sang 4:135–140
2. Wilson L (1954) Sperm agglutinins in human semen and blood. Proc Soc Exp Biol Med 85:652–655
3. Taylor PJ, Collins JA (1992) Unexplained infertility. Oxford University Press, Oxford, UK, pp 128–131
4. Helmerhorst FM, Finken MJJ, Erwich JJ (1999) Detection assays for antisperm antibodies: what do they test? Hum Reprod 14:1669–1671
5. Lombardo F, Gandini L, Dondero F et al (2001) Antisperm immunity in natural and assisted reproduction. Hum Reprod Update 7:450–456

6. Bronson RA, Cooper G, Hjort T et al (1985) Anti-sperm antibodies, detected by agglutination, immobilization, microcytotoxicity and immunobead-binding assays. J Reprod Immunol 8:279–299

7. WHO Reference Bank for Reproductive Immunology (1977) Auto- and iso-antibodies to antigens of the human reproductive system. 1. Results of an international comparative study. Clin Exp Immunol 30:173–180

8. Collins JA, Burrows EA, Yeo J et al (1993) Frequency and predictive value of antisperm antibodies among infertile couples. Hum Reprod 8:592–598

9. Francavilla F, Catignani P, Romano R et al (1984) Immunological screening of a male population with infertile marriages. Andrologia 16:578–586

10. Hargreave TB, Haxton M, Whitelaw J et al (1980) The significance of serum sperm-agglutinating antibodies in men with infertile marriages. Brit J Urol 52:566–570

11. Menge AC, Medley NE, Mangione CM et al (1982) The incidence and influence of antisperm antibodies in infertile human couples on sperm-cervical mucus interactions and subsequent fertility. Fertil Steril 38:439–446

12. Meinertz H, Hjort T (1986) Detection of autoimmunity to sperm: mixed antiglobulin reaction (MAR) test or sperm agglutination ? A study on 537 men from infertile couples. Fertil Steril 46:86–91

13. Clarke GN, Elliott PJ, Smaila C (1985) Detection of sperm antibodies in semen using the immunobead test: a survey of 813 consecutive patients. Am J Reprod Immunol Microbiol 7:118–123

14. Sinisi AA, Di Finizio B, Pasquali D et al (1993) Prevalence of antisperm antibodies by SpermMAR test in subjects undergoing a routine sperm analysis for infertility. Int J Androl 16:311–314

15. Broderick GA, Tom R, McClure RD (1989) Immunological status of patients before and after vasovasostomy as determined by the immunobead antisperm antibody test. J Urol 142:752–755

16. Fisch H, Laor E, BarChama N et al (1989) Detection of testicular endocrine abnormalities and their correlation with serum antisperm antibodies in men following vasectomy. J Urol 141: 1129–1132

17. Jarow JP, Goluboff ET, Chang TS et al (1994) Relationship between antisperm antibodies and testicular histologic changes in humans after vasectomy. Urology 43:521–524

18. Matson PL, Junk SM, Masters JR et al (1989) The incidence and influence upon fertility of antisperm antibodies in seminal fluid following vasectomy reversal. Int J Androl 12:98–103

19. Eggert-Kruse W, Christmann WM, Gerhard I et al (1989) Circulating antisperm antibodies and fertility prognosis: a prospective study. Hum Reprod 4:513–520

20. Witkin SS, David SS (1988) Effect of sperm antibodies on pregnancy outcome in a subfertile population. Am J Obstet Gynecol 158:59–62

21. Rumke PH, Van Amstel N, Messer EN et al (1974) Prognosis of fertility of men with sperm agglutinins in the serum. Fertil Steril 25:393–398

22. Ayvaliotis B, Bronson RA, Rosenfeld D et al (1985) Conception rates in couples where autoimmunity to sperm is detected. Fertil Steril 43:739–741

23. Abshagen K, Behre HM, Cooper TG et al (1998) Influence of sperm surface antibodies on spontaneous pregnancy rates. Fertil Steril 70:355–356

24. Meinertz H, Linnet L, Fogh-Andersen P et al (1990) Antisperm antibodies and fertility after vasovasostomy: a follow-up study of 216 men. Fertil Steril 54:315–321

25. Francavilla F, Santucci R, Barbonetti A et al (2007) Naturally-occurring antisperm antibodies in men: interference with fertility and clinical implications. An update. Front Biosci 12:2890–2911

26. D' Cruz OJ, Haas GG (1990) Lack of complement activation in the seminal plasma of men with antisperm antibodies associated in vivo on their sperm. Am J Reprod Immunol 24:51–57

27. Petersen BH, Lammel CJ, Stites DP et al (1980) Human seminal plasma inhibition of complement. J Lab Clin Med 96:582–591

28. Bronson RA, Cooper GW, Rosenfeld DL (1984) Autoimmunity to spermatozoa: effect on sperm penetration of cervical mucus as reflected by postcoital testing. Fertil Steril 41:609–614
29. Haas GG (1986) The inhibitory effect of sperm-associated immunoglobulins on cervical mucus penetration. Fertil Steril 46:334–337
30. Mathur S, Williamson HO, Baker ME et al (1984) Sperm motility on post coital testing correlates with male autoimmunity to sperm. Fertil Steril 41:81–87
31. Aitken RJ, Parsow JM, Hargreave TB et al (1988) Influence of antisperm antibodies on human sperm function. Br J Urol 62:367–373
32. Clarke GN (1988) Immunoglobulin class and regional specificity of antispermatozoal autoantibodies blocking cervical mucus penetration by human spermatozoa. Am J Reprod Immunol Microbiol 16:135–138
33. Kremer J, Jager S (1980) Characteristics of anti-spermatozoal antibodies responsible for the shaking phenomenon with special regard to immunoglobulin class and antigen-reactive sites. Int J Androl 3:143–152
34. Wang C, Baker HW, Jennings MG et al (1985) Interaction between human cervical mucus and sperm surface antibodies. Fertil Steril 44:484–488
35. Bronson RA, Cooper GW, Rosenfeld DL et al (1987) The effect of an IgA_1 protease on immunoblobulins bound to the sperm surface and sperm cervical mucus penetrating ability. Fertil Steril 47:985–991
36. Price RJ, Boettcher B (1979) The presence of complement in human cervical mucus and its possible relevance to infertility in women with complement-dependent sperm-immobilizing antibodies. Fertil Steril 32:61–66
37. D'Cruz OJ, Haas GG, Lambert H (1990) Evaluation of antisperm complement-dependent immune mediators in human ovarian follicular fluid. J Immunol 144:3841–3848
38. Acosta AA, van der Merwe JP, Doncel G et al (1994) Fertilization efficiency of morphologically abnormal spermatozoa in assisted reproduction is further impaired by antisperm antibodies on the male partner's sperm. Fertil Steril 62:826–833
39. Chang TH, Jih MH, Wu TCJ (1993) Relationship of sperm antibodies in women and men to human in vitro fertilization, cleavage, and pregnancy rate. Am J Reprod Immunol 30:108–112
40. Clarke GN, Lopata A, McBain JC et al (1985) Effect of sperm antibodies in males on human in vitro fertilization (IVF). Am J Reprod Immunol Microbiol 8:62–66
41. Ford WCL, Williams KM, McLaughlin EA et al (1996) The indirect immunobead test for seminal antisperm antibodies and fertilization rates at in-vitro fertilization. Hum Reprod 11:1418–1422
42. Matson PL, Junk SM, Spittle JW et al (1988) Effect of antispermatozoal antibodies in seminal plasma upon spermatozoal function. Int J Androl 11:101–106
43. Rajah SV, Parslow JM, Howell RJ et al (1993) The effects on in-vitro fertilization of autoantibodies to spermatozoa in subfertile men. Hum Reprod 8:1079–1082
44. Vazquez-Levin MH, Notrica JA, de Fried EP (1997) Male immunologic infertility: sperm performance on in vitro fertilization. Fertil Steril 68:675–681
45. Culligan PJ, Crane MM, Boone WR et al (1998) Validity and cost-effectiveness of antisperm antibody testing before in vitro fertilization. Fertil Steril 69:894–898
46. Mandelbaum SL, Diamond MP, DeCherney AH (1987) Relationship of antisperm antibodies to oocyte fertilization in in vitro fertilization-embryo transfer. Fertil Steril 47:644–651
47. Sukcharoen N, Keith J (1995) The effect of the antisperm auto-antibody-bound sperm on in vitro fertilization outcome. Andrologia 27:281–289
48. Vujisic S, Lepej SZ, Jerkovic L et al (2005) Antisperm antibodies in sperm, sera and follicular fluids of infertile patients: relation to reproductive outcome after in vitro fertilization. Am J Reprod Immunol 54:13–20
49. De Almeida M, Gazagne I, Jeulin C et al (1989) In-vitro processing of sperm with autoantibodies and in-vitro fertilization results. Hum Reprod 4:49–53

50. Lähteenmäki A (1993) In-vitro fertilization in the presence of antisperm antibodies detected by the mixed antiglobulin reaction (MAR) and the tray agglutination test (TAT). Hum Reprod 8:84–88
51. Palermo G, Devroey P, Camus M et al (1989) Assisted procreation in the presence of a positive direct mixed antiglobulin reaction test. Fertil Steril 52:645–649
52. Francavilla F, Romano R, Santucci R et al (1997) Occurrence of the interference of sperm-associated antibodies on sperm fertilizing ability as evaluated by the sperm-zona pellucida binding test and by the TEST-Yolk Buffer enhanced sperm penetration assay. Am J Reprod Immunol 37:267–274
53. Francavilla F, Santucci R, Romano R et al (1988) A direct immunofluorescence test for the detection of sperm surface bound antibodies. Comparison with sperm agglutination test, indirect IF test and MAR test. Andrologia 20:477–483
54. Hellstrom WJG, Overstreet JW, Samuels SJ et al (1988) The relationship of circulating anti-sperm antibodies to sperm surface antibodies in infertile men. J Urol 140:1039–1044

Tests for Sperm Antibodies

3.2

A. Agarwal and T. M. Said

3.2.1
Introduction

Research in the area of antisperm-antibodies (ASA) began in the nineteenth century when it was reported that sperm could be antigenic if injected into a foreign species. Thereafter, it was reported that sperm were also antigenic when injected into the same species [1]. The presence of ASA coating the spermatozoa can significantly interfere with fertility; this may be due to immobilization of the spermatozoa, impaired cervical mucus penetration, inhibition of capacitation, and disturbance in sperm–ovum interaction. Furthermore, some ASA have been identified as cytotoxic leading to cell death [2]. Although ASA can be detected in serum, they do not necessarily impair fertility unless they are found within the reproductive tract or are detectable on living spermatozoa [3].

There has been significant concern regarding the inconsistency between different testing methodologies and their association with clinical scenarios of infertility. There is wide variation regarding this association depending upon which test(s) are employed, the study methodology used, and the patient population under study. A relatively recent review argues that the use of widespread immune testing in clinical practice cannot be supported by existing data. Moreover, the resulting therapies are similarly of unconfirmed benefit and may cause harm [4]. Nevertheless, the routine use of ASA testing appears to be cost-effective considering the expenses encountered during in vitro fertilization (IVF) cycles [5]. Proper testing for ASA allows the determination of antibodies on the sperm surface, which may be associated with low IVF success rates. In these cases, intracytoplasmic sperm injection has been shown to yield higher fertilization rates [6]. Thus a simple test for ASA may prevent a failed IVF cycle and outline the correct treatment option,

Several methods have been described for the detection of ASA. These include the tube slide agglutination test (TSAT), gelatin agglutination test (GAT), sperm immobilization test (SIT), immunobead test (IBT), and mixed antiglobulin reaction (MAR) test using

A. Agarwal (✉)
Cleveland Clinic Lerner College of Medicine, Case Western Reserve University, 9500 Euclid Avenue, Cleveland, OH, 44195, USA
e-mail: agarwaa@ccf.org

W. K. H. Krause and R. K. Naz (eds.), *Immune Infertility*,
DOI: 10.1007/978-3-642-01379-9_3.2, © Springer Verlag Berlin Heidelberg 2009

sensitized erythrocytes. Despite the multiplicity of testing methods, the World Health Organization (WHO) Special Programme of Research Development and Research Training in Human Reproduction has consistently recommended the inclusion of only the MAR test or the IBT in the assessment of human semen [7].

3.2.2
Detection of Sperm Antibody Classes

ASA IgM has been detected in the circulation of men; however, no traces of the IgM molecules were detected in the male genital tract. Therefore, testing for the IgM class does not appear to be of value in the context of male fertility evaluation [8]. On the other hand, 1% of the serum IgG has been documented in the male genital tract. Seminal IgG results from either transudation from circulation or from local antibody production [9]. Similarly, IgA class in human semen is the result of local production as seminal plasma IgA is of the secretory IgA type [10].

3.2.3
Testing Methods

Tests developed to detect and quantitate antibodies to sperm may be categorized into three groups on the basis of the antigen source: (a) sperm extract assays such as immunodiffusion or immunoelectrophoresis; (b) fixed sperm assays such as immunofluorescence, mixed antiglobulin tests, enzyme linked immunoassays, and radioimmunoassay; (c) live sperm assays such as macroagglutination, microagglutination, cytotoxicity, or sperm/cervical mucus interaction tests [11]. Only the MAR test and the IBT are routinely performed by diagnostic laboratories and appear to correlate well with immunological infertility [7]. Other historical tests of interest are also reviewed below to highlight the development of ASA testing.

3.2.3.1
Macro/Microagglutination and Immobilization

Many decades ago, a macroscopic protocol has been described to identify ASA in serum. The GAT is conducted by suspending the semen from a donor known not to have ASA with the complement-inactivated serum of the suspected subfertile patient in a gelatin mix. Clumping of sperm agglutinates at the bottom of the gelatin mix is interpreted as positive [12]. As the test is known to reveal false positive results because of the presence of debris in seminal plasma and the clinical relevance of ASA in serum is now hugely debated, the GAT no longer plays a role in the diagnosis of immunological infertility. Similarly the TSAT is no longer recommended as a testing modality. During TSAT, a sample of donor semen is mixed with complement-inactivated patient serum and the sperm agglutination is noted using a microscopic drop [13].

The SIT procedure resembles the TSAT but small volumes of rabbit or guinea pig serum are added as a source of complement. During microscopic assessment, the number of motile sperms is determined and the test is considered positive if more than half of counted sperms are found to be nonmotile [14]. In addition to the disadvantages noted above for the GAT and the TSAT, SIT lacks the ability to detect IgA as fixation of complement and initiation of the cascade sequence are possible only if the antibodies are IgG and IgM [15].

3.2.3.2
Enzyme-Linked Immunosorbent Assay and Immunofluorescence

The enzyme-linked immunosorbent assay (ELISA) has been adapted to quantitatively assess the presence of ASA. ELISA combines the specificity of the antigen–antibody reaction with the continuous degradation of chromogenic substrate by an enzyme to amplify the sensitivity of the reaction. Numerous materials and methods have been used for the ELISA procedure: solid phase materials (silicon rubber, glass); carriers (tubes, beads, disks); enzymes (alkaline phosphatase, horseradish peroxidase); substrates (p-nitrophenyl phosphate) and wash solutions [16]. Other variables of the assay include sperm concentration, type of sperm fixation, blocking agents, and serum and seminal plasma dilutions. The complexity, instrumentation, and expense of the ELISA have all hampered its widespread use in the workup of male immunological infertility.

The use of flow cytometry to detect sperm-bound antibodies and to quantitate the sperm antibody load (antibody molecules/spermatozoa) has been reported. After staining washed sperm samples, dead sperm are excluded with fluorescein-isothiocyanate-conjugated F(ab′)2 fragments of anti-IgG and IgA antibodies by the use of calibration standards. The sperm antibody load can be used to compare different patients or to follow up with the same patient as flow cytometry has the potential reliability and objectivity to quantitate sperm antibodies [17]. Similar to ELISA, flow cytometry is not currently widely used for the detection of ASA because of its complexity, expense and instrumentation requirement, which may not be available in standard andrology laboratories. In the same context, agglutinin assays with radiolabeled antibodies to detect and quantify ASA are of limited use. This method is also limited by an inability to determine specific ASA location, expense, and reliance on skilled labor [18]. However, it is to be noted that there is a close correlation between radiolabeled agglutinin assay test results and IBT [19].

3.2.3.3
Mixed Antiglobulin Reaction Test

The MAR test was initially developed to detect surface ASA [20]. It is on the basis of modification of the famed Coombs test described in1956 by Coombs et al. [21]. The initial version of the assay was simple and consisted of mixing three ingredients as single drop and covering it with a cover slip. The semen sample is mixed with a suspension of group O,

Rh-positive, human red cells of $R_1 R_2$ type, sensitized with human IgG in addition to undiluted, monospecific anti-IgG antiserum of rabbit or goat. The reaction is then observed after 10 min of incubation. The red cells are coated with IgG, as well as the sperm cells, if they have antibodies on them. The added anti IgG antiserum will then link together the two kinds of cells. Agglutination will be seen as mixed clumps of spermatozoa and red blood cells with a slow "shaky" movement when observed under a light microscope.

Results of the MAR test are noted as percentages of motile spermatozoa incorporated into the mixed agglutinates. The site of attachment can also be noted. No interpretation of the test is given unless agglutination of red blood cells and the presence of sufficient motile spermatozoa are observed. A MAR test is considered positive when >10% agglutination is seen, but is considered to be of clinical significance when only >80% agglutination is present.

The advantages of the MAR test are that it can be applied directly to fresh, untreated semen samples and results can be obtained within a few minutes. Therefore, the assay is considered quick, simple, and repeatable. The MAR test correlates with most other sperm antibody tests e.g., SIT and IBT [20]. Although MAR test is considered an ideal method for screening of ASA, it has certain limitations [22]. The assay cannot be used in patients with oligozoospermia, asthenozoospermia, and azoospermia, it is difficult to quantitate, it must be performed on a fresh sample, and it can be influenced by debris, semen viscosity, mucus, and microbial factors.

Commercially available sperm MAR kits are on the basis of an antiserum against human IgG to induce mixed agglutination between antibody-coated sperm and latex beads conjugated with human IgG [23]. The SpermMar kit is a superior alternative to erythrocyte MAR as it is time and cost effective; also, it can be applied to fresh, untreated semen samples (Fig. 3.2.1). One formulation of the kit contemplates the assessments of IgA and IgG classes. The advantage of the sperm MAR compared to erythrocyte MAR is the convenience of the kit, as it has proven to be time and cost-effective. The preparation of IgG sensitized erythrocytes is not always available, and also unwashed spermatozoa can be used [24]. The disadvantage of the sperm MAR (IgG labeled) is that indirect sperm MAR, i.e., using serum samples and donor spermatozoa, is difficult to interpret. The indirect MAR is usually considered in cases with azoospermia. In these cases, ASA should rather be detected using another method. Nevertheless, the assay can be successfully used for the routine evaluation of male partners of infertile couples if included routinely in semen analysis [24].

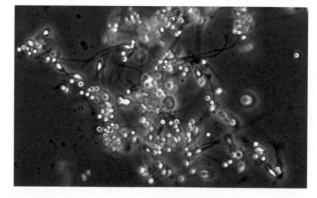

Fig. 3.2.1 Positive mixed antiglobulin reaction (MAR) test. Raw semen sample with latex beads coated with IgG seen bound to sperm surfaces, mainly tails (phase contrast, ×40)

3.2.3.4
Immunobead Test

The IBT has been described as a relatively simple procedure, inexpensive and easy to perform. Similar to the MAR test, it is very convenient, utilizing only a bench centrifuge, light microscope, commercially available beads (latex beads coated with antihuman IgG, IgA, and IgM) and takes less than 30 min to perform [25]. Spermatozoa are washed to discard any free immunoglobulins which may be in the seminal plasma and which, if present, would alter the assay results (Fig. 3.2.2).

IBT allows determination of the antibody class attached to spermatozoa, the localization on the spermatozoa, and the proportions of spermatozoa coated with antibody [25]. Sperm concentrations are usually adjusted to $10–25 \times 10^6$ motile sperm/mL to optimize the microscopic assessment of sperm. Adjustments are occasionally necessary if the sample is oligozoospermic or asthenozoospermic. Separation of sperm from seminal plasma is usually done using sperm preparation techniques. The IBT can also be conducted indirectly on reproductive fluids, seminal plasma, follicular fluid, cervical mucus, and serum. The immunoglobulin class detected can be of clinical importance. The direct and indirect IBT are therefore reliable, specific tests for the detection of sperm bound antibodies and sperm antibodies in reproductive fluids and serum [23].

Immunobead Reaction

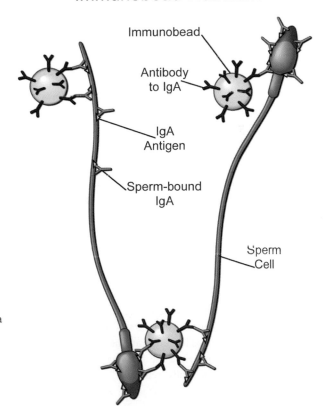

Fig. 3.2.2 Immunobeads are polyacrylamide spheres with covalently bound rabbit antihuman immunoglobulins. Test is considered positive if ≥20% of motile spermatozoa have immunobead binding and is considered clinically significant when at least 50% of the motile spermatozoa are coated with immunobeads

The intra-assay reproducibility of the indirect IBT was evaluated by testing aliquots of antisperm-antibody-positive sera from two patients against the same donor sperm sample. The inter-assay reproducibility was also evaluated by testing a positive serum sample first with different sperm samples from the same donor and second with sperm samples from different donors. The results of those experiments showed that the indirect IBT has very low intra-assay variation and a high inter-assay variability [26].

3.2.3.5
Tests for Cervical Mucus

Both IgG and IgA can be found in the cervical mucus. The presence of ASA in cervical mucus can be assessed by using in vivo or in vitro sperm–mucus interaction tests. The in vivo post coital test (PCT) shows poor results in the presence of ASA; however technical problems may also be responsible; therefore, caution is urged when attributing poor PCT to immunologically hostile mucus. The PCT is conducted by sampling the cervical mucus several hours after intercourse and examining it for the presence of spermatozoa. The presence of less than 10 sperm/HPF could be interpreted as a poor result. Most importantly, the presence of a distinctive "shaking" pattern of sperm motility is suggestive of the presence of ASA [27].

The in vitro sperm-cervical mucus contact (SCMC) test could also be used to evaluate the presence of ASA in cervical mucus. In this assay, aliquots of cervical mucus and liquefied semen are mixed and examined for the characteristic "shaking" pattern of sperm motility. The test is considered positive if more than 25% of spermatozoa display the shaking pattern of motility. In a study on 17 couples who repeatedly demonstrated unexpected poor PCTs, 15 of them revealed a positive SCMC test [28]. Therefore, the SCMC test is considered to be a reliable screening test for the detection of ASA among infertile couples.

3.2.4
Comparison of ASA Tests

The comparison between the MAR test and the IBT is of interest as both assays appear to be the most commonly used [7]. The two testing protocols are designed to detect immunoglobulins on the sperm surfaces. Indirect tests for ASA using the commercial MAR test have been applied to a panel of sera whose reactions in the TSAT, GAT, and SIT are well characterized. The results from MAR tests were compared directly with those obtained from IBT carried out at the same time. Results from screening tests performed on 30 sera confirmed complete correspondence among the GAT, MAR, and IBT. When sera were titrated, the IBT proved slightly more sensitive than the GAT, while the MAR test was slightly more sensitive than the IBT [23].

Another comparison between the IBT and the MAR test showed a high degree of agreement, but the former was less accurate than the latter. Also, the MAR tests for the secretory IgA present in semen, while the IBT may cross react with nonsecretory IgA present in serum [29]. A similar study reported that the standard MAR protocol (direct test of unwashed semen) was found to be more sensitive than IBT on washed sperm. The MAR does not require washing the spermatozoa free of seminal plasma, which makes it easier and faster than the IBT. It requires less semen volume and could be applied to samples with a lower sperm concentration compared to the IBT [30, 31]. In contrast, when the MAR test was performed on washed sperm or with an indirect antibody transfer from serum or seminal plasma, the results gave mostly low values for bead binding in comparison with IBT. Therefore, the MAR test is mostly suitable in direct assays employing unwashed ejaculates and it can be easily incorporated into routine semen analysis as a screening test, but the positive results should be confirmed by IBT [32].

Cross-inhibition studies have revealed high specificity between positive IBT and the presence of membrane-bound immunoglobulin. Good correlations have been reported also between the IBT and other immunoassays such as PCT and sperm-cervical mucus compatibility assays [33]. Poor correlations between the IBT and sperm agglutination test have been reported but may reflect the observation that sperm agglutination may occur because of nonimmunological factors [25].

It is of importance to note that there are several pitfalls associated with comparisons between the different methods of ASA detection. Many methods rely on subjective determinations and variable specimen preparations. False-positive results may occur with agglutination tests in the absence of ASA. In addition, sensitivity and specificity vary for each of the testing modalities [34].

3.2.5
Interpretation and Significance of ASA Tests

There is sufficient evidence to support the hypothesis that ASA play a role in selected couples with unexplained infertility. Both the prevalence and magnitude of this role remain controversial. Conflicting outcomes may result from variable specimen preparation, different testing methods, subjective test interpretation, and natural biologic variation [35]. In the clinical context of male infertility, the MAR test and the IBT are currently being used for the detection of ASA. The existing consensus indicates that a semen sample is to be considered immunocompromised if more than 50% of spermatozoa show binding in the MAR test or the IBT [7]. The identification of ASA in a given sample does not necessarily indicate other inherent defects. An attempt made to correlate results of MAR test with other defects in the seminal fluid revealed a significant correlation between a positive MAR test and spontaneous sperm autoagglutination [36]. No correlations were observed, however, between test positivity and concentration, motility and sperm morphologic features, the macroscopic aspects studied, or increased concentration of leukocytes.

Contradictory findings were identified in a different trial that correlated the results of the IgG MAR test with the semen analysis parameters of 1,176 infertile males [37]. The test was only positive in 3.1% of the cases. The positive IgG MAR test proved to correlate significantly both with the number and motility of the spermatozoa. Whether the detection of ASA is associated with other deficiencies in the semen analysis or not should not infringe on the importance of the assay, which appears to be of significant value in identifying the etiology of infertility.

Men presenting with a history of infertility were evaluated in terms of ASA levels. MAR test results were found as positive in 48 (10%) of 484 men with normal sperm counts, 18 (23%) of 78 with low sperm motility, and 19 (15%) of 128 with low counts. Therefore, the MAR test may be considered as a part of the routine semen analysis, as the presence of IgG ASA can be established in about 10% of men who might otherwise be passed as normal. In support, the evaluation of patients whose infertility remains unexplained (by routine physical and laboratory investigations) exhibits significantly elevated ASA levels in 18% of males compared to that in fertile individuals. Thus, the identification of autoimmune imbalance may help to resolve some cases of unexplained infertility [38].

3.2.6
Conclusions

The assessment of ASA in the context of infertility has not been devoid of controversies. It was rightly noted that "neither a specific antigen(s) nor a superior antibody detection assay exists, although both are requisite to an understanding of the significance of antisperm antibody production a for the purpose of infertility reduction" [39]. The only valid current indication of conducting an ASA assay appears to be unexplained infertility. However, routine ASA screening in couples with unexplained infertility is limited because there is no well-accepted consensus about which assay should be used. Most of the data support the use of either IBT or MAR to evaluate whether IgG or IgA ASA are present. The MAR test is easier to perform but is not suitable for testing of serum or plasma using an indirect approach.

References

1. Li TS (1974) Sperm immunology, infertility, and fertility control. Obstet Gynecol 44(4): 607–623
2. Naz RK, Menge AC (1994) Antisperm antibodies: origin, regulation, and sperm reactivity in human infertility. Fertil Steril 61(6):1001–1013
3. Dondero F, Gandini L, Lombardo F, Salacone P, Caponecchia L, Lenzi A (1997) Antisperm antibody detection: 1. Methods and standard protocol. Am J Reprod Immunol 38(3):218–223
4. Kallen CB, Arici A (2003) Immune testing in fertility practice: truth or deception? Curr Opin Obstet Gynecol 15(3):225–231
5. Bronson R (1999) Detection of antisperm antibodies: an argument against therapeutic nihilism. Hum Reprod 14(7):1671–1673
6. Clarke GN, Bourne H, Baker HW (1997) Intracytoplasmic sperm injection for treating infertility associated with sperm autoimmunity. Fertil Steril 68(1):112–117
7. World Health Organization (1999) WHO laboratory manual for the examination of human semen and sperm-cervical mucus interaction. Cambridge University Press, Cambridge
8. Rumke P (1974) The origin of immunoglobulins in semen. Clin Exp Immunol 17(2):287–297

9. Haas GG Jr, Cunningham ME (1984) Identification of antibody-laden sperm by cytofluorometry. Fertil Steril 42(4):606–613

10. Witkin SS, Zelikovsky G, Good RA, Day NK (1981) Demonstration of 11S IgA antibody to spermatozoa in human seminal fluid. Clin Exp Immunol 44(2):368–374

11. Alexander N, Ackerman S, Windt M-L (1990) Immunology. In: Acosta A, Swanson R, Ackerman S, Kruger T, van Zyl J, Menkveld R (eds) Human spermatozoa in assisted reproduction. Williams and Wilkins, Baltimore, pp 208–222

12. Kibrick S, Belding DL, Merrill B (1952) Methods for the detection of antibodies against mammalian spermatozoa. II. A gelatin agglutination test. Fertil Steril 3(5):430–438

13. Franklin RR, Dukes CD (1964) Antispermatozoal antibody and unexplained infertility. Am J Obstet Gynecol 89:6–9

14. Isojima S, Tsuchiya K, Koyama K, Tanaka C, Naka O, Adachi H (1972) Further studies on sperm-immobilizing antibody found in sera of unexplained cases of sterility in women. Am J Obstet Gynecol 112(2):199–207

15. Bronson RA, Cooper GW, Rosenfeld DL (1982) Correlation between regional specificity of antisperm antibodies to the spermatozoan surface and complement-mediated sperm immobilization. Am J Reprod Immunol 2(4):222–224

16. Ackerman SB, Wortham JW, Swanson RJ (1981) An indirect enzyme-linked immunosorbent assay (ELISA) for the detection and quantitation of antisperm antibodies. Am J Reprod Immunol 1(4):199–205

17. Ke RW, Dockter ME, Majumdar G, Buster JE, Carson SA (1995) Flow cytometry provides rapid and highly accurate detection of antisperm antibodies. Fertil Steril 63(4):902–906

18. Haas GG Jr, D'Cruz OJ (1989) A radiolabeled antiglobulin assay to identify human cervical mucus immunoglobulin (Ig) A and IgG antisperm antibodies. Fertil Steril 52(3):474–485

19. Haas GG Jr, Lambert H, Stern JE, Manganiello P (1990) Comparison of the direct radiolabeled antiglobulin assay and the direct immunobead binding test for detection of sperm-associated antibodies. Am J Reprod Immunol 22(3–4):130–132

20. Jager S, Kremer J, van Slochteren-Draaisma T (1978) A simple method of screening for antisperm antibodies in the human male. Detection of spermatozoal surface IgG with the direct mixed antiglobulin reaction carried out on untreated fresh human semen. Int J Fertil 23(1):12–21

21. Coombs RR, Marks J, Bedford D (1956) Specific mixed agglutination: mixed erythrocyte platelet anti-globulin reaction for the detection of platelet antibodies. Br J Haematol 2(1):84–94

22. Mathur S, Williamson HO, Landgrebe SC, Smith CL, Fudenberg HH (1979) Application of passive hemagglutination for evaluation of antisperm antibodies and a modified Coomb's test for detecting male autoimmunity to sperm antigens. J Immunol Methods 30(4):381–393

23. Kay DJ, Boettcher B (1992) Comparison of the SpermMar test with currently accepted procedures for detecting human sperm antibodies. Reprod Fertil Dev 4(2):175–181

24. Sinisi AA, Di Finizio B, Pasquali D, Scurini C, D'Apuzzo A, Bellastella A (1993) Prevalence of antisperm antibodies by SpermMARtest in subjects undergoing a routine sperm analysis for infertility. Int J Androl 16(5):311–314

25. Franco JG Jr, Schimberni M, Stone SC (1987) An immunobead assay for antibodies to spermatozoa in serum. Comparison with traditional agglutination and immobilization tests. J Reprod Med 32(3):188–190

26. Franco JG Jr, Schimberni M, Rojas FJ, Moretti-Rojas I, Stone SC (1989) Reproducibility of the indirect immunobead assay for detecting sperm antibodies in serum. J Reprod Med 34(4): 259–263

27. Mortimer D (1994) Clinical relevance of diagnostic procedures. Practical laboratory andrology. Oxford University Press, New York, pp 241–267

28. Franken DR, Slabber CF, Grobler S (1983) The SCMC test: a screening test for spermatozoal antibodies. Andrologia 15(3):270–273

29. Mahmoud A, Comhaire F (2000) Antisperm antibodies: use of the mixed agglutination reaction (MAR) test using latex beads. Hum Reprod 15(2):231–233

30. Ackerman S, McGuire G, Fulgham DL, Alexander NJ (1988) An evaluation of a commercially available assay for the detection of antisperm antibodies. Fertil Steril 49(4):732–734
31. Rasanen M, Lahteenmaki A, Saarikoski S, Agrawal YP (1994) Comparison of flow cytometric measurement of seminal antisperm antibodies with the mixed antiglobulin reaction and the serum tray agglutination test. Fertil Steril 61(1):143–150
32. Hellstrom WJ, Samuels SJ, Waits AB, Overstreet JW (1989) A comparison of the usefulness of SpermMar and immunobead tests for the detection of antisperm antibodies. Fertil Steril 52(6):1027–1031
33. Pretorius E, Franken DR, Shulman S, Gloeb J (1986) Sperm cervical mucus contact test and immunobead test for sperm antibodies. Arch Androl 16(3):199–202
34. Haas GG Jr, D'Cruz OJ, DeBault LE (1991) Comparison of the indirect immunobead, radio-labeled, and immunofluorescence assays for immunoglobulin G serum antibodies to human sperm. Fertil Steril 55(2):377–388
35. Mazumdar S, Levine AS (1998) Antisperm antibodies: etiology, pathogenesis, diagnosis, and treatment. Fertil Steril 70(5):799–810
36. Cerasaro M, Valenti M, Massacesi A, Lenzi A, Dondero F (1985) Correlation between the direct IgG MAR test (mixed antiglobulin reaction test) and seminal analysis in men from infertile couples. Fertil Steril 44(3):390–395
37. La Sala GB, Torelli MG, Salvatore V, Dessanti L, Dall'Asta D, Cantarelli M, Alboni P (1987) The direct IgG-MAR test (mixed antiglobulin reaction test): results and correlations with seminal analysis in 1176 men from infertile couples. Acta Eur Fertil 18(6):385–390
38. Fichorova RN, Boulanov ID (1996) Anti-seminal plasma antibodies associated with infertility: I. Serum antibodies against normozoospermic seminal plasma in patients with unexplained infertility. Am J Reprod Immunol 36(4):198–203
39. Cunningham DS, Fulgham DL, Rayl DL, Hansen KA, Alexander NJ (1991) Antisperm antibodies to sperm surface antigens in women with genital tract infection. Am J Obstet Gynecol 164(3):791–796

Impact on Fertility Outcome

3.3

3.3.1
Introduction

Many different factors may cause human infertility, which is a serious problem for many people (about 15–20%) wishing to have children. Impairment of semen quality in men, anovulation, endometriosis, as well as adhesions inside and outside Fallopian tubes in women are frequent causes of decreased fertility. The presence of antibodies to spermatozoa in men as well as in women is also considered as an immunological problem of conception.

Sperm have been known to be antigenic for more than a century. The presence of anti-sperm antibodies (ASA) has long been suggested since the antigenicity of spermatozoa was first demonstrated by Landsteiner and Metchnikoff in 1899 [1, 2]. Positive levels of human ASA were first reported in 1969 when Fjallbrandt [3] demonstrated that antibodies obtained either from infertile patients or from immunized rabbits were able to produce agglutination and thereby block in vitro penetration of human spermatozoa into female cervical mucus. The principle of sperm agglutination depends on specificity of sperm antibody to sperm antigen coating sperm head, midpiece, tail, or tail tip.

The immune response against sperm cells (spermatozoa) is genetically determined [e.g., 4]. ASA occur in both men and women, and also in homosexual men [5]. It is supposed that testicular trauma (e.g., biopsy, torsion, accident during sports activity), varicocele, testicular cancer, infection such as orchitis during mumps, and vasectomy are associated with autoimmunity to spermatozoa in up to 70% of men [e.g., 1]. The majority of cases of sperm autoimmunity are spontaneous and idiopathic. Rational access for the origin of autoimmune ASA in men is the disturbance of haematotesticular barrier. In infertile women, ascendant and frequent isoimmunization during long lasting, unprotected coital experience is suspected.

Z. Ulcova-Gallova
Department of Obstetrics and Gynecology, Charles University and Faculty Hospital, Alej Svobody 80, Plzen-Lochotin, 326 00, Czech Republic
e-mail: ulcova@fnplzen.cz

W. K. H. Krause and R. K. Naz (eds.), *Immune Infertility*,
DOI: 10.1007/978-3-642-01379-9_3.3, © Springer Verlag Berlin Heidelberg 2009

Seminal plasma, as a natural medium for spermatozoa has many immunological properties influencing the fertilization capacity of reproductive cells. In the past, clinical significance of ASA in human infertility was supported by many investigators and authors
[e.g., 6–11].

3.3.2
Influences of ASA on Infertility Prognosis

The most valuable sign for infertility prognosis appears to be the local ASA activity (in
seminal plasma in men and in cervical ovulatory mucus, endometrial, peritoneal, and follicular fluids in women). Our daily experience [e.g., 12, 13, 16, 20] shows that infertile
women are able to produce local immune response to spermatozoa more often and earlier
than to serum. Their systemic reaction as ASA activity is proven later and, from that point,
ASA are detected in both ovulatory cervical mucus and serum.

Generally, high titers of ASA are able to block initial stages of the reproductive
process. Infertile patients with immunological cause are less likely to conceive because
in some the ASA not only interfere with sperm migration, but also inhibit the fertilization process at various stages, and exhibit negative effect on the early embryo development. ASA can affect the mechanisms of transport of spermatozoa within the female
genital tract, may alter sperm capacitation or acrosome reaction, can interfere with egg
fertilization, or have postfertilization effects on the zygote and preimplantation embryo
[e.g.,6, 7].

The reason for detection of ASA is to determine clinically significant sperm antibody
titers and to estimate their role in iso-/autoimmune reactions leading to infertility. The
levels of ASA also depend on character of spermiogrammes. We noticed the relationship
between sperm antibodies in seminal plasma and proteins of acute phase of inflammation [6]. Sperm-agglutinating antibodies are much more frequent in IgG and IgA class in
seminal plasma and in IgG, as well as in IgM and IgE in sera. Interindividual findings of
seminal levels of lactoferrin, albumin, C3, and C4 were reported [6, 7]. Secretory immunity plays an important role in male infertility. Infertile men have significantly higher
levels of lysozyme, C3, alpha-1-antitrypsin, alpha-2-macroglobulin, and beta-2-micro-
globulin in their seminal plasma. Immunological changes in seminal plasma caused by
local inflammatory reactions and characterized especially by the presence of ASA or
pathological levels of seminal protein in acute phase of inflammation decrease sperm
function. Contemporary trends in andrology also clarify the pathology of acrosomal
functions [14].

As reported earlier [15], ASA effectively block fertilization. Some mechanisms, such
as the inhibition of sperm binding because of sperm agglutination, sperm immobilization
or cytotoxic reaction, the inhibition of sperm penetration through the zona pellucida, and
the fusion of the sperm plasma membrane with the vitelline membrane of the oocyte, have
been described. ASA may also block implantation or inhibit the development of early
embryos [e.g., 16].

3.3.3
Steroid Treatment of ASA

Recent evidence and simple field experience suggest that immunocompetent cells in immunological antisperm mechanisms could be influenced by condom blocking effect, oral corticosteroids [17–20], local hydrocortisone application to ectocervix [16, 21], or plasmapheresis [22]. One of our earlier studies [6] showed good therapeutic effect of oral prednisone in infertile men with ASA in seminal plasma that was associated with reduced fertility. It succeeded to reduce sperm-agglutinating levels in seminal plasma. Treatment scheme of oral prednisone adopted in 19 selected patients with high titers of ASA in seminal plasma only was as follows: prednisone at dose of 20 mg (in the morning)-20 mg (at noon) – 20 mg (in the evening) daily for the first week, 20-10-10 mg for the second week, 15-10-5 mg for the third week, 10-5-5 mg for the fourth and fifth weeks, 5-5-5 mg for the sixth and seventh weeks, and 5-5-0 mg for the eighth to 12th weeks. The levels of sperm-agglutinating antibodies estimated by direct MAR-test (mixed anti immunoglobulin reaction test) in IgG, sIgA, IgM, and IgE before the prednisone treatment, and after 2, 4, and 6 weeks during the above mentioned scheme of therapy are shown in Fig. 3.3.1. Individual decrease of ASA level is well recognizable after 6 weeks of the treatment. Patients JK1, JH, PK, JK3, and FR became fathers. Reduction in activity and levels of sperm antibodies was observed especially in immunoglobulin class A and G. The dynamics of seminal ASA as mean values of MAR-tests can be also seen in Fig. 3.3.1. After 6 weeks of prednisone treatment individual sensibility to corticosteroids was observed. ASA were not detected any more in ten patients, the wives of patients JK1, JH, and JK3 became pregnant by the end of their husbands' treatment, and the wives of PK and FR became pregnant in the sixth month. Impact of immunosuppressive treatment of immunocompetent cells creating ASA is evident from the fertility outcome.

Increased pregnancy rate after various schemes of prednisone dosages is referred between 11 and 56 % [e.g., 2, 3, 20, 23, 24]. On every consultation of our patients, blood pressure was measured and anamnestic data were screened. No unwanted systemic effects were registered during the oral prednisone treatment, although some nonspecific side effects such as aseptic necrosis hip, exacerbation of incipient duodenal ulcers or cardiovascular effects were described [25].

Highly individualized sensitivity and mechanisms responsible for the influence of immunocompetent cells creating ASA are supposed to exist. In treated patients, we monitored the ASA in seminal plasma three times during the corticosteroid therapy. When the pregnancy is not observed at the time of the husbands' treatment, in vitro fertilization (IVF) is planned, as a logical way in long lasting "unexplained" infertility, in three stimulated ovulations of the wives. Our experience shows that in some men better treatment is the parenteral administration of corticosteroids timed 24 or 12 h (depending on the levels of ASA) before the collection of semen for IVF.

As we know, ASA impair sperm transport within the female genital tract. Sperm penetration and progressive motility through cervical mucus are stopped or decreased [15, 26]. When all sperm cells are coated with antibodies, the cervical ovulatory mucus

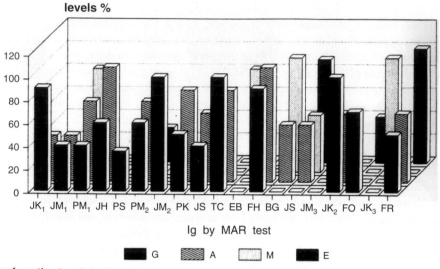

before the treatment

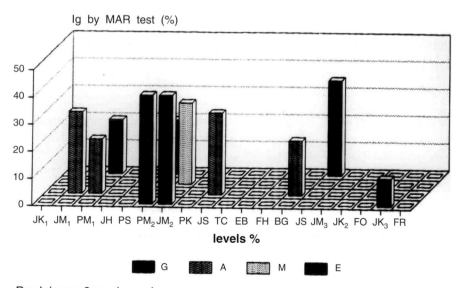

Prednisone 6 weeks and more

Fig. 3.3.1 The effect of prednisone on immunocompetent cells in men with positive sperm-agglutinating antibodies in seminal plasma

has no motile spermatozoa [15]. ASA are detected not only in semen, but also in ovulatory cervical mucus owing to ascendant female immunization by sperm antigens. IgG and/or IgA have been found in the cervix uteri [21, 27]. Sperm head directed antibodies [15], mainly those in IgA class, and/or IgA and IgG class antibodies directed against antigens on the principal piece of the sperm tail severely impair the ability of spermatozoa to penetrate mucus [28]. In the second mechanism of sperm transport impairment, complement-mediated IgG and/or IgM antibodies are able to activate the complement cascade, which results in target cell lysis [8]. Complement-mediated sperm immobilization within cervical mucus does not act immediately after sperm penetration into the cervical mucus, but requires 4–8 h. High decrease of sperm immobilization was observed in IgG. Practically all antibodies that are formed against sperm are designed to immobilize them.

Next mechanism of interference with fertilization by ASA acts via antibody dependent cell-mediated cytotoxicity [29] which impairs the process of capacitation (calcium dependent biochemical and structural changes and acrosomal reaction – exposure to enzymes such as acrosin, trypsin like proteinase, and hyaluronidase allowing contact with egg plasma membrane) [14, 30]. Sperm–egg interaction could be also influenced by the attack of ASA, which can alter fertilization by affecting the ability of spermatozoa to bind to the zona pellucida, as well as to the egg plasma membrane. Evidence suggests that ASA may interfere with sperm recognition of the zona pellucida in humans also [4]. The isotypes of ASA bound to the head may be important in determining the degree of impairment of sperm-zona pellucida binding. It was found [31] that IgA sperm antibodies were more inhibitory than IgG. Mahoney et al. [32] found that antibodies directed against the sperm head can affect zona binding, but not in every case. This suggests that impairment of zona pellucida binding depends on the antigens against which antibodies are directed, that is, whether they are the functional epitopes of a zona receptor ligand.

3.3.4
ASA Influences on Pregnancy Rate

The presence of ASA in the IVF culture-medium results in an impairment of fertilization. Immunoglobulins of the IgA class appeared to be more effective in impairing fertilization than IgG. More critical examination of the results of IVF in women with isoimmunity to sperm revealed both diminished fertilization rate and diminished embryonic cleavage rate, as well as reduced chance of pregnancy as shown by the study of Vasquez-Levin [33]. On the other hand, significant pregnancy rates can be achieved despite the presence of ASA. These antibodies cannot be eliminated from the egg by washing. Pagidas et al. [34] claimed that IVF is not significantly affected by the presence of ASA in female sera used to supplement the culture media or by antibodies bound to inseminated sperm. Inhibition of IVF fertilization may be caused by a synergistic effect of IgG and/or IgA classes of ASA.

In IVF trials other authors did not find any differences between antibody-positivity and antibody-negativity in the outcome of the IVF-embryo transfer attempt [35].

Menge and Naz [9] suggested three mechanisms by which ASA can affect embryo survival. The first mechanism consists of the possibility that sperm surface antigens are incorporated into the zygotic membrane at fertilization. Fertilization involves the possibility of sperm made oolemma plasma membranes moving to a mixture of antigens. The second mechanism proposed is that similar epitopes are present on spermatozoa and embryos. Several common antigens have been found. The last proposed mechanism to account for postfertilization reproductive loss mediated by ASA is via an indirect effect of antibodies on embryo development.

A woman whose partner has ASA following a vasectomy often makes antibodies of her own [10]. In humans, clinical evidence of an association between early pregnancy loss and immunity to sperm is not definitely clear. Approximately 15% of women produce antibodies to sperm in the cervical mucus and in the blood. Over 50% of men with low sperm motility have been found to carry these antibodies in semen plasma and in serum. Sperm cells have unique surface antigens that elicit an immune response.

Beer also speculates [10] about the rising incidence of ASA in women. It may be due to delaying pregnancy until late in life, by which time they will probably have had several sexual relationships. This increases the risk of developing an immune sensitization. When ASA develop in a woman, they agglutinate and/or immobilize sperm from her partner or any sperm donor and we speak about nonpartner-specific ASA in such a case. Beer studied [10] ASA levels in over 100 prostitutes. ASA were measured and compared with those of 40 age-matched women. More than 40% of prostitutes had ASA compared with just 5% among the control group. Over 60% of these women who had never used any form of contraception became infertile within 9 years.

The same author also observed [10] that ASA can be associated with antibodies to phospholipids. There is strong indication that the woman will have anti-DNA antibodies in addition to elevated levels of circulating natural killer cells and CD19+/5+ B-cells that produce the ASA. Such a problem can manifest itself as repeated IVF failures when embryo is implanted, but later it leads to very early miscarriage. Immunotherapy is an effective way of treating women with antibodies to sperm who experience this problem. A number of autoimmune and/or isoimmune conditions of the reproductive system are associated with poor fertility. Several topics [e.g., 13, 18, 22, 39] have described the relationship between ASA and pregnancy prognosis. Also allergies to heavy metals can negatively influence reproduction, because in sensitive persons they are able to alter the immune reactions including production of autoantibodies. The altered immune reaction can then cause infertility. In patients with metal intolerance diagnosed by the MELISA test, the release of metal ions from dental materials can be one of the stimulating factors which may adversely affect fertility [11]. An Italian group [23] studied the presence of ASA in 190 patients with testicular cancer 1 month after orchiectomy and before radiotherapy or chemotherapy. The results support the hypothesis that testicular cancer might not be a possible cause of antisperm autoimmunization and infertility. Marconi et al. [24] did not find any relationship between ASA detected by mixed agglutination reaction or immunobead test and chronic inflammation and infection of the seminal tract.

3.3.5
Conclusion

Earlier published incidence of ASA in an infertile population is 9% of the men and 15% of the women has to be considered [25]. ASA play an important role in the etiology of immune infertility. Circulating and local ASA may be markers for disorders of the reactivity of the immune system and may be involved in iso- and autoimmune processes. ASA testing is important in cases with explained or unexplained infertility, but without pregnancy success after repeated procedures of IVF. Today effort is necessary to define sperm antigens with significance for fertility. The association of the ASA with infertility demands their detection and the couples have to be treated appropriately. As these antibodies can induce infertility, they have the potential to induce the development for contraceptive purposes in humans [36–44].

Acknowledgment   This paper was supported by a grant of the Ministry of Education, Charles University MSM 002 162 0812.

References

1. Landsteiner K (1899) Zur Kenntnis der spezifisch auf Blutkoprochen wirkenden Sera. Zbl bakt 25:546–551
2. Metchnikoff S (1900) Etudes sur la spermatoxine. Ann Inst Pasteur 14:561–577
3. Fjallbrant B (1969) Cervical mucus penetration by human spermatozoa treated with anti-spermatozoal antibodies from rabbit and man. Acta Obstet Gynecol Scand 48:71–77
4. O'Rand MG (1977) The presence of sperm specific isoantigens on the egg following fertilization. J Exp Zool 202:267–293
5. Wolf H, Schill WB (1985) Antisperm antibodies in infertile and homosexual men; relationship to serologic and clinical findings. Fertil Steril 44:673–677
6. Ulcova-Gallova Z (1997) Immunological findings in seminal plasma from men of infertile couples. Andrologia 2:5–9
7. Shulman S, Bronson P (1969) Immunochemical studies on human seminal plasma. J Reprod Fertil 18:481–491
8. Isojima S, Tsuchiya K, Koyama K, Tahala C, Naka O, Adachi H (1972) Further studies on sperm-immobilizing antibody found in sera of unexplained cases of sterility in women. Am J Obstet Gynecol 112(2):199–207
9. Menge AC, Naz RK (1988) Immunologic reactions involving sperm cells and preimplantation embryo. Am J Reprod Immunol Microbiol 18:17–20
10. Beer AE, Kantecki J, Reed J (2006) Is your body baby-friendly?. AJR, Windsor, p 483. ISBN 0-9785078-0-0
11. Podzimek S, Prochazkova J, Bultasova L, Bartova J, Ulcova-Gallova Z, Mrklas L, Stejskal VD (2005) Sensitization to inorganic mercury could be a risk factor for infertility. Neuro Endocrinol Lett 26:277–282
12. Bronson RA, Fusi FF (1995) The reproductive immunology of fertilization failure. Assist Reprod Rev 5:14–25
13. Eggert-Kruse W, Christmann M, Bernard I, Pohl S, Klina K, Runnebaum B (1989) Circulating antisperm antibodies and fertility prognosis: a prospective study. Hum Reprod 4:513–520

14. Peknicova J, Chladek D, Hozak P (2005) Monoclonal antibodies against sperm intra-acrosomal antigens as markers for male infertility diagnostics and estimation of spermatogenesis. Am J Reprod Immunol 53(1):42–49

15. Bronson RA, Cooper GW, Rosenfeld D (1984) Sperm antibodies: their role in infertility. Fertil Steril 42:171–175

16. Ulcova-Gallova Z, Mraz L, Planickova E, Macku F, Ulc I (1990) Three years experience with local hydrocortisone treatment in women with immunological cause of infertility. Ztrb fur Gynacol 112:867–873

17. Alexander JN, Sampson JH, Fugham DL (1983) Pregnancy rates in patients treated for anti-sperm antibodies with prednisone. Int J Fertil 28:63–66

18. D`Almeida M, Soufir JC (1977) Corticosteroid therapy for male with autoimmune infertility. Lancet 2:815–821

19. Hendry WF, Stedronska J, Hughes L (1979) Steropid treatment of male subfertility caused by antisperm antibodies. Lancet 1:498–502

20. Ulcova-Gallova MT (1994) Effect of prednisone therapy on infertile men with spermantibodies in seminal plasma. Andrologia 2:7–13

21. Ulcova-Gallova Z, Mraz L, Planickova E, Macku F, Ulc I (1988) Local hydrocortisone treatment of spermagglutination antibodies in infertile women. Int J Fertil 33:421–426

22. Ulcova-Gallova Z, Opatrny K, Krauz V, Panzner P, Zavazal V (1990) Plasmapheresis–a new therapeutic method of immunological infertility. Cas Lek Cesk 129:104–112

23. Paoli D, Gilio B, Piroli E, Gallo M, Lombardo F, Dondero F, Lenzi A, Gandini L (2008) Testicular tumors as a possible cause of antisperm autoimmune response. Fertil Steril 25:123–134

24. Marconi M, Nowotny A, Pantke P, Diemer T, Weidner W (2008) Antisperm antibodies detected by mixed agglutination reaction and immunobead test are not associated with chronic inflammation and infection of the seminal tract. Andrologia 40(4):227–234

25. Shulman S, Shulman J (1982) Methylprednisolone treatment of immunologic infertility in male. Fertil Steril 38:5–12

26. Alexander NJ (1984) Antibodies to human spermatozoa impede sperm penetrationof cervical mucus or hamster eggs. Fertil Steril 41:433–439

27. Kremer J, Jager S (1980) Characteristics of anti-spermatozoal antibodies responsible for the shaking phenomena with special regard to immunoglobulin class and antigen-reactive sites. Int J Androl 3:143–152

28. Wang C, Gordon Baker HW, Jennins MG, Burger HG, Lutjen P (1985) Interaction between human cervical mucus and sperm surface antibodies. Fertil Steril 44:484–488

29. D`Cruz OJ, Haas GG Jr (1995) Beta2 integrin (C11b/CD18) is the primary adhesive glycoprotein complex involved in neutrophil-mediated immune injury to human sperm. Biol reprod 53: 1118–1130

30. Yanagimachi R (1988) Sperm-egg vision. Curr Top Membr Transp 32:3–43

31. Tsukui S, Noda Y, Yano J, Fukuda A, Mori T (1986) Inhibition of sperm penetration through human zona pellucida by antisperm antibodies. Fertil Steril 46:92–96

32. Mahoney MC, Alexander NJ, Bronson RA (1991) Inhibition of human sperm-zona pellucida tight binding in the presence of antisperm antibody positive polyclonal patient sera. J Reprod Immunol 19:287–291

33. Vasquez-Levin M, Kaplan P, Guzan I, Grunfeld I, Garrisi GJ, Navot D (1991) The effect of female antisperm antibodies on in vitro fertilization, earlyembryonic development and pregnancy outcome. Fertil Steril 56:84–90

34. Pagidas K, Hemmings R, Falkone T, Miron P (1994) The effect of antisperm auto antibodies in male or in female partners undergoing in vitro fertilization-embryo transfer. Fertil Steril 62: 363–369

35. Sukcharoen N, Keith J (1995) The effect of the antisperm autoantibody-bound sperm on in vitro fertilization outcome. Andrologia 27:281–289

36. Chamley LW, Clarke GN (2007) Antisperm antibodies and conception. Semin Immunopathol 29(2):169–184
37. Alexander NJ, Anderson DJ (1979) Vasectomy: consequences of autoimmunity to sperm antigens. Fertil Steril 32:253–259
38. Jung SM, Matson PL, Yovich JM, Yovich TJ (1986) The fertilization of human oocytes by spermatozoa from men with antispermatozoal antibodies in semen. J In Vitro Fertil Embry Transf 3:350–357
39. Kobayashi S, Bessho T, Shigeta M, Koyama K, Isojima S (1990) Correlation between quantitative antibody titers of sperm immobilizing antibodies and pregnancy rates by treatment. Fertil Steril 54:1107–1113
40. Mathur S, Baker ER, Williamson HO (1981) Clinical significance of sperm antibodies in infertility. Fertil Steril 36:486–495
41. Nakov LS (1998) Genetics of the immune response against sperm antigens. Cent Eur J Immunol 2:16–24
42. Rumke P (1954) The presence of sperm antibodies in the serum of two patients with oligozoospermia. Vox Sang 4:135–140
43. Shulman S (1972) Immunological barrier to fertility. Obstet Gynecol Survey 27:553–606
44. Shulman S, Harlin B, Davis P, Reyniak JV (1978) Immune infertility and new approaches to treatment. Lancet 1:309–319

Sperm Antibodies and Assisted Reproduction

3.4

Jerome H. Check

3.4.1
Potential Mechanism of How Antisperm Antibodies (ASA) Impair Infertility

Antisperm antibodies (ASA) present in males or female partners have been demonstrated to be a cause of human infertility [1]. These ASA may inhibit fertility by preventing sperm from progressing through the cervical mucus [2–6]. Other data show that ASA may contribute to infertility by disrupting sperm–oocyte recognition and fusion [7,8] inhibiting the sperm from undergoing capacitation [9], or acrosome reaction [10], or binding to the zona pellucida [11–13]. There are even data suggesting that ASA directed to specific sperm cell membrane antigens that are essential for oocyte division can inhibit the ability of a fertilized oocyte to cleave into an embryo [14].

3.4.2
Strategies for Treating Infertility Related to Antisperm Antibodies

For males or females with ASA, there may be multiple antibodies directed against different sperm antigens, or there may be antibodies directed against a single antigen. Thus, some antibodies may only be immobilizing antibodies and thus contribute to infertility by inhibiting the progression through the cervical mucus, but once the sperm reach the oocyte the fertilization process is not effected. This type of ASA problem should theoretically respond to intrauterine insemination (IUI) merely by bypassing the cervical mucus.

If there are no sperm immobilizing the ASA present, but only those inhibiting fertilization or postfertilization events leading to infertility, the couple should have a normal postcoital test if the semen parameters and mucus quality are normal and the testing is

J. H. Check
Department of Obstetrics and Gynecology, Division of Reproductive Endocrinology & Infertility,
The University of Medicine and Dentistry of New Jersey, Robert Wood Johnson Medical School
at Camden, Camden, NJ, USA
e-mail: laurie@ccivf.com

W. K. H. Krause and R. K. Naz (eds.), *Immune Infertility*,
DOI: 10.1007/978-3-642-01379-9_3.4, © Springer Verlag Berlin Heidelberg 2009

performed at the right time [2,15,16]. The use of simple IUI would not be expected to correct the infertility problem assuming a sufficient concentration of ASA to inhibit fertilization and/or postfertilization events. For this paradigm of the presence of only antibodies preventing fertilization and no sperm progression through cervical mucus, if the ASA existed in the male partner the ideal method (and maybe the only treatment option) might be in vitro fertilization (IVF) with intracytoplasmic sperm injection (ICSI). On the other hand, if the sperm were coated with ASA and if the antibodies could be eluted from the sperm or the adverse function of the antibodies negated without damaging the sperm, IUI could be also an effective therapy.

One cannot assume that if there are immobilizing antibodies present then the presence of ASA inhibiting fertilization are absent. There is a probability, when ASA are measured, that they may be directed against antigens that lead to immobilization in the mucus and also inhibit fertilization. Thus, one cannot assume that simple IUI would necessarily be effective if the postcoital test is poor.

The presence of sperm immobilizing ASA or ASA inhibiting fertilization does not necessarily cause infertility depending on the percentage of sperm that are coated with them or the concentration of the ASA per sperm. Similarly ASA in the female reproductive tract would not necessarily cause infertility if the concentration of ASA was low. Furthermore, demonstration of ASA in the serum of women does not necessarily mean that they are present in the reproductive tract. Finally, there may be a sufficient percentage of sperm coated with ASA with sufficient concentration per sperm, yet not associated with infertility, because the antibodies are directed against sperm antigens not essential for mobilization through cervical mucus or the fertilization process.

Thus, faced with the paradigm of the presence of sperm coating at least 50% of the sperm as determined by a test measuring ASA bound to the sperm, e.g., direct immunobead (IBT) assay [17,18] or the mixed antiglobulin reaction (MAR) test [19,20] and with a poor postcoital test, the practical options to the infertile couple and treating physicians is to try IUI alone, try IUI with attempts to elute or neutralize the action of the attached sperm, go directly to IVF, or do IVF with ICSI. Another option that could be offered is to treat the male with high-dosage glucocorticoids for a week each month or a lower dosage chronically; however, because of somewhat limited success and significant risk of complications, e.g., avascular necrosis, this treatment option is rarely offered in the modern era with safer assisted reproductive techniques available.

Some of the decisions about which treatment to perform in the above paradigm could be governed by the patient's finances and insurance. Some mandated insurance coverage requires three or four IUI cycles before allowing IVF to be performed unless it can be demonstrated that IVF-ET, with or without ICSI, is the only treatment option. A medical consultant for the insurance company, with knowledge that IUI can be effective, may require this therapy first even if the patient/physician preference is to go directly to IVF with ICSI.

If the infertile couple cannot afford IVF-ET and ICSI, they may decide to try less-expensive IUI, gambling that this will work. If it is not successful, then the couple has added the expense of IUI to the IVF that will next be performed. Though pregnancies have been reported by merely performing standard IUI [21] or by having the male partner dilute some of the antibodies that attach at the time of ejaculation by ejaculating into media [22], in the author's opinion the couple should be advised that there are data suggesting techniques which elute or damage the antibodies by enzymatic cleavage prior to IUI may improve the chance of IUI working [23–26]. Though most infertility centers have the availability of IVF with ICSI, only a minority have, or choose to use, techniques of eluting or enzymatic cleavage of ASA prior to IUI and this fact could effect decisions for treatment. Not all infertility centers believe that pretreatment of sperm prior to IUI improves the efficacy above IUI alone but this has not been the author's experience [23].

In the paradigm of the presence of ASA bound to sperm associated with a poor postcoital test where the decision has been to proceed to IVF immediately or at least after a few failed IUI cycles, since, besides the immobilizing ASA there may be concomitant ASA that would prevent fertilization, one could argue that there would be no reason why conventional oocyte insemination rather than ICSI should be performed since one is taking a chance on fertilization failure. However, if one could demonstrate normal fertilization and embryo cleavage by conventional oocyte insemination there would be certain advantages of the former over ICSI. First, ICSI adds an additional expense and if the couple is not insured the savings could be helpful. Second, if normal fertilization could be demonstrated the couple may be content to try some IUI cycles provided IVF was their first treatment option or go back and try a few more IUI cycles aimed with the knowledge that if one could get the sperm into the uterine cavity, conception would be possible. The third reason is that there are some recent data suggesting a higher chance of pregnancy if the oocytes are fertilized in the conventional manner vs. ICSI [27]. In circumstances, where the knowledge of conventional fertilization could influence subsequent decisions on the type of therapy, one could suggest fertilization of half of the oocytes with conventional insemination and half with ICSI so that if there is no or marked decreased fertilization with conventional oocyte insemination, hopefully ICSI will provide enough embryos.

When faced with the paradigm of ASA bound to a sufficient percentage of the sperm (at least 70%) but with a normal postcoital test, the decision could be to do nothing about the presence of ASA assuming some other correctable infertility factor could be found. IUI with untreated sperm would not seem likely to improve fertility outcome in this circumstance. However, one could choose to have IUI performed with enzymatically treated sperm or sperm treated to elute the antibodies from the sperm. In case immobilizing ASA do not exist but ASA that could inhibit fertilization may be present, if no other infertility factor is identified, and the ASA are assumed to be contributing, another option besides IUI with treated sperm would be to have IVF with ICSI.

3.4.3
The Use of In Vitro Fertilization and Intracytoplasmic Sperm Injection for Antisperm Antibodies Counting Sperm

If an evaluation of the effect of ASA on the outcome following conventional insemination is small enough to fortuitously select males mostly with immobilizing ASA, or if one chooses for selection males with weakly positive ASA, one could conclude that conventional oocyte insemination is sufficient and ICSI is not necessary. For example, a study by Vujisic et al. concluded that the presence of ASA on the sperm was not associated with

IVF outcome in the couples where the male partner had good quality semen characteristics [28]. However, in that study, ASA detected by MAR test, IgG was considered present if it is more than 20% and only four patients had ASA >75%; the total study consisted of 14 patients with positive ASA [28].

Besides the possibility of low concentration of ASA bound to the sperm and ASA limited to immobilizing ASA, another factor that may allow normal fertilization is the location of the sperm. Mandelbaum et al. found no correlation between ASA binding to the sperm tail tip and the fertilization of inseminated metaphase II oocytes [29].

Thus, with these caveats it is not surprising that during the decade following the first publication of the adverse effect of ASA bound to sperm on fertilization rates by Junk et al. [30], there were some small studies finding no reduction in fertilization rates with IVF without ICSI [28,31]. Nevertheless, the majority of studies did find that ASA bound to sperm does reduce the fertilization rate [29,32–37].

In contrast to conventional oocyte insemination with IVF, most data show that ICSI allows normal fertilization rates [38–41]. The data also suggested normal pregnancy rates [38–41]. However, some studies have suggested a higher miscarriage rate from the transfer of embryos where the oocytes were fertilized by ICSI with sperm coated with ASA [38,40]. Lahteenmaki et al. found miscarriages in 38% (5/13) of couples with sperm positive for ASA vs. a zero rate in the controls [40]. Check et al. found only a 14% miscarriage rate in pregnancies achieved by sperm with <50% binding by direct IBT vs. 25% for those with >80% binding [38]. In contrast, Clarke did not find an increased miscarriage rate [39].

3.4.4
The Use of In Vitro Fertilization and Intracytoplasmic Sperm Injection for Antisperm Antibodies in the Female Partner

The incidence of ASA in the female partner with sufficient levels to cause a poor postcoital test is much less common than ASA bound to sperm causing a poor postcoital test [42,43]. Immobilizing ASA in the female partner should be found in the cervical mucus and should be diagnosed by mucous testing, e.g., the indirect IBT.

Despite studies showing that ASA bound to sperm is a much more common cause of the poor postcoital test than ASA in the female partner, when prevalence of ASA in the sera of males vs. females were compared, one study reported ASA in 7% of men and 13% of women [44]. Similar findings were reported by Pattinson and Mortimer – 10% for men and 15% for women [45]. Another study found that ASA were present in the sera of 77% of women with unexplained infertility vs. only 5% of controls [46].

The majority of males who test positive for ASA by direct IBT have poor postcoital tests and those who do have normal postcoital tests achieve a higher pregnancy rate even with normal intercourse [2]. The majority of males with significant levels of ASA bound to sperm have abnormal postcoital tests [2]. This suggests that most of the time when couples have poor post-coital tests with the male partner's sperm coated with ASA. Immobilizing autoantibodies must frequently co-exist with immobilizing ASA since simple IUI is not effective. It is likely that ASA in women would show similar percentages of immobilizing ASA as found in males. This suggests that the ASA in serum of women may not be likely to be found in reproductive secretions, e.g., cervical mucus, or may be present in a lower concentration so that they are less likely to contribute to the infertility process in the majority of women showing them present in the sera. Support for this concept was provided by a study from Daitoh et al. showing normal fertilization rates and high pregnancy and implantation rates in women with ASA [47].

One caveat is the protein source for the oocyte insemination medium. Today, most IVF centers use albumin. However, for those still using the female's partners' sera there is a possibility that fertilization rates could be impaired if there were ASA in the serum.

Women demonstrating ASA in cervical mucus with sufficient level to impair sperm progress could be treated simply with IUI. However, the possibility exists that ASA are also directed against sperm antigens that impair the fertilization process, so it may be more prudent to pretreat the sperm [23,26]. Failure to conceive with IUI would then be followed by IVF-ET but ICSI would usually not be required because attachment of antibodies by contact with female fluids would be bypassed.

3.4.5
The Future

As mentioned previously, the biggest dilemma facing the physician and patient is how to determine if the ASA detected is contributing to the infertility and if so were they merely immobilizing the sperm in the mucus or just impairing fertilization or both. Knowledge of this would help to determine when to quickly directly proceed to IVF with ICSI.

One limitation of the direct IBT or MAR test is that they fail to determine the concentration of ASA per sperm. Nevertheless, at present the best method to study the pathologic importance of these ASA is to determine the percentage of sperm showing ASA attachment by the above tests. Generally, the higher the percentage, the greater the likelihood that these ASA are pathological.

Some studies suggest that ASA that prevent fertilization are more likely head-related [48,49]. Others find decreased percentage of sperm binding to the zona pellucida with ASA directed to sperm head [50,51]. Thus, on the basis of these data one might consider IVF with ICSI sooner if IgG or IgA is detected against sperm head.

However, other researchers do not agree that localization of ASA influences the mechanism of infertility [29,31,52]. Probably, the best method for determining the most appropriate therapy for ASA will be with the detection of antibodies to specific sperm antigens to which there is knowledge as to what role these antigens play in the fertilization process [53,54].

Until the time of establishing which antigens are not important and which impair only sperm motility vs. the actual fertilization process, the best choice at present to observe subfertile sperm based on the presence of ASA is by way of detecting a high percentage of sperm with IgG and/or IgA on any part of the sperm except the tail tip.

The decision on whether to try IUI or IVF should be based on insurance coverage, financial considerations and previous treatments (e.g., a couple, with previous failed fertilization detecting that a possible etiology was sperm coated with ASA, may prefer to go straight to IVF with ICSI).

The expertise of a given center with IUI methods could be a deciding factor. The author does not have any personal experience with the method of eluting ASA from sperm with FA-1 antigens [26]. However, the author does have experience with treating sperm coated with ASA with the protein digestive enzyme chymotrypsin [23,55, Fig. 3.4.1]. Though

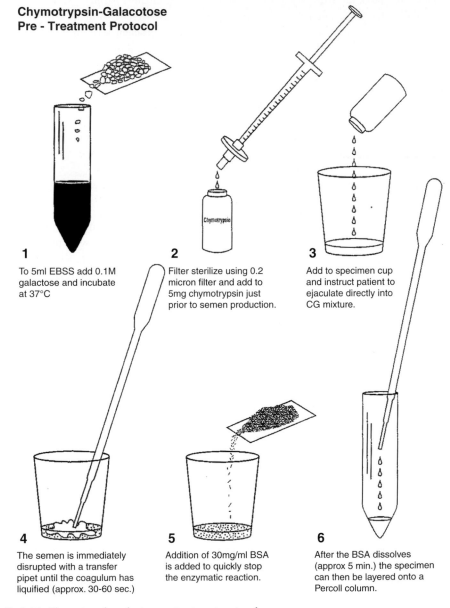

Chymotrypsin-Galacotose Pre - Treatment Protocol

1
To 5ml EBSS add 0.1M galactose and incubate at 37°C

2
Filter sterilize using 0.2 micron filter and add to 5mg chymotrypsin just prior to semen production.

3
Add to specimen cup and instruct patient to ejaculate directly into CG mixture.

4
The semen is immediately disrupted with a transfer pipet until the coagulum has liquified (approx. 30-60 sec.)

5
Addition of 30mg/ml BSA is added to quickly stop the enzymatic reaction.

6
After the BSA dissolves (approx 5 min.) the specimen can then be layered onto a Percoll column.

Fig. 3.4.1 Chymotrypsin-galactose pretreatment protocol

improved pregnancy rates with the treatment of sperm with chymotrypsin-galactose prior to conventional oocyte insemination during IVF has been reported to improve pregnancy rates [55], if one is going so far as to do IVF it is probably wiser to just do ICSI than pre-treat the sperm and then do conventional IVF.

The author's IVF center is located in a state where there is a mandate for IVF coverage. However, not all women evaluated are from the state of New Jersey or are covered under the mandate (or possibly were covered but exhausted their insurance coverage). Given the choice of IUI with chymotrypsin-galactose vs. IVF with ICSI after being apprised of our previous success rates with both procedures (higher expectations per cycle for IVF with ICSI) – in data submitted for the 2009 International Congress of Andrology in Barcelona, Spain – we found that there were 258 cycles of IUI with chymotrypsin-galactose-treated sperm vs. 167 cycles of IVF with ICSI over the last 10 years in women aged $\leq$42 whose male partners had >80% of the sperm coated by ASA as determined by the direct IBT. Thus, IUI cycles with pretreated sperm were chosen by a slight majority of couples (60.7%) compared with IVF with ICSI.

These data showed a clinical (gestational sac present, by ultrasound) pregnancy rate of 13.1% per IUI cycle (34/258) with a miscarriage rate of 14.8% (5/34). With IVF and ICSI, the clinical pregnancy rate per embryo transfer was 40.7% (68/167) ($p < 0.01$, chi-square), the miscarriage rate being 19.1% (13/68). These miscarriage rates are slightly higher than our normal rates in this age group with sperm not associated with ASA. Thus, these data suggest that if ASA does influence successful implantation once fertilization takes place the presence of ASA may increase the miscarriage rate only slightly if at all.

Most of the time, ASA do not adversely affect semen parameters [56]. The extra expense of the test is well worth doing this test routinely when performing the initial semen analysis because this abnormality is not that rare and failure to identify this problem could lead to many expensive frustrating treatment cycles that do not offer the couple maximum efficacy.

References

1. Naz RK, Menge AC (1994) Antisperm antibodies: origin, regulation, and sperm reactivity in human infertility. Fertil Steril 61:1001–1013
2. Check JH, Bollendorf A (1992) Effect of antisperm antibodies on postcoital results and effect of intrauterine insemination on pregnancy outcome. Arch Androl 28:25–31
3. Clarke GN (1988) Immunoglobulin class and regional specificity of antispermatozoal autoantibodies blocking cervical mucus penetration by human spermatozoa. Am J Reprod Immunol Microbiol 16:135–138
4. Eggert-Kruse W, Hofsab A, Haury E, Tilgen W, Gerhard I, Runnebaum B (1991) Relationship between local anti-sperm antibodies and sperm–mucus interaction in vitro and in vivo. Hum Reprod 6:267–276
5. Menge AC, Beitner O (1989) Interrelationships among semen characteristics, antisperm antibodies and cervical mucus penetration assays in infertile human couples. Fertil Steril 51: 486–492

6. Steen Y, Forssman L, Lonnerstedt E, Jonasson K, Wassen AC, Lycke E (1994) Anti-sperm IgA antibodies against the equatorial segment of the human spermatozoon are associated with impaired sperm penetration and subfertility. Int J Fertil 39:52–56

7. Fann CH, Lee CYG (1992) Monoclonal antibodies affecting sperm–zona binding and/or zona-induced acrosome reaction. J Reprod Immunol 21:175–187

8. Wolfe JP, DeAlmeida M, Ducot B, Rodrigues D, Jouannet P (1995) High levels of sperm-associated antibodies impair human sperm oolemma interaction after subzonal insemination. Fertil Steril 63:584–590

9. Randoh R, Yamano S, Kamada M, Daitoh T, Aono T (1992) Effect of sperm-immobilizing antibodies on the acrosome reaction of human spermatozoa. Fertil Steril 57:387–392

10. Tasdemir I, Tasdemir M, Fukuda J, Kodama H, Matsui T, Tanaka T (1995) Effect of sperm-immobilizing antibodies on the spontaneous and calcium-ionophore (A23187) induced acrosome reaction. Int J Fertil 40:192–195

11. Liu DY, Clarke GN, Baker HWG (1991) Inhibition of human sperm–zona pellucida and sperm–oolemma binding by antisperm antibodies. Fertil Steril 55:440–442

12. Mahony MC, Alexander NJ (1991) Sites of antisperm antibody action. Hum Reprod 6: 1426–1430

13. Zouari R, De Almeida M (1993) Effect of sperm associated antibodies on human sperm ability to bind to zona pellucida and to penetrate zona-free hamster oocytes. J Reprod Immunol 24:175–186

14. Naz RK (1992) Effects of antisperm antibodies on early cleavage of fertilized ova. Biol Reprod 46:130–139

15. Check JH (1991) The importance of the postcoital test. Am J Obstet Gynecol 164:932

16. Check JH, Nowroozi K, Wu CH, Liss J, Dietterich C (1986) The use of pelvic sonography and serum estradiol and progesterone assays in diagnosis and treatment of cervical factor. Infertility 9:247–256

17. Bronson R, Cooper G, Rosenfeld D (1984) Sperm antibodies: their role in infertility. Fertil Steril 42:171–183

18. Clark GN, Elliott PJ, Smaila C (1985) Detection of sperm antibodies in semen using the immunobead test: a survey of 813 consecutive patients. Am J Reprod Immunol 7:118–123

19. Hendry WF, Stedronska J (1980) Mixed erythrocyte-spermatozoa antiglobulin reaction (MAR Test) for the detection of antibodies against spermatozoa in infertile males. J Obstet Gynecol 1:59–62

20. Jager S, Kremer J, van Slochteren-Draaisma T (1978) A simple method of screening for anti-sperm antibodies in the human male. Int J Fertil 23:12–21

21. Agarwal A (1992) Treatment of immunological infertility by sperm washing and intrauterine insemination. Arch Androl 29:207–213

22. Windt ML, Menkveld R, Kruger TF, van der Merwe JP, Lombard CJ (1989) Effect of rapid dilution of semen on sperm-bound autoantibodies. Arch Androl 22:227–231

23. Bollendorf A, Check JH, Katsoff D, Fedele A (1994) The use of chymotrypsin/galactose to treat spermatozoa bound with anti-sperm antibodies prior to intra-uterine insemination. Hum Reprod 9:484–488

24. Bronson RA, Cooper GW, Rosenfeld DL, Gilbert JV, Plaut AG (1987) The effect of an IgA protease on immunoglobulins bound to the sperm surface and sperm cervical mucus penetrating ability. Fertil Steril 47:985–991

25. Kutteh WH, Kilian M, Ermel LD, Mosteck YT (1995) Antisperm antibodies in infertile women: subclass distribution of immunoglobulins (Ig) A antibodies and removal of IgA sperm-bound antibodies with a specific IgA1 protease. Fertil Steril 63:63–70

26. Menge AC, Christman GM, Ohl DA, Naz RK (1999) Fertilization antigen-1 removes anti-sperm autoantibodies from spermatozoa of infertile men and results in increased rates of acrosome reaction. Fertil Steril 71:256–260

27. Check JH, Bollendorf A, Wilson C, Summers-Chase D, Horwath D, Yuan W (2007) A retrospective comparison of pregnancy outcome following conventional oocyte insemination vs. intracytoplasmic sperm injection for isolated abnormalities in sperm morphology using strict criteria. J Androl 28:607–612

28. Vujisic S, Lepej SZ, Jerovic L, Emedi I, Sokolic B (2005) Antisperm antibodies in semen, sera and follicular fluids of infertile patients: Relation to reproductive outcome after in vitro fertilization. Am J Reprod Immunol 54:13–20

29. Mandelbaum SL, Diamond SP, DeCherney AH (1987) Relationship of antisperm antibodies to oocyte fertilization in in vitro fertilization-embryo transfer. Fertil Steril 47:644–651

30. Junk SM, Matson PL, Yovich JM (1986) The fertilization of human oocyte by spermatozoa from men with antispermatozoal antibodies in semen. J In Vitro Fert Embryo Transf 3:350–352

31. Sukcharoen N, Keith J (1995) The effect of the antisperm auto-antibody-bound sperm on in vitro fertilization outcome. Andrologia 27:281–289

32. Acosta AA, van der Merwe JP, Doncel G et al (1994) Fertilization efficiency of morphologically abnormal spermatozoa in associated reproduction is further impaired by antisperm antibodies on the male partner's sperm. Fertil Steril 62:826–833

33. Chang TH, Jih MH, Wu TC (1993) Relationship of sperm antibodies in women and men to human in vitro fertilization, cleavage, and pregnancy rate. Am J Reprod Immunol 30:108–112

34. DeAlmeida M, Gazagne I, Jeulin C et al (1989) In-vitro processing of sperm with autoantibodies and in vitro fertilization results. Hum Reprod 4:49–53

35. Lahteenmaki A (1993) In vitro fertilization in the presence of antisperm antibodies detected by the mixed antiglobulin reaction, MAR, and the tray agglutination test, TAT. Hum Reprod 8:84–88

36. Matson PL, Junk SM, Spittle JW et al (1988) Effects of antisperm antibodies in seminal plasma upon sperm function. Int J Androl 11:101–106

37. Rajah SV, Parslow J, Howell RJ et al (1993) The effects on in vitro fertilization of autoantibodies to spermatozoa in subfertile men. Hum Reprod 8:1079–1082

38. Check ML, Check JH, Katsoff D, Summers-Chase D (2000) ICSI as an effective therapy for male factor with antisperm antibodies. Arch Androl 45:125–130

39. Clarke GN, Bourne M, Baker HWG (1997) Intracytoplasmic sperm injection for treating infertility associated with sperm autoimmunity. Fertil Steril 68:112–117

40. Lahteenmaki A, Reima I, Hovatta O (1995) Tretment of severe male immunological infertility by intracytoplasmic sperm injection. Hum Reprod 10:2824–2828

41. Nagy ZP, Verheyen G, Liu J et al (1995) Results of 55 intracytoplasmic sperm injection cycles in the treatment of male-immunological infertility. Hum Reprod 10:1775–1780

42. Check JH, Bollendorf A, Katsoff D, Kozak J (1994) The frequency of antisperm antibodies in the cervical mucus of women with poor postcoital tests and their effect on pregnancy rates. Am J Reprod Immunol 32:38–42

43. Check JH, Nowroozi K, Adelson HG, Bollendorf A, Chern R, Press M (1990) An in vivo technique for screening immunologic factors in the etiology of the unexplained poor postcoital test. Int J Fertil 35:215–221

44. Haas GG Jr, Cines DB, Schreiber AD (1980) Immunologic infertility: identification of patients with antisperm antibodies. N Engl J Med 303:722–727

45. Pattinson HA, Mortimer D (1987) Prevalence of sperm surface antibodies in the male partners of infertile couples as determined by immunobead screening. Fertil Steril 48:466–469

46. Nip MMC, Taylor PV, Rutherford AJ, Hancock KW (1995) Autoantibodies and antisperm antibodies in sera and follicular fluids of infertile patients: relation to reproductive outcome after in vitro fertilization. Hum Reprod 10:2564–2569

47. Daitoh T, Kamada M, Yamano S, Murayama S, Kobayashi T, Maegawa M (1995) High implantation rate and consequently high pregnancy rate by in vitro fertilization-embryo transfer treatment in infertile women with antisperm antibody. Fertil Steril 63:87–91

48. Clarke GN, Lopata A, McBain JC, Baker HW, Johnston WI (1985) Effect of sperm antibodies in males on human in vitro fertilization (IVF). Am J Reprod Immunol Microbiol 8:62–66

49. Yeh WR, Acosta AA, Seltman HJ, Doncel G (1995) Impact of immunoglobulin isotype and sperm surface location of antisperm antibodies and fertilization rates in-vitro in the human. Fertil Steril 63:1287–1292

50. Bronson RA, Cooper GW, Rosenfeld DL (1982) Sperm-specific isoantibodies and autoantibodies inhibit the binding of human sperm to the human zona pellucida. Fertil Steril 38:724–729

51. Mahony MC, Blackmore PF, Bronson RA, Alexander NJ (1991) Inhibition of human sperm-zona pellucida tight binding in the presence of antisperm antibody positive polyclonal patient sera. J Reprod Immunol 19:287–301

52. Ford WC, Williams KM, McLaughlin EA, Harrison S, Ray B, Hull MG (1996) The indirect immunobead test for seminal antisperm antibodies and fertilization rates at in-vitro fertilization. Hum Reprod 11:1418–1422

53. Domagala A, Pulido S, Kurpisz M, Herr JC (2007) Application of proteomic methods for identification of sperm immunogenic antigens. Mol Hum Reprod 13:437–444

54. Francavilla F, Santucci R, Barbonetti A, Francavilla S (2007) Naturally-occurring antisperm antibodies in men: interference with fertility and clinical implications. An update. Front Biosci 12:2890–2911

55. Katsoff D, Check JH, Bollendorf A, Benfer K (1995) Chymotrypsin-galactose treatment of sperm with anitsperm antibodies results in improved pregnancy rates following in vitro fertilization. Am J Reprod Immunol 33:149–154

56. Check JH, Adelson HG, Bollendorf A (1991) Effect of antisperm antibodies on computerized semen analysis. Arch Androl 27:61–63

Treatment of Immune Infertility

3.5

Rajesh K. Naz

3.5.1
Discussion

Antisperm antibodies (ASA) can cause infertility. The incidence of antisperm immunity in infertile couples is 9–36%, depending on the reporting center [1–4]. ASA reactive with sperm antigens that are involved in fertilization and expressed on the surface for antibody binding are more relevant to infertility. Also, these antibodies have to be present in the genital tract secretions of a female partner or bound on the sperm surface in a male partner in sufficient amount to cause infertility effects. The kinetics, valency, and class/subclass of antibodies play an important role in defining the significance of ASA in infertility.

Although there are several articles written on various aspects of immunoinfertility, there are only a few covering the therapeutic treatment modalities for male and female immune infertility. The aim of this chapter is to review the conventional treatment methods for immune infertility, discuss their relative merits and limitations, and describe the recent novel perspectives that are being investigated.

3.5.2
Treatment of Immune Infertility

Although the understanding of etiology of ASA has increased, the therapeutic measures have not made the same strides [5]. Various treatment methods available at present can be divided broadly into four categories: immunosuppressive therapies, assisted reproductive technologies (ART), laboratory techniques, and novel recent perspectives using defined sperm antigens.

R. K. Naz
Center for Research in Reproductive Sciences (CRRS), West Virginia University, School of Medicine, 2085 Robert C. Byrd Health Sciences Center North, Morgantown, WV, USA
e-mail: Rnaz@hsc.wvu.edu

W. K. H. Krause and R. K. Naz (eds.), *Immune Infertility*,
DOI: 10.1007/978-3-642-01379-9_3.5, © Springer Verlag Berlin Heidelberg 2009

3.5.2.1
Immunosuppressive Therapies

The method of immunosuppression that has been most commonly used is corticosteroid therapy. Pregnancy rates of 6–50% have been reported after corticosteroid therapy [6]. However, almost all the studies reported in the literature for the effect of steroid treatment on immunosuppression of ASA titers lack appropriate placebo controls, have employed different doses and regimens of various immunosuppressive drugs, and have used different laboratory techniques to monitor the ASA titers to examine the effect of drug treatment. These factors make it difficult to compare and conclude whether or not immunosuppression is effective in the treatment of immunoinfertility.

Two of the clinical trials had appropriate placebo controls and are worth describing here. One study conducted a 6-month randomized trial using high dose of prednisolone given through cycle days 1–10 of the female partner, which was then tapered rapidly for the next 2 days [7]. The steroid treatment group resulted in a pregnancy rate of 31% compared with 9% in the placebo group. Another prospective, double-blind, placebo-controlled study included 43 men who had ASA bound to sperm [8]. Of these, 24 were given methylprednisolone and 19 received placebo for three cycles. There was a statistically significant decrease in sperm-associated IgG, but not IgA, in the steroid treatment group and not in the placebo group. However, in spite of decrease in the antibody titer, there was no statistically significant difference in pregnancy outcome between the two groups.

The efficacy of steroid treatment, if any, must be judged against the potential adverse effects. The steroid therapy could cause several side effects [9]. The potential adverse effects and lack of effectiveness in many cases have decreased the enthusiasm for use of steroids for the treatment of immunologic infertility. As an alternative, cyclosporine was tested in a cohort of men with ASA. After treatment, a pregnancy rate of 33% was observed [10]. Since this study did not have placebo controls, no definite conclusions can be drawn.

3.5.2.2
Assisted Reproductive Technologies (ART)

Recently ART have been used to treat ASA. Several studies have examined the use of intrauterine insemination (IUI), gamete intrafallopian transfer (GIFT), in vitro fertilization (IVF), and intracytoplasmic sperm injection (ICSI) procedures for the treatment of immune infertility in men and women as discussed below.

3.5.2.2.1
IUI Procedure

IUI has been found to be useful for the treatment of ASA-positive infertile men and women. Theoretically, it should circumvent problems related to sperm transport in the female genital tract, especially sperm passage through the cervical canal/mucus. However, in women having ASA in the cervical mucus, pregnancy rates after IUI were identical to women who did not have ASA, if the male partner did not have ASA or male factor infertility [11]. In two other studies of female sperm immunity, IUI treatment did not increase the pregnancy rates per couple or per cycle [12, 13]. However, the pregnancy outcome significantly improved after including the ovarian hyperstimulation treatment along with IUI.

IUI also has been found to enhance pregnancy rates in some cases of ASA-positive infertile men. A 56% pregnancy rate has been reported after IUI procedure in ASA-positive infertile men, who had a poor postcoital test, compared with an 83% pregnancy rate in ASA-negative infertile men, who also had a poor postcoital test [14]. In another study, after IUI the pregnancy outcomes in 19 couples having male immune infertility were compared with 86 couples having other diagnoses. No pregnancy was seen in 110 IUIs in the ASA-positive group (0%) vs. a 26% pregnancy rate per couple and 5.6% cycle fecundity in the control group [15]. From the Cleveland Clinic Foundation, Agarwal compared 42 ASA-positive couples with 117 ASA-negative infertile couples who were treated with sperm washing and IUI over a 2-year period [16]. There were 15 pregnancies in the ASA-positive group compared with 37 for the entire group.

Another study compared IUI with oral steroid therapy [17]. This study included 46 couples in which the male partner had ASA. The immune infertile men received either 20 mg/day of prednisolone for days 1–10 followed by 5 mg/day for days 11 and 12 of the cycle and timed intercourse, or underwent IUI with no steroid treatment for three cycles. The couple was switched to the other group if not pregnant. The pregnancy rate before switching for the IUI group was 16.7%, and for the steroid group was 0%. After switching, one more pregnancy occurred in the IUI group and one in the steroid group. This study concluded that IUI is better than low-dose steroid therapy for treating male immune infertility.

It is not clear, theoretically speaking, how IUI can circumvent male immune infertility. Washing the sperm in the incubation medium should not elute the antibodies bound to the sperm surface proteins, unless a) these antibodies are directed against the adsorbed seminal plasma proteins that are shed off during capacitation/acrosome reaction, b) the antibodies are of low binding affinity, which does not seem to be the case in immunoinfertilty, and/or c) the swim-up sperm used for IUI are not coated with antibodies such as non-swim-up sperm, which also seems highly unlikely.

There are mixed reports on simple sperm washing on ASA elution from various laboratories. Adeghe [18] found that washing decreased IgG bound on the sperm surface. Another group [19] did not find the similar positive effects, nor did Haas et al. [20] even after subjecting the sperm to multiple washings. Antibodies were also not reduced by passing sperm through percoll gradient [21].

3.5.2.2.2
GIFT Procedure

In GIFT procedure, sperm and eggs are mixed in vitro and then transferred to the fallopian tubes for fertilization. Theoretically speaking, there is not a strong rationale to how it will help either the ASA-positive infertile men or women. Nevertheless, in one study, GIFT was performed in 16 immune infertile couples. This group achieved pregnancy rates of

43% per couple and 24% per cycle [22]. This study did not include any control group, and the pregnancy rates are comparable to those that are reported after GIFT in patients having other etiologies.

3.5.2.2.3
IVF Procedure

Several studies have shown decreased rates of oocyte fertilization in IVF in immune infertile patients [23]. An inverse relationship between ASA titers and fertilization rates has been reported [24]. In a study, 33 ASA-positive infertile couples were subjected to 47 IVF cycles [25]. The couples with high ASA titers had lower fertilization rates than those with lower ASA titers. In contrast, there are also studies that found fertilization to be identical in ASA-positive and ASA-negative populations [26]. Interestingly, there are also studies reporting increased rates of IVF outcome including implantation and pregnancy rates in ASA-positive infertile women compared to women with tubal factor infertility [27]. In IVF procedure, generally albumin, instead of female partner's serum, is used as a protein source in the insemination medium that circumvents the antibodies if present in the female partner. Thus, theoretically speaking, IVF can take care of female but not male immune infertility. Fertilization and pregnancies have been achieved using oocytes from ASA-positive infertile women where the men had normal semen analysis, and were free of ASA [28, 29]. In ASA-positive infertile men, both the class/subclass specificity and subcellular localization of the antibodies on sperm have been correlated with various degrees of fertilization failure rates in IVF [4]. ASA that bind to the sperm head may decrease fertilization more than ASA bound to midpiece or tail regions of the sperm cell. In the IVF procedures involving immunoinfertile couples, it was found that the couples who had ASA bound to the head region of the sperm cell showed more fertilization failure than those having ASA bound to the tail region. Yeh et al. [30] reported that IgA significantly reduces fertilization rates in IVF procedure only when it was associated with IgM and was present on the sperm head. Equality of embryos obtained after IVF using sperm from ASA-positive men is generally poor compared to sperm from ASA-negative men [31, 32].

3.5.2.2.4
ICSI Procedure

IVF with ICSI have become a routine and widely acceptable procedure in the clinics. In the ICSI procedure, a single sperm is injected into the cytoplasm of the oocyte. ICSI has been tried using sperm of ASA-positive infertile men. Two of these studies are worth mentioning here. One study subjected 29 infertile ASA-positive couples to ICSI; 22 of them were tested before in IVF procedure and had poor fertilization rate (6%) [31]. After ICSI, the fertilization (79%) and cleavage (89%) rates in the ASA-positive group were similar to those (68 and 93%, respectively) in the ASA-negative group. Surprisingly, 46% of the pregnancies in the ASA-positive group ended in spontaneous pregnancy loss compared with none in the ASA-negative group. In contrast, another study did not demonstrate any difference in pregnancy rates (30%) between the ASA-positive and ASA-negative groups undergoing ICSI procedure [30].

Some ASA can have deleterious postfertilization effects on developing preimplantation embryos [33–36]. ASA can affect early embryonic development if (a) an oocyte is fertilized with a sperm cell, which carries these specific antibodies into the ooplasm and/or (b) these antibodies are cross-reactive with the antigens present on the developing embryos. Some of these antigens and antibodies have been characterized and the cDNA encoding for a few of these antigens has also been cloned and sequenced [37]. Using the ICSI procedure in immunoinfertile men, one can achieve higher fertilization rates than using the IVF procedure; however, the fertilized zygotes show higher degeneration and mortality, and decreased embryonic development.

3.5.2.3
Laboratory Techniques

Several innovative laboratory techniques have been investigated and can broadly be classified into two categories: (1) methods that prevent binding of ASA to sperm or elute the bound ASA from sperm surface and (2) methods that separate ASA-free sperm from ASA-coated sperm. Although these methods have been explored extensively, owing to conflicting findings, these techniques have not been accepted as the methods for treatment in the clinics. Some of these reports and their findings are discussed below.

It was erroneously thought that ASA bind to sperm during and/or just after ejaculation and the antibodies are mostly present in the secretions of prostate and seminal vesicles. On the basis of this notion, the antibodies and the sperm are present and ejaculated in different fractions of the semen. To avoid binding of antibodies to sperm, splitting the semen into various fractions during ejaculation were attempted in various laboratories. However, it has been proven ineffective in decreasing ASA binding to sperm [38]. Collection of semen into insemination medium containing high concentrations of fetal cord/ maternal serum has also been investigated to examine if it would decrease the antibody binding to sperm. Two studies [39, 40] observed that semen collection into serum-supplemented medium results in increased fertilization rates in IVF procedure, and one of these studies also showed an increase in pregnancy rates. We conducted a study to investigate at which site of the male genital tract the antibodies percolate from serum to bind to sperm [41]. I^{125}-labeled antibodies to sperm-specific FA-1 antigen were injected intravenously into male mice. The results indicate that the antibodies preferentially transude into epididymis (especially corpus or caudal regions) and vas deferens to bind to sperm cells and not into testes. These findings indicate that in men ASA bind to sperm before ejaculation via transudation through epididymis, vas deferens, and probably rete testis.

The immunomagnetic separation technique has been tried to separate the antibodies bound on the sperm surface [42]. The sperm with antibodies are tagged with anti-immunoglobulin antibodies coupled to magnetic microspheres, and then magnetic field is applied. However, limited success in isolating sufficient number of ASA-free sperm of good motility makes this procedure theoretically interesting but clinically unacceptable.

Bronson suggested that protease treatment may be utilized to destroy antibodies on the sperm surface [43]. Kutteh and associates reported that IgA1 protease treatment was effective in reducing IgA on sperm [44]. In another study, incubation of sperm with chymotrypsin before IUI resulted in a 25% cycle fecundity vs. 3% in controls [45]. However, this needs to be examined whether or not the treatment with proteolytic enzymes affect proteins, especially the oocyte binding receptors present on the sperm surface.

The use of immunobeads has been suggested as a treatment to remove the sperm-bound antibodies. It has been reported that simple incubation of ASA-positive sperm from immunoinfertile men with immunobeads results in a time-dependent decrease in antibody concentration on sperm surface [46], and even enhanced pregnancies [47]. The explanation that the antibodies are removed from the sperm surface after incubation with immunobeads is not widely accepted, and it is generally believed that the immunobeads just select ASA-positive sperm, leaving ASA-free sperm. Theoretically, there is not a strong rationale why and how incubation with immunobeads should elute antibodies from sperm surface.

3.5.2.4
Novel Recent Perspectives Using Defined Sperm Antigens

Several sperm antigens have been defined from various laboratories that may be involved in fertilization and fertility [48]. Our laboratory showed that one of these, namely fertilization antigen-1 (FA-1) is an exciting molecule because it is involved in human immunoinfertility, and thus will be discussed here.

3.5.2.4.1
Immunoelution of Antibodies with FA-1 Antigen

FA-1 antigen is a well-defined novel sperm-specific surface molecule that is evolutionarily conserved on sperm of various mammalian species including humans [49]. Antibodies to FA-1 antigen inhibit human sperm–zona interaction and also block human sperm capacitation/ acrosome reaction by inhibiting tyrosine phosphorylation [50]. The cDNA encoding for mouse FA-1 and human FA-1 have been cloned and sequenced [51, 52] and vaccination of female mice with recombinant FA-1 antigen causes a long-term reversible contraception by raising sperm-specific immune response [53].

FA-1 antigen is involved in human immunoinfertility in both men and women. The antibodies are found in sera as circulating antibodies and also locally in genital tract secretions, such as seminal plasma of men and cervical mucus and vaginal secretions of women [54, 55]. The lymphocytes from immunoinfertile but not fertile men and women are sensitized against FA-1 antigen and proliferate upon incubation with the antigen in vitro [56]. The presence of these antibodies inhibits fertilization in the IVF procedure. The involvement of FA-1 antigen in human involuntary immunoinfertility has been confirmed in several laboratories by leading investigators working in the field of antisperm antibodies. On the basis of these findings, a clinical trial was conducted at the University of Michigan Medical School to determine whether immunoadsorption with the human sperm FA-1 antigen would remove autoantibodies from the surface of sperm cells of immunoinfertile men and thus increase their fertilizing capacity [57]. Adsorption with FA-1 antigen increased immunobead-free swimming sperm on an average of 50% and 76% for IgA and IgG antisperm antibodies, respectively. The acrosome reaction rates increased significantly and showed improvement in 78% of the sperm samples after FA-1 adsorption. The IUI of FA-1-treated antibody-free sperm resulted in normal pregnancies and healthy babies, indicating that the antigen treatment does not have a deleterious effect on implantation, and embryonic and fetal development. This study needs to be extended to a larger number of ASA-positive infertile men and constitutes an exciting therapeutic modality using well-defined sperm antigens.

3.5.3
Conclusion

In conclusion, although various methods have been tried, none have provided a satisfactory means of treating immune infertility. Almost all the methods have yielded contradictory results, with the findings of one clinic reporting a positive outcome and another contradicting it. This may be due to how immune infertility was defined in one clinic vs, another. As discussed earlier, any immunoglobulin that binds to sperm should not be defined as "antisperm" antibody unless it has a functional significance. This, along with the kinetics, valencey, titer, class/subclass, and circulating/ local nature of the immunoglobulin, plays an important role in defining the significance of ASA in the immunoinfertility. The ASA present in a female partner may be bypassed by ART such as IVF/ ICSI procedures. However, embryos obtained after IVF are of poor quality and there are more spontaneous abortions/miscarriages after ICSI using sperm from ASA-positive men in several studies. The sperm-bound antibodies present in a male partner are difficult to be removed even by invasive and expensive reproductive technologies. The antibodies have to be of low affinity to elute them from the sperm surface by simple washing techniques. The developing knowledge of local immunity and sperm antigens that have a role in fertility will help to better define immunoinfertility and develop better methods for treatment. The animal models as discussed above constructed using defined sperm antigens will help to elucidate the mechanisms involved in the physiology and pathophysiology of immunoinfertility and may assist to solve the controversy and confusion regarding the significance of ASA in infertility and in the development of novel treatment modalities.

Acknowledgments   This work was supported by NIH grant HD24425 to RKN. The excellent typing assistance provided by Sarah Davis is gratefully acknowledged.

References

1. Ayvaliotis B, Bronson R, Rosenfeld D et al (1985) Conception rates in couples where autoimmunity to sperm is detected. Fertil Steril 43:739–742
2. Collins JA, Burrows EA, Yeo J et al (1993) Frequency and predictive value of antisperm antibodies among infertile couples. Hum Reprod 8:592–598

3. Menge AC, Medley NE, Mangione CM et al (1982) The incidence and influence of antisperm antibodies in infertile human couples on sperm-cervical mucus interactions and subsequent fertility. Fertil Steril 38:439–446

4. Ohl D, Naz RK (1995) Infertility due to antisperm antibodies. J Urol 46:591–602

5. Naz RK (2004) Modalities for treatment of antisperm antibody mediated infertility: novel perspectives. Am J Reprod Immunol 51:390–397

6. Turek PJ, Lipshultz LI (1994) Immunologic infertility. Urol Clin North Am 21:447–468

7. Hendry WF, Hughes L, Scammell G et al (1990) Comparison of prednisolone and placebo in subfertile men with antibodies the spermatozoa. Lancet 335:85–88

8. Haas GG Jr, Manganiello P (1997) A double-blind, placebo-controlled study of these of methyl-prednisolone in infertile men with sperm-associated immunoglobulins. Fertil Steril 47:295–301

9. Pearce G, Tabensky DA, Delmas PD et al (1998) Corticosteroid-induced bone loss in men. J Clin Endocrinol Metab 83:801–806

10. Bouloux PM, Wass JA, Parslow JM et al (1986) Effect of cyclosporine A in male autoimmune infertility. Fertil Steril 46:81–85

11. Check JH, Bollendorf A, Katsoff D et al (1994) The frequency of antisperm antibodies in the cervical mucus of women with poor postcoital tests and their effect on pregnancy rates. Am J Reprod Immunol 32:38–42

12. Gregoriou O, Vitoratos N, Papdias C et al (1991) Intrauterine insemination as a treatment of infertility in women with antisperm antibodies. Int J Gynecol Obstet 35:151–156

13. Margalloth EJ, Sauter E, Bronson RA et al (1988) Intrauterine insemination as treatment for antisperm antibodies in the female. Fertil Steril 50:441–446

14. Check JH, Bollendorf A (1992) Effect of antisperm antibodies on postcoital results and effect of intrauterine insemination on pregnancy outcome. Arch Androl 28:25–31

15. Francavilla F, Romano R, Santucci R et al (1992) Failure of intrauterine insemination in male immunolocial infertility in cases in which all spermatozoa are antibody-coated. Fertil Steril 58:587–592

16. Agarwal A (1992) Treatment of immunological infertility by sperm washing and intrauterine insemination. Arch Androl 29:207–213

17. Lahteenmaki A, Veilahti J, Hovatta O (1995) Intra-uterine insemination versus cyclic, low-dose prednisolone in couples with male antisperm antibodies. Hum Reprod 10:142–147

18. Adeghe AJ (1987) Effect of washing on sperm surface autoantibodies. Br J Urol 60:360–363

19. Windt ML, Menkveld R, Kruger TF et al (1989) Effect of sperm washing and swim-up on antibodies bound to sperm membrane: use of immunobead/sperm cervical mucus contact tests. Arch Androl 22:55–59

20. Haas GG, D'Cruz OJ, Denum BM (1988) Effect of repeated washing on sperm-bound immunoglobulin G. J Androl 9:190–196

21. Almagor M, Margalioth EJ, Yaffe H (1992) Density differences between spermatozoa with antisperm autoantibodies and spermatozoa covered with antisperm antibodies from serum. Hum Reprod 7:959–961

22. Van der Merwe JP, Kruger TF, Windt ML et al (1990) Treatment of male sperm autoimmunity by using the gamete intrafallopian transfer procedure with washed spermatozoa. Fertil Steril 53:682–687

23. Junk SM, Matson PL, Yovich JM et al (1986) The fertilization of human oocytes by spermatozoa from men with antispermatozoal antibodies in semen. J In Vitro Fertil Embryo Transf 3:350–352

24. Ford WCL, Williams KM, McLaughlin EA et al (1996) The indirect immunobead test for seminal antisperm antibodies and fertilization rates at in-vitro fertilization. Hum Reprod 11:1418–1422

25. Lahteenmaki A (1993) In-vitro fertilization in the presence of antisperm antibodies detected by the mixed antiglobulin reaction (MAR) and the tray agglutination test (TAT). Hum Reprod 8:84–88

26. de Almeida M, Herry M, Testart J et al (1987) In-vitro fertilization results from thirteen women with anti-sperm antibodies. Hum Reprod 2:599–602
27. Daitoh T, Kamada M, Yamano S et al (1995) High implantation rate and consequently high pregnancy rate by in vitro fertilization-embryo transfer treatment in infertile women with antisperm antibody. Fertil Steril 63:87–91
28. Acosta AA, Van Der Merwe JP, Doncel G et al (1994) Fertilization efficiency of morphologically abnormal spermatozoa in assisted reproduction is further impaired by antisperm antibodies on the male partner's sperm. Fertil Steril 62:826–833
29. Zouari R, DeAlmeida M, Rodrigues D et al (1993) Localization of antibodies on spermatozoa and sperm movement characteristics are good predictors of in vitro fertilization success in cases of male autoimmune infertility. Fertil Steril 59:606–612
30. Yeh WR, Acosta A, Seltman HJ et al (1995) Impact of immunoglobulin isotype and sperm surface location of antisperm antibodies on fertilization in vitro in the human. Fertil Steril 62:826–833
31. Lahteenmaki A, Reima I, Hovatta O (1995) Treatment of severe male immunological infertility by intracytoplasmic sperm injection. Hum Reprod 10:2824–2828
32. Lombardo F, Gandini L, Dondero F et al (2001) Antisperm immunity in natural and assisted reproduction. Hum Reprod Update 7:450–456
33. Ahmad K, Naz RK (1991) Antibodies to sperm surface antigens and the c-myc proto-oncogene product inhibit early embryonic development in mice. Biol Reprod 45:814–850
34. Ahmad K, Naz RK (1992) Effects of human antisperm antibodies on development of preimplantation embryos. Arch Androl 29:9–20
35. Menge AC, Naz RK (1988) Immunologic reactions involving sperm cells and preimplantation embryos. Am J Reprod Immunol Microbiol 18:17–20
36. Naz RK (1992) Effects of antisperm antibodies on early cleavage of fertilized ova. Biol Reprod 46:130–139
37. Javed AA, Naz RK (1992) Human cleavage signal-1 protein: cDNA cloning, transcription and immunological analysis. Gene 112:205–211
38. Lenzi A, Gandini L, Claroni F et al (1988) Immunological usefulness of semen manipulation for artificial insemination homologous (AIH) in subjects with antisperm antibodies bound to sperm surface. Andrologia 20:314–321
39. Byrd W, Kutteh WH, Carr BR (1994) Treatment of antibody-associated sperm with media containing high serum content: a prospective trial of fertility involving men with high antisperm antibodies following intrauterine insemination. Am J Reprod Immunol 31:84–90
40. Elder KT, Wick KL, Edwards RG (1990) Seminal plasma anti-sperm antibodies and IVF: the effect of semen sample collection into 50% serum. Hum Reprod 5:179–184
41. Naz RK, Bhargava KK (1990) Antibodies to sperm surface fertilization antigen (FA-1): their specificities and site of interaction with sperm in male genital tract. Mol Reprod Dev 26:175–183
42. Foresta C, Varotto A, Caretto A (1990) Immunomagnetic method to select human sperm without sperm surface-bound autoantibodies in male autoimmune infertility. Arch Androl 24:221–225
43. Bronson RA, Cooper GW, Rosenfeld DL et al (1987) The effect of an IgA1 protease on immunoglobulins bound to the sperm surface and sperm cervical mucus penetrating ability. Fertil Steril 47:985–991
44. Kutteh WH, Kilian M, Ermel LD et al (1994) Antisperm antibodies (ASAs) in infertile males: subclass distribution of IgA antibodies and the effect of an IgA1 protease on sperm-bound antibodies. Am J Reprod Immunol 31:77–83
45. Bollendorf A, Check JH, Katsoff D et al (1994) The use of chymotrypsin/ galactose to treat spermatozoa bound with anti-sperm antibodies prior to intra-uterine insemination. Hum Reprod 9:484–488

46. Gould JE, Brazil CK, Overstreet JW (1994) Sperm immunobead binding decreases with in vitro incubation. Fertil Steril 62:167–171

47. Grundy CE, Robinson J, Guthrie KA et al (1992) Establishment of pregnancy after removal of sperm antibodies in vitro. Br Med J 304:292–293

48. Naz RK (2002) Molecular and immunological characteristics of sperm antigens involved in egg binding. J Reprod Immunol 53:13–23

49. Naz RK, Alexander NJ, Isahakia M et al (1984) Monoclonal antibody to a human sperm membrane glycoprotein that inhibits fertilization. Science 225:342–344

50. Naz RK, Ahmad K, Kumar R (1991) Role of membrane phosphotyrosine proteins in human spermatozoal function. J Cell Sci 99:157–165

51. Naz RK, Zhu X (2002) Molecular cloning and sequencing of cDNA encoding for human FA-1 antigen. Mol Reprod Dev 63:256–268

52. Zhu X, Naz RK (1997) Fertilization antigen-1: cDNA cloning, testis-specific expression, and immunocontraceptive effects. Proc Natl Acad Sci USA 94:4704–4709

53. Naz RK, Zhu X (1998) Recombinant fertilization antigen-1 causes a contraceptive effect in actively immunized mice. Biol Reprod 59:1095–1100

54. Menge AC, Naz RK (1988) Immunoglobulin (Ig) G, IgA, and IgA subclass antibodies against fertilization antigen-1 in cervical secretions and sera of women of infertile couples. Fertil Steril 60:658–663

55. Naz RK (1987) Involvement of fertilization antigen (FA-1) in involuntary immunoinfertility in humans. J Clin Invest 80:1375–1383

56. Naz RK, Chaudhry A, Witkin SS (1990) Lymphocyte proliferative response to fertilization antigen in patients with antisperm antibodies. Am J Obstet Gynecol 163:610–613

57. Menge AC, Ohl DA, Naz RK et al (1999) Fertilization antigen (FA-1) removes antisperm autoantibodies from sperm of infertile men resulting in increased rates of acrosome reaction. Fertil Steril 71:256–260

Section IV

Immune Contraception

Immunization with Sperm Antigens to Induce Contraception

4.1

4.1.1
Introduction

There are several limited options available for contraception [1–4]. Besides the availability of these contraceptive methods, the world population has exceeded 6.67 billion and will grow by 1 billion every 12 years at the current rate [5]. Also, the unintended pregnancies continue to impose a major public health issue. In the U.S. alone, half the pregnancies are unintended which result in over 1 million elective abortions each year [6, 7]. In over half of these unintended pregnancies, the women were using some method of contraception. The 2004 Institute of Medicine (IOM) report indicates that between 1995 and 2000 more than one quarter of 1.2 billion pregnancies were unwanted [8]. Thus, there is an urgent need for a better method of contraception that is reversible, nonsteroidal, nonbarrier, intercourse-independent, acceptable, and effective. An ideal contraceptive method should be highly effective, safe, and inexpensive, have a prolonged duration of action, be rapidly reversible, easily accessible, require infrequent administration, and can be used privately [1]. A contraceptive vaccine (CV) can fulfill most of these properties of an ideal contraceptive. The development of a vaccine for contraception is an exciting proposition because the developed and most of the developing nations have an infrastructure for mass immunization.

Various targets have been explored for the development of a CV. These can broadly fall in three categories: vaccines inhibiting gamete production (gonadotropin releasing hormone (GnRH), follicle-stimulating hormone (FSH), and lueteinizing hormone, (LH)), gamete function (Zona pellucida (ZP) proteins and sperm antigens), or gamete outcome (human chorionic gonadotropin (hCG)) [9, 10]. GnRH based vaccines are effective in several species and can be used for both males and females. However, they are not acceptable for human use because they affect sex steroids causing impotency. They have been

R. K. Naz
Centre for Research in Reproductive Sciences (CRRS), West Virginia University, School of Medicine, Robert C. Byrd Health Sciences Center North, Morgantown, WV, USA
e-mail: Rnaz@hsc.wvu.edu

W. K. H. Krause and R. K. Naz (eds.), *Immune Infertility*,
DOI: 10.1007/978-3-642-01379-9_4.1, © Springer Verlag Berlin Heidelberg 2009

197

taken over by pharmaceutical companies for fertility control in domestic pets, farm, and wild animals, and for noncontraceptive purposes such as prostatic hypertrophy and carcinoma [11, 12]. FSH-based vaccines can inhibit spermatogenesis in males of several species and can potentially provide a male contraceptive. However, they cause oligospermia rather than azoospermia [13]. LH/LH receptor-based vaccines are effective in both males and females [14, 15]. However, they affect sex steroids, so are not acceptable for humans. Thus, disadvantages of CVs targeting gamete production are that they affect sex steroids and/or show only a partial effect in reducing fertility. CVs targeting gamete functions are better choices. Vaccines based on ZP proteins are quite efficacious in producing contraceptive effects [16]. However, they induce oophoritis which affects sex steroids [17]. They have been successfully used for controlling wild and zoo animals such as deer, horses, elephants, and dogs [18]. Sperm antigens constitute a promising and exciting target for CVs and at the present time no disadvantages are known. Vaccines targeting gamete outcome primarily focus on the hCG molecule. The hCG-based vaccines have undergone phase I and II clinical trials in women and demonstrated efficacy and lack of immunopathology [19]. However, there is variability of immune response among vaccinated women. The present article will focus on the development of CV based upon sperm antigens.

4.1.2
Discussion

4.1.2.1
Rationale for Sperm Vaccine Development

There is a strong rationale for the development of a sperm based vaccine. Sperm are immunogenic in both males and females. Immunization of several species of animals and humans with sperm/testis preparations develop antisperm antibodies (ASA) leading to infertility [20, 21]. In 1932, Baskin injected 20 fertile women, who had at least one prior pregnancy, with their husband's sperm [22]. These women developed ASA and no conception was reported for up to 1 year of observation. A U.S. patent was issued for this spermatoxic vaccine in 1937 (US patent number 2103240). Over 70% of men develop ASA after vasectomy [23] and there is limited success in the regain of fertility even after successful surgical re-anastomosis in vaso-vasostomy attributed to the presence of ASA [3]. Up to 2–30% cases of infertility may be associated with the presence of ASA in the male or female partner of an infertile couple [24]. These ASA are causative factors of infertility since disappearance of them cause regain of fertility [25]. These findings provide evidence that spermatozoa can generate an immune response in both men and women that can lead to a contraceptive state. However, the whole sperm cannot be used for the development of contraceptive vaccine because there are numerous antigens present on the surface and internally in sperm that are shared with somatic cells. Thus, the immunization with the whole sperm can cause immunopathological consequences in other tissues and organs. The utility of a sperm antigen is contingent upon sperm-specific expression, surface expression accessible to antibody binding, and its role in fertilization/fertility. Also, the sperm antigen, alone or after conjugation with appropriate carrier protein, should be able to raise high titer and long lasting antibody response in circulation and locally in the genital tract. If it is also involved in human immunoinfertility then it is an especially attractive candidate. An ideal sperm antigen for immunocontraception should have tissue-specific expression on sperm surface and be involved in sperm–zona pellucida binding and human immunoinfertility.

4.1.2.2
Sperm Antigens

Various methodologies of genomics and proteomics have been used to delineate sperm antigens that have a role in fertilization/ fertility and can be used for the contraceptive vaccine development. Recently, using gene knockout technology, >100 novel testis/sperm genes/proteins have been identified that have a crucial role in various aspects of fertility [26, 27]. Some of these gene knockouts cause a defect in testis development and endocrine milieu, some in spermatogenesis, some in mating behavior, some in sperm structure/function/motility, and others in fertilization. The majority of these knockouts also demonstrated an effect on nonreproductive organs concomitant with an effect on fertility. We did an extensive database analysis of these genes/proteins to examine how many of these have the characteristics required for the contraceptive vaccine development as discussed above. The knockouts of only a few genes/proteins induced a specific effect on fertility without a serious side effect. Majority of them are not expressed on the sperm surface, and thus are not amenable to antibody binding. Although these can provide ideal targets for pharmacological inhibition for contraception, they are not suitable for contraceptive vaccine development. The gene knockout technology is a powerful approach to identify suitable novel targets and the list of gene knockout mice is ever growing.

The molecules involved in sperm–oocyte membrane fusion have been actively examined for some time. Various candidates have been proposed that include DE, CD46, equatorin Sperad, and $SAMP_{32}$ [28]. CD46 gene knockout mice do not show a defective sperm–oocyte fusion [29]. ADAM family proteins have drawn considerable attention because they have a putative fusion peptide ($ADAM_1$) and disintegrin domains ($ADAM_2$ and $ADAM_3$) [30]. However, $ADAM_1$, $ADAM_2$, and $ADAM_3$ gene knockout mice did not show a defect in sperm–oocyte membrane fusion, but show impairment in sperm–zona binding [31]. CD9 present on the oocyte plasma membrane seems to be essential for fusion with the sperm cell [32]. It was thought that integrins $\alpha6$ and β_1 present on sperm are involved in binding to oocyte CD9 for sperm–oocyte fusion [33]. However, gene knockout of these molecules did not inhibit fertility [34]. Recently, a very interesting gene knockout was reported. The gene knockout mice of a sperm gene, designated as *Izumo*, are healthy but all males are sterile [29, 35]. *Izumo* is named after a Japanese shrine dedicated to marriage. Male mice produce normal looking sperm that bind to and penetrate the ZP but are incapable of fusing with the oocyte membrane. Human sperm also express Izumo protein. Izumo protein is not detectable on ejaculated sperm but becomes detectable after sperm cell undergoes acrosome reaction. Izumo antigen seems to be an interesting molecule and its utility in the contraceptive vaccine development needs to be investigated. Since it is not exposed until the sperm cell undergoes acrosome reaction, the antibodies have to be present at that particular time and space for binding to Izumo antigen. Our laboratory recently demonstrated that immunization with Izumo peptides causes a reduction in fertility of female mice [36].

Several sperm genes/antigens have been delineated, and cloned and sequenced, and antibodies to some of these antigens affect sperm function/fertilization in vitro, and the immunization with only a few of them have shown to cause a contraceptive effect in vivo in any animal model. Notable among these are lactate dehydrogenase-C_4 (LDH-C_4) [37], PH-20 [38], SP-17 [39], SP-10 [40], FA-1 [41–44], and YLP$_{12}$ [45, 46]. Most of these active immunization studies, except related to PH-20 antigen, were carried out in the mouse model. At the present time, no sperm antigen has undergone Phase I / II clinical trial in humans. Two studies have examined the effect of sperm antigen vaccination in nonhuman primate model. One study reported reduced fertility of female baboons after immunization with LDH-C_4 [47]. However, a study by another group found no effect on fertility in female monkeys after vaccination with LDH-C_4 [48]. The reason for this discrepancy is not clear at the present time. Male monkeys were immunized with an epididymal protein, designated as epididymal protein inhibitor (Eppin) [49]. After immunization, 78% of the monkeys who developed high anti-Eppin antibody titers became infertile, and 71% of them recovered fertility after immunization was stopped. To maintain high antibody titers, booster injections with Freund's adjuvant have to be given every 3 weeks for almost the whole duration of study of 691 days. The potential immunopathological effects of immunization were not examined. This interesting study indicates that antisperm CV can also be developed for men.

Antibodies to several sperm antigens inhibit sperm–oocyte interaction/fertilization in vitro. However, the active immunization with many of these molecules does not inhibit fertility in vivo. Also, the gene knockouts of many of these molecules do not inhibit fertility. For example, although antibodies to fertilin/PH-30 inhibit fertilization in vitro [28], the active immunization with fertilin/PH-30 does not affect fertility in vivo [50]. Similarly, although antibodies to sperm integrins $\alpha6$ and β_1 inhibit sperm–oocyte fusion in vitro [33], the gene knockouts of these molecules do not affect the fertility in vivo [34]. These differences in in vitro and in vivo effects may be due to the a) class/subclass, valency, affinity, and kinetics of the antibodies generated in vivo, b) antibodies have to be present in time and space to bind to the appropriate molecules, and/or c) there may be redundancy of some of these molecules.

Another problem that the sperm vaccinologists are facing at the present time is to find an appropriate animal model to examine the efficacy of a sperm antigen. The most used animal model is the mouse. However, up until now, no one has reported 100% block in fertility after immunization with any single antigen in the mouse model. Even immunizations with the whole sperm or their solubilized preparations do not cause a total block in fertility in mice, male, or female. The maximum reduction in fertility after immunization with any antigen/sperm preparation is up to 70–75% (Table 4.1.1). Very few, if any, knockout of a single gene has made mice totally infertile. The recently reported *Izumo* gene knockout did make the male mice almost totally infertile [29]. It needs to be seen whether the 70–75% reduction in fertility in the mouse model translates to 100% reduction in humans or not. The female mouse ovulates several eggs every cycle and a woman ovulates normally one egg every cycle. So there are differences between the mouse and man. Over

Table 4.1.1 Effect of immunization with sperm peptides on fertility

Peptide	Gender	a.a. (n)	Fertility reduction (%)	Reference
Mouse				
rFA-1	Female	Whole molecule	71	[9, 52]
YLP$_{12}$	Female	12	70	[45, 51]
P10G	Female	10	>70	[39]
A9D	Female	9	50	[39]
SP56	Female	16	>70	[36]
Primates				
LDH-C4-bC5-19	Female	15	62	[47]
LDH-C4-bC5-19	Female	15	0	[48]
rEppin	Male	Whole molecule	78	[49]

70–75% reduction in fertility in the mouse model may translate to 100% block in humans. Maybe that it is the inherent nature of the mouse model in which it is difficult to make mice completely infertile. However, after active immunization or deleting a single gene, one does find a few mice that are totally infertile. Vaccinations with multiple sperm epitopes (peptide and DNA) enhances the efficacy but still does not cause 100% contraceptive effect [36, 51, 52].

The phage display technology is a novel and innovative tool for delineating specific binding peptide sequences to various ligands and antibodies. It was first reported by George Smith in 1985 [53]. This technology is being widely used in several laboratories at the present time. The peptide sequences are presented on the surface of filamentous phage to examine their interaction with specific ligands/antibodies. The DNA encoding any peptide sequence get incorporated into genome of the phage capsid protein and the encoded peptide is expressed and displayed on phage surface as fusion protein. We used this technology and the 2D gel electrophoresis/matrix-assisted laser desorption mass spectrometry (MALDI MS) to delineate the peptide sequences that are involved in human immunoinfertility [54–57] and the peptide sequences present on human sperm cell that are involved in binding to human ZP [46].

Besides antibodies, various cytokines can also affect sperm function and fertility either positively or negatively. For example, interferon-γ and tumor necrosis factor-α can negatively alter sperm motility and function [58], and interleukin-6 can enhance sperm capacitation and acrosome reaction [59]. A sperm cell has receptors for many of these cytokines such as interferon-γ and interferon-α [60]. These factors are present in the seminal plasma and the levels are modulated to various degrees in infertility. Immunization with the whole sperm preparation or specific sperm antigens can raise many cytokines besides antibodies that can affect sperm function [61].

4.1.2.3
Passive Immunization and scFv Antibodies

The progress in the development of CV against various targets including sperm has been hampered by the following facts. These include (1) delineating the appropriate fertility-related antigen(s), (2) variability of the immune response among the vaccinated individuals,

(3) attainment and maintenance of high titer of antibodies for bioefficacy, (4) time lag to achieve reasonably good antibody titers after the first injection, and (5) uncertainty regarding how long the antibody titer will remain in the circulation to exercise the contraceptive effects. The last four concerns are associated with the active immunization studies involving CV. It is envisaged that these four concerns may be taken care of using the passive immunization approach [62]. Passive immunization approach has been successful for protection against various immunological and infectious diseases [63, 64].

Several of these antibodies have become treatment modalities in the clinics [63, 65, 66]. Phage display technology has been widely used to obtain a variety of engineered antibodies, including single chain variable fragments (scFv) antibodies against several antigens [67–71]. ScFv is an antibody fragment that plays a major role in the antigen-binding activity, and is composed of variable heavy (VH) and variable light (VL) chains connected by a peptide linker. The most widely used peptide linker is a repeat of a 15-residue sequence of glycine and serine $(Gly_4Ser)_3$. The affinity and stability of the scFv antibodies produced in bacteria are comparable with those of the native antibodies and are maintained by a strong disulfide bond. ScFv antibodies can be produced on a large scale using specially modified bacterial hosts and have an advantage over the whole immunoglobulin (Ig) molecule. ScFv antibodies lack the Fc portion that eliminates unwanted secondary effects associated with Fc, and due to its small size can be easily absorbed into tissues and gene manipulated [72]. The mouse monoclonal antibody can elicit strong antimouse antibody reaction, chimeric antibody can cause antichimeric response, and xenogenic complementarity-determining regions (CDRs) of humanized antibodies can also evoke an anti-idiotypic response, when injected into humans [73–75]. Antibodies must be of human origin if to be used in humans. The potential poor immunogenicity and toxicity of an antigen and ethical issues, limit immunizing humans to obtain human antibodies. However, the phage display technology can be used to obtain these antibodies against target antigens if they exist involuntarily in humans, such as ASA in immunoinfertile men and women, and vasectomized men.

We recently did a study to obtain fertility-related scFv human antibodies that can be used for CV immunoinfertility. Peripheral blood leukocytes (PBL) were obtained from antisperm antibody-positive immunoinfertile and vasectomized men, activated with human sperm antigens in vitro, and cDNA was prepared from their RNA and PCR-amplified using several primers based on all the available variable regions of VH and VL chains [76]. The amplified VH and VL chains were ligated and the scFv repertoire was cloned into pCANTAB5E vector to create a human scFv antibody library. Panning of the library against specific antigens yielded several clones, and the four strongest reactive (designated as AFA-1, FAB-7, YLP20, and AS16) were selected for further analysis. These clones were shown to have novel sequences with unique CDRs when a search was performed in the immunogenetic database. ScFv antibodies were expressed, purified, and analyzed for human sperm reactivity and effects on human sperm function (Table 4.1.2). AFA-1 and FAB-7 scFv antibodies, having IgG3 heavy and IgK3 light chains, recognized human sperm FA-1 antigen, which is involved in human sperm function and fertilization. The third, YLP20 scFv antibody, reacted with a sperm protein of 48 ± 5 kDa, which contains the dodecamer sequence, YLPVGGLRIGG. The fourth antibody, AS16, reacted with a 18 kDa

Table 4.1.2 Sperm-specific human cFv antibodies

scFv antibody	Sperm antigen recognized	Molecular mass (kDa)	Acrosome-reacted sperm
AFA-1	FA-1	~50	36 ± 7[a]
FAB-7	FA-1	~50	44 ± 6[a]
YLP20	YLP_{12}	~48	42 ± 3[a]
AS16	SAGA	18 (major)	Not done
		37, 55, 100 (minor)	
CAB-3 control	None	None	74 ± 5

[a]Significantly different compared to control, $p < 0.01$ to < 0.001 [76]

sperm protein (major band) and was found to be a human homolog of the mouse monoclonal recombinant antisperm antibody (RASA) [77]. These antibodies inhibited human sperm capacitation/acrosome reaction in a concentration-dependent manner. This is the first study to report the use of phage display technology to obtain human antisperm scFv antibodies of defined antigen specificities from immunoinfertile/vasectomized men. These antibodies will find clinical applications in the development of novel immunocontraceptives and specific diagnostics for immunoinfertility in humans. The contraceptive effect of these antibodies in vivo is currently being investigated.

4.1.3
Conclusions

In conclusion, development of CV targeting sperm is an exciting proposition and may provide a valuable alternative to the presently available methods. As limitation with other vaccines, the progress in CV development has been delayed due to variability of immune response after vaccination. The multiepitope vaccines may enhance the efficacy and obliterate the concern of the inter-individual variability of the response. Also, this concern may be addressed by the passive immunization approach using preformed human antibodies. Several antibodies are being tried as therapeutic agents. At the present time, >100 antibodies are in clinical trials and ~20 FDA-approved monoclonal antibodies are available in the market for various clinical conditions, including cancer and infectious diseases. Over 80% of these antibodies are genetically engineered [78, 79]. The scFv antibodies that we have synthesized in vitro using cDNAs from antisperm antibody-positive immunoinfertile and vasectomized men may provide a useful, once-a-month immunocontraceptive. These human antibodies are sperm-specific and inhibit sperm function in vitro. Their immunocontraceptive potential in vivo is presently being investigated.

Acknowledgments   This work is supported by the NIH grant HD24425. The excellent typing assistance provided by Sarah Davis is gratefully acknowledged.

References

1. Contraception online (2004) Baylor College of Medicine. Huston Texas. htttp://www.contra-ceptiononline.org/
2. Harper MJK (2005) In search of a second contraceptive revolution. Sex Reprod Menopause 3:59–67
3. Silber SJ, Grotjan HE (2004) Microscopic vasectomy reversal 30 years later: a summary of 4010 cases by the same surgeon. J Androl 25:845–859
4. Upadhyay U (2004) New contraceptive choices. Pop Rep M 19. Johns Hopkins Bloomberg School of Public Health, Baltimore, MD. The INFO Project
5. Anonymous (2008) World POP clock projection US census bureau http://www.factfinder.census.gov
6. Grow DR, Ahmed S (2000) New contraception methods. Obstet Gynecol Clin North Am 27:901–916
7. Henshaw SK (1998) Unintended pregnancy in the United States. Fam Plann Perspect 30:24–29
8. Institute of Medicine (2004) In: Nass SJ, Strauss JF III (eds) New frontiers in contraceptive research. A blue print for action. National Academies Press, Washington DC
9. Naz RK (2005) Contraceptive vaccines. Drugs 65:593–603
10. Naz RK, Gupta SK, Gupta JC et al (2005) Recent advances in contraceptive vaccine development. Hum Reprod 20:3271–3283
11. Ferro VA, Stimson WH (1999) Antigonadotropin releasing hormone vaccines and their potential use in treatment of hormone responsive cancers. Bio Drugs 12:1–12
12. Simms MS, Scholfield DP, Jacobs E et al (2000) Anti-GnRH antibodies can induce castrate levels of testosterone in patients with advanced prostate cancer. Br J Cancer 83:443–446
13. Moudgal NR, Murthy GS, Prasanna Kumar KM et al (1997) Responsivness of human male volunteers to immunization with ovine follicile stimulating hormone vaccine:results of a pilot study. Hum Reprod 12:457–463
14. Saxena BB, Clavio A, Singh M et al (2002) Modulation of ovarian function in female dogs immunized with bovine luteinizing hormone receptor. Reprod Domest Anim 37:9–17
15. Thau RB, Wilson CB, Sundaram K et al (1987) Long-term immunization against the beta-subunit of ovine luteinizing hormone (oLH beta) has no adverse effects on pituitary function in rhesus monkeys. Am J Reprod Immunol Microbiol 15:92–98
16. Aitken JR (2002) Immunocontraceptive vaccines for human use. J Reprod Immunol 57:273–287
17. Tung KSK, Lou Y, Bagavant H (1999) Zona pellucida chimeric peptide vaccine. In: Gupta S (ed) Reproductive immmunology. Narosa, New Delhi, pp 303–308
18. Kirkpatrick JF, Turner J (2002) Reversibility of action and safety during pregnancy of immunization against porcine zona pellucida in wild mares (Equus Caballus). Reprod Suppl 60:197–202
19. Talwar GP, Singh O, Pal R et al (1994) A vaccine that prevents pregnancy in women. Proc Natl Acad Sci U S A 91:2532–2536
20. Allardyce RA (1984) Effect of ingested sperm on fecundity in the rat. J Exp Med 159:1548–1553
21. Menge AC (1970) Immune reactions and infertility. J Reprod Fertil Suppl 10:171–185
22. Baskin MJ (1932) Temporary sterilization by injection of human spermatozoa: a preliminary report. Am J Obstet Gynecol 24:892–897
23. Liskin L, Pile JM, Quillan WF (1983) Vasectomy safe and simple. Popul Rep 4:61–100
24. Ohl D, Naz RK (1995) Infertility due to antisperm antibodies. J Urol 46:591–602
25. Bronson RG, Cooper G, Rosenfeld D (1984) Sperm antibodies: their role in infertility. Fertil Steril 42:171–182

26. Naz RK, Rajesh C (2005) Novel testis/sperm-specific contraceptive targets identified using gene knockout studies. Front Biosci 10:2430–2446
27. Naz RK, Rajesh P (2005) Gene knockouts that cause female infertility: search for novel contraceptive targets. Front Biosci 10:2447–2459
28. Stein KK, Primakoff P, Myles D (2004) Sperm–egg fusion: events at the plasma membrane. J Cell Sci 117:6269–6274
29. Inoue N, Ikawa M, Nakanishi T et al (2003) Disruption of mouse CD46 causes an accelerated spontaneous acrosome reaction in sperm. Mol Cell Biol 23:2614–2622
30. Nishimura H, Kim E, Nakanishi T et al (2004) Possible function of the ADAM1a/ADAM2 fertilin complex in the appearance of $ADAM_3$ on the sperm surface. J Biol Chem 279: 34957–34962
31. Cho C, Bunch DO, Faure JE et al (1998) Fertilization defects in sperm from mice lacking fertilin beta. Science 281:1857–1859
32. Le Naour F, Rubinstein E, Jasmin C et al (2000) Severly reduced female fertility in CD9-deficient mice. Science 287:319–321
33. Almeida EAC, Huovila APJ, Sutherland AE et al (1995) Mouse egg intergin $\chi_6\beta_1$ functions as a sperm receptor. Cell 81:1095–1104
34. He ZY, Brakebusch C, Fässler R et al (2003) None of the integrins known to be present on the mouse egg or to be ADAM receptors are essential for sperm–egg binding and fusion. Dev Biol 233:204–213
35. Inoue N, Ikawa M, Isotani A et al (2005) The immunoglobin superfamily protein izumo is required for sperm to fuse with eggs. Nature 434:234–238
36. Naz RK (2008) Immunocontraceptive effect of Izumo and enhancement by combination vaccination. Mol Reprod Dev 75:336–344
37. Goldberg E, Herr JC (1999) LDH-C_4 as a contraceptive vaccine. In: Gupta S (ed) Reproductive immunology. Narosa, New Delhi, India, pp 309–315
38. Primakoff P, Lathrop W, Woolman L et al (1988) Fully effective contraceptive in male and female guinea pigs immunized with the sperm protein PH20. Nature 335:543–547
39. Lea IA, Van Lierop MJC, Widgren EE et al (1998) A chimeric sperm peptide induces antibodies and strain-specific reversible infertility in mice. Biol Reprod 59:527–536
40. Herr JC, Flickinger CJ, Homyk M (1990) Biochemical and morphological characterization of intra-acrosomal antigen SP-10 from human sperm. Biol Reprod 42:181–189
41. Menge AC, Christman GM, Ohl DA et al (1999) Fertilization antigen-1 removes antisperm autoantibodies from spermatozoa of infertile men and results in increases rates of acrosome reaction. Fertil Steril 71:256–260
42. Naz RK, Zhu X (2002) Molecular cloning and sequencing of cDNA encoding for human FA-1 antigen. Mol Reprod Dev 63:256–268
43. Naz RK, Ahmad K, Menge AC (1993) Antiidiotypic antibodies to sperm in sera of fertile women that neutralize antisperm antibodies. J Clin Invest 92:2331–2338
44. Zhu X, Naz RK (1997) Fertilization antigen-1: cDNA cloning, testis specific expression, and immunocontraceptive effects. Proc Natl Acad Sci U S A 94:4704–4709
45. Naz RK, Chauhan SC (2002) Human sperm-specific peptide vaccine that causes long-term reversible contraception. Biol Reprod 62:318–324
46. Naz RK, Zhu X, Kadam A (2000) Identification of human sperm peptide sequence involved in egg binding for immunocontraception. Biol Reprod 7:21–26
47. O'Hearn PA, Liang ZG, Bambra CS et al (1997) Colinear synthesis of an antigen-specific B-cell epitote with a promiscuous tetanus toxin T-cell epitote: a synthetic peptide immunocontraceptive. Vaccine 15:1761–1766
48. Tollner TL, Overstreet JW, Branciforte D et al (2002) Immunization of female cynomolgus macaques with a synthetic epitope of sperm-specific lactate dehydrogenase results in high antibody titers but does not reduce fertility. Mol Reprod Dev 62:257–264

49. O'Rand MG, Widgren EE, Sivashanmugam P et al (2004) Reversible immunocontraception in male monkeys immunized with eppin. Science 306:1189

50. Hardy CM, Clarke HG, Nixon B et al (1997) Examination of the immunocontracptive potential of recombinant rabbit fertilin subunits in rabbit. Biol Reprod 57:879–886

51. Naz RK (2006) Effect of sperm DNA vaccine on fertility of female mice. Mol Reprod Dev 73:918–928

52. Naz RK (2006) Effect of fertilization antigen (FA-1) DNA vaccine on fertility of female mice. Mol Reprod Dev 73:1473–1479

53. Smith G (1985) Filamentous fusion phage:novel expression vectors that display cloned antigens on the virion surface. Science 228:1315–1317

54. Auer J, Pignot-Paintrand I, De Almeida M (1995) Identification of human sperm surface glycoproteins by sperm-membrane specific autoantibodies. Hum Reprod 10:551–557

55. Naz RK (2005) Search for peptide sequences involved in human antisperm antibody- mediated male immunoinfertility by using phage display technology. Mol Reprod Dev 72:25–30

56. Pillai S, Wright DR, Gupta A et al (1996) Molecular weights and isoelectric points of sperm antigens relevant to autoimmune infertility in men. J Urol 155:1928–1933

57. Shetty J, Naaby-Hansen S, Shibahara H et al (1999) Human sperm proteome: immunodominant sperm surface antigens identified with sera from infertile men and women. Biol Reprod 61:61–69

58. Naz RK, Kumar R (1991) Transforming growth factor β_1 enhances expression of 50 kDa protein related to 2′-5′ oligoadenylate synthetase in human sperm. J Cell Physiol 146:156–163

59. Naz RK, Kaplan P (1995) Interleukin-6 enhances the fertilizing capacity of human sperm by increasing capacitation and acrosome reaction. J Androl 15:228–233

60. Naz RK, Chauhan SC, Rose LP (2000) Expression of alpha and gamma interferon receptors in the sperm cell. Mol Reprod Dev 56:189–197

61. Naz RK, Mehta K (1989) Cell-mediated immune responses to sperm antigens: effects on mouse sperm and embryos. Biol Reprod 41:533–542

62. Naz RK, Rajesh C (2004) Passive immunization for immunocontraception:lessons learned from infectious diseases. Front Biosci 9:2457–2465

63. Casadevall A (1999) Passive antibody therapies: progress and continuing challenges. Clin Immunol 93:5–15

64. Zeitlin L, Cone RA, Moench TR et al (2000) Preventing infectious diseases with passive immunization. Microbes Infect 2:701–708

65. Dunman PM, Nessin M (2003) Passive immunization as prophylaxis: when and where will this work? Curr Opin Pharmacol 20:351–360

66. Riethmuller G, Schneider-Gadicke E, Johnson JP (1993) Monoclonal antibodies in cancer therapy. Curr Opin Immunol 5:732–739

67. Park KJ, Lee SH, Kim TI et al (2007) A human scFv antibody against TRAIL receptor 2 induces autophagic cell death in both TRAIL-sensitive and TRAIL-resistant cancer cells. Cancer Res 67:7327–7334

68. Rader C, Barbas CF (1997) Phage display of combinatorial antibody libraries. Curr Opin Biotechnol 8:503–508

69. Ye Z, Hellstrom I, Hayden-Ledbetter M et al (2002) Gene therapy for cancer using single-chain Fv fragments specific for 4–1BB. Nat Med 8:343–348

70. Zhang W, Matsumoto-Takasaki A, Kusada Y et al (2007) Isolation and characterization of phage-displayed single chain antibodies recognizing nonreducing terminal mannose residues. 2. Expression, purification, and characterization of recombinant single chain antibodies. Biochemistry 46:263–270

71. Zhou Y, Drummond DC, Zou H et al (2007) Impact of single-chain Fv antibody fragment affinity on nanoparticle targeting of epidermal growth factor receptor expressing tumor cells. J Mol Biol 371:934–947

72. Yokota T, Milenic DE, Whitlow M et al (1992) Rapid tumor penetration of a single-chain Fv and comparison with other immunoglobulin forms. Cancer Res 52:3402–3408
73. Koren E, Zuckerman LA, Mire-Sluis AR (2002) Immune response to therapeutic proteins in humans-clinical significance, assessment and prediction. Curr Pharm Biotechnol 3:349–360
74. Mirick GR, Bradt BM, Denardo SJ et al (2004) A review of human anti-globulin antibody (HAGA, HAMA, HACA, HAHA) responses to monoclonal antibodies. Not four letter words. Q J Nucl Med Mol Imaging 48:251–257
75. Sidhu SS, Fellouse FA (2006) Synthetic therapeutic antibodies. Nat Chem Biol 2:682–688
76. Samuel AS, Naz RK (2008) Isolation of human single chain variable fragment antibodies against specific sperm antigens for immunocontraceptive development. Hum Reprod 23: 1324–1337
77. Norton E, Diekman AB, Westbrook VA et al (2001) RASA, a recombinant single chain variable fragment (scFv) antibody directed against the human sperm surface: implications for novel contraceptives. Hum Reprod 16:1854–1860
78. Hollinger P, Hudson PJ (2005) Engineered antibody fragments and the rise of single domains. Nat Biotech 23:1126–1136
79. Marasco WA, Sui J (2007) The growth and potential of human antiviral monoclonal antibody therapeutics. Nat Biotech 25:1421–1434

Immunocontraception in Wildlife Animals

4.2

Katarina Jewgenow

4.2.1
Immunocontraception in Wildlife Species

4.2.1.1
Captive Population

Not only is there a need for reproduction control in captive animals, but also exotic animals in captivity serve as models for the establishment of contraceptive approaches for wildlife. Because improved animal husbandry and veterinary care has led to a low adult mortality and an increase in longevity, especially in large ungulates, carnivores, and even species managed in breeding programmes, high quality enclosures are overcrowded. This results in the demand for population control. Prevention of offspring (sterilization or contraception) is an alternative to the elimination of captive animals (euthanasia or transfer to other institutions) [1].

In addition, as zoos usually do not share the same limitations as wildlife managers, it is possible to apply a wider variety of contraceptive techniques, or even allow research on contraceptive approaches which would not be possible in wildlife animals. Therefore, not surprisingly the first anti-fertility vaccinations were applied to captive wildlife animals [2–4]. Two types of experimental immunocontraceptive vaccines have been broadly applied to exotic captive animals. They contain either porcine zona pellucida (PZP) proteins extracted from pig ovaries [5, 6] or synthetic conjugated gonadotropin releasing hormone (GnRH) peptides [7–9]. These vaccines require repeated injections and are limited to captive or small populations of free-ranging wild animals.

K. Jewgenow
Leibniz Institute for Zoo and Wildlife Research, PF 60110310252, Berlin, Germany
e-mail: jewgenow@izw-berlin.de

W. K. H. Krause and R. K. Naz (eds.), *Immune Infertility*,
DOI: 10.1007/978-3-642-01379-9_4.2, © Springer Verlag Berlin Heidelberg 2009

4.2.1.2
Wildlife Population

Reproductive control is important for the management of certain wildlife, which ironically may also be endangered species, particularly in the increasingly common situation in which the size and the nature of habitat are restricted by man's encroachment [10]. Additionally, some wildlife species have adapted successfully to changing environmental conditions and concentrated in large populations significantly impacting on their habitats or their prey species; they have served as reservoirs of infectious diseases, making them "pest species." The challenge is to develop acceptable and sustainable methods to reduce and maintain populations of these animals at levels that minimize their impact on environment.

4.2.1.2.1
Pest Species

Pest mammals have severe economic, environmental, and social impacts throughout the world [11]. Methods of immunocontraception are being investigated for small rodents, in particular for rabbits and house mice, and for overabundant marsupial species, like brushtail possum in New Zealand [12]. Most small rodent species are characterized by high reproductive rate. Therefore, fertility control needs to be adapted to their reproduction strategy (r-strategy) which is characterized by a high rate of reproduction, high juvenile mortality, and strongly fluctuating population sizes within fluctuating habitats. Population models which were developed to predict possible outcomes of fertility control showed that at least 80% of females will need to be infertile and that this infertility will have to be permanent [13]. Virally vectored immunocontraception (VVIC) has been proposed as an economic way to achieve this [14, 15]. Although VVIC may have the advantage of being self-regulating depending on the density of the target species [16], biological safety and regulatory concerns must be addressed in future before VVIC can be applied for field testing [11, 17, 18].

4.2.1.2.2
Alien Species

Alien species is any species that has spread beyond its natural range into new locations as a result of human activity. Invasive alien species are species that have some advantage over native species. These advantages are often enhanced when aliens move into ecological niches and thrive because, outside their natural environments, they are not held back by natural predators, parasites, disease, or competition in the way that native species are. Therefore, there is a major need to control population sizes in nonindigenous animals and/ or imported species such as the grey squirrel [19] and several deer species in Europe [20], or fox in Australia [21]. In the case of some alien species, a full eradication from their new habitats might be considered.

4.2.1.3
Over-Abundant Wildlife

Over-abundance of wildlife often has nothing to do with biological carrying capacity, when population reduces the rate at which food resources are replenished. Wildlife is considered to be overabundant (ecological over-abundance) when a population is so dense that it threatens the persistence of other species or it becomes unacceptable to humans (societal over-abundance). In this respect, a number of wildlife species have become overabundant on a local or regional scale throughout the world. Traditionally, overabundant wildlife is controlled by hunting and trapping, but this may be restricted or infeasible in parks and suburban areas. Application of wildlife fertility control is suggested for use in urban or suburban areas (e.g., for deer species and wild boars) and in situations where immigration is limited and lethal control is restricted (e.g., for elephants in national parks).

4.2.1.4
Transmitters of Zoonoses

Zoonoses are infectious diseases that can be transmitted between humans and animals, both wild and domestic. Approximately 75% of recently emerging infectious diseases that affect humans are diseases of animal origin, and approximately 60% of all human pathogens are zoonotic. During the last 30 years, new epidemiological patterns have emerged as free-ranging wildlife have become progressively more involved in the epidemiology of both common and emerging infectious diseases of humans and domestic animals. This has been seen in rabies, bovine tuberculosis, and more recently in wild-boar classical swine fever [22]. Offensive lethal control, however, failed to control badgers, wild boar, and foxes for tuberculosis, classical swine fever, and rabies, respectively. Culling these species reduced their populations to a logarithmic part of their growth curve, such that any losses due to culling were very quickly replaced by individuals who normally would have died because of population density pressures. Consequently, immunocontraception in combination with disease vaccination is being discussed as an alternative strategy to lethal control.

4.2.2
Development of Immunocontraceptive Vaccines for Wildlife Species

4.2.2.1
Porcine Zona Pellucida (PZP)

The most widely tested immunocontraceptive vaccine for wildlife species is on the basis of developing antibodies to zona pellucida, which surrounds the mammalian egg. The PZP antigens are isolated from porcine ovaries obtained from slaughter house material. When PZP is injected into females other than pigs, the target species will produce antibodies against the antigen. These antibodies attach to the zona pellucida of ovulated eggs and cause steric hindrance which then blocks fertilization. Long-term application or hyperactive immune response, however, can cause ovarian failure and permanent sterilization.

The initial PZP vaccine was on the basis of multiple-shot boosting [23]. Since then several technologies have been developed to achieve efficiency with a single immunization [24, 25]. PZP has been shown to be effective in a wide variety of ungulates [3, 4, 26–29], equines [5, 30–32], elephants [10, 33–35], and some carnivores [28, 36, 37].

Despite a high individual variability in immune response observed [38], the biological efficacy of PZP depends on species-specific antigentiy and immunogenity of PZP [2, 39, 40], and therefore must be validated before it can be applied for contraceptive population control in a particular species.

4.2.2.2
Gonadotropin-Releasing Hormone (GnRH) Vaccine

Vaccination against GnRH entails the administration of a modified form of the GnRH hormone in order to stimulate the production of anti-GnRH antibodies, which bind and inactivate the endogenous GnRH. The hormone (GnRH) stimulates the pituitary to secret the gonadotropins LH and FSH. Therefore, immunization against GnRH disrupts the reproductive axis by depression of gonadotropin production in order to inhibit follicle growth, ovulation, or spermatogenesis. In addition, vaccination against GnRH is the most promising alternative to castration for reducing male aggressive behaviour in captive adult animals [41]. The molecular structure of GnRH is conserved among mammalian species. Therefore, anti-GnRH vaccines can be applied in a wide range of animals.

Recent studies on the use of GnRH vaccination for suppression of fertility, aggression, and sexual behaviour have shown promising results in several domestic species, such as sheep [42], pigs [43], cattle [44], and horses [45]. GnRH vaccination has also been suggested for application in fertility control of overabundant wildlife, such as wild boar [8], white-tailed [9] or black-tailed deer [46], and ground squirrel [47]. Suppression of steroid production by GnRH vaccines, however, might be combined with effects which are characteristically seen for castration: changes in secondary sex characteristics, like antler growth in deer or the mane in lions; therefore, these effects should be taken into account. In addition, safety trials should be performed to assure that nonreproductive functions of the hypothalamus and pituitary gland are retained in treated animals.

4.2.2.3
Other Antigens for Immuncontraception

Most currently available methods for immunocontraception interact at some point with the sequence of hormone synthesis or are involved in essential reproductive events, like ovulation, spermatogenesis, sperm or egg transport, or implantation. New molecular technologies are applied to generate vast peptides libraries that are screened for their potential impact on fertility.

A variety of proteins derived from sperm and oocytes have been experimentally assessed for their immunocontraceptive potential in wildlife species [21, 48, 49]. In particular, sperm antigens are suggested to act as species-specific immunogenes, an essential prerequisite for oral vaccines applied in free-ranging wildlife. In this respect, a promising strategy appears to be the construction of immunogens that include repeated peptides from proteins involved in fertilization [50–52]. Fertilization-related antigens are isolated from germ cell plasma membranes [53] or are identified from cDNA libraries of oocytes or sperm cells [54]. Besides sperm–egg receptors, many other biologically active components of reproduction are considered for contraceptive vaccines [55, 56], but none of them has been used yet for contraception in exotic species.

4.2.3
Delivery Methods

Fertility management is not yet a practical reality in wildlife management. Before it can be implemented it must meet the demands on risk assessment of health and behavioural effects in the target species, as well as of any potential effects on nontarget species [57]. Immunocontraception in wildlife requires acceptable and safe application (e.g., humane use, environmental safety, and target specificity), and knowledge of how to apply it strategically (e.g., where, when, how often, and how intensively) [58]. The species-specific application can be achieved either through vaccine compound itself or by the delivery method. Vaccine-developing strategy includes the identification of an antifertile antigen and the development of an effective vaccine composition including acceptable carriers, adjuvants, and delivering systems [59]. The following delivery methods had been used or suggested for wildlife species.

4.2.3.1
Parenteral Immunisation

Attempts to use immunocontraceptive vaccines to stop breeding in wildlife animals date back to late 1980. Initial studies showed that pregnancies could be prevented by multiple-shot vaccines [5, 60] containing PZP and Freund's adjuvants. These were followed by studies showing that these vaccines could be remotely delivered effectively to free-ranging animals (horses, deer, and elephants), but the requirement for repeated initial shots and annual boosters limited their practical application. During the following years the formulation of vaccines was improved steadily. Now vaccines are effective for several years with a single treatment [6, 61]. Multiple booster treatment were replaced by microsphere particles or polymer-based controlled-release pellets [25, 27, 62] containing the antigen and the adjuvant. Immunogenity of antigens was increased by tagging them to another protein, and incorporation of different adjuvants [25, 63, 64]. The replacement of Freund's adjuvant was aimed to prevent local and systemic side effects described in several wildlife animals [65, 66]. Beside the progress made in delivery procedure, the parenteral immunization requires an individual approach to the animal and is therefore limited to captive or small populations of free-ranging wild animals.

4.2.3.2
Oral Delivery via Baits

Alternative immunocontraceptive vaccines are actively being developed to enable large numbers of wild animals to be targeted by oral delivery of baits, when a single animal's treatment will be not effective or possible (pest or alien species). The distribution of baits and collection of remaining baits could be handled in a way similar to that of the rodendicide baits [11]. It is proposed that vaccines which will be delivered orally in a bait will stimulate a mucosal immune response to the foreign antigen(s). Such a vaccine requires a detailed understanding of reproductive-tract mucosal immunity in target species. Oral contraceptive vaccines under consideration include viral or bacterial vectors and microencapsulated antigens [21]. Although baits are increasingly used in wildlife management to deliver vaccines for disease control, a contraceptive oral vaccine is not available yet. In addition, safety requirements are concerned with the transmissibility of the antigen in case of viral or bacterial vectors, the reversibility of the intervention within an individual animal and in animal populations, as well as the species specificity of the antigen used [67].

4.2.3.3
Plant Based Contraceptives

An alternative approach to protein production using bacteria or virus presents the plant-based immunocontraception especially for herbivore animals. Female possums vaccinated with immunocontraceptive antigens showed reduced fertility, and possums fed with potato-expressed heat labile toxin-B (LT-B) expressed mucosal and systemic immune responses to the antigen. This demonstrated that immunocontraception was effective in possums and that oral delivery in edible plant material might be possible. Prior to attempts at large scale production, more effective immunocontraceptive antigen—adjuvant formulations are probably required before plant-based immunocontraception can become a major tool for immunocontraceptive control of overabundant vertebrate pests [68].

4.2.3.4
Virally-Vectored Immunocontraception (VVIC)

One approach to deliver immunocontraceptive vaccines are self-disseminating agents such as viruses. This approach employs live, genetically modified viruses to deliver immunocontraception and has proved successful under laboratory conditions. Under field condition a virus may have the advantage of being self-regulating depending on the density of the target species [16] and can be species specific if the viral vector is species specific

[18, 69–71]. However, despite a large number of studies on VVIC [49, 56, 71–73], so far no product has been developed for field testing. The ability of an immunocontraceptive virus to control populations is not only compromised by several factors such as sufficient transmission rate, competition with field strains of virus or its ability to induce infertility in the presence of field strains [74], there are also safety and regulatory concerns about maintaining the species specificity of the viral vector and other potential unexpected changes in such a genetically modified virus. Once released, a vector cannot be recalled and may spread to regions where the original target species is not a pest [17]. These constraints indicate that it is very unlikely that VVIC will be applied in near future [75].

4.2.4
Problems Connected with IC

4.2.4.1
Animal Welfare and Health Issues

Potential adverse effects of contraception may include harmful effects on pregnant animals, inhibition of parturition or dystocia, changes in ovarian structure or function, changes in sex ratio, changes in lactation or mammary glands, impact on fertility of young, changes in testicular structure or function, changes in secondary sex characteristics, changes in bodyweight, changes in behaviour, changes in annual breeding season, other physiologic and pathologic changes, and abscesses or inflammatory reactions [76]. The impact of contraception on animal welfare is intensively monitored in captive animals [65], but is difficult to assess in free-ranging wildlife.

Contraceptives that disrupt endocrine function have the potential to disturb metabolic homeostasis and thereby cause disease. Antibodies that target sperm or egg proteins have the potential to incite immune-mediated damage in organs producing gametes. Long lived animals which never had a chance to reproduce may express tumour or cyst development within the uterus, as reported for nonreproducing captive elephants and rhinoceros [77]. All potential risks need to be assessed and then weighted against benefits of contraception, but unfortunately the number of studies on animal behaviour and physiology are still scarce and inconsistent.

The use of PZP in seasonal breeders may result in delayed breeding and birth of offspring outside optimal breeding season [78]. In addition, PZP does not suppress the ovarian activity; therefore, treated animals may express recurrent or persistent oestrus. Especially in carnivores, the permanent exposure to endogenous steroids might cause the same pathological effects as shown for exogenous steroids [79].

The GnRH vaccination in male cervids causes delayed antler growth and retention of velvet [80]. Active immunization against GnRH in pigs also caused damage to cells in the hypothalamus, other than those producing GnRH [81], but similar safety studies have not been conducted in exotic animals. Treatment of domestic pigs with GnRH vaccine was also associated with higher food consumption and higher deposition of subcutaneous fat

[82]; a similar increase in body weight was observed in wild boars [8], whereas male lambs immunized against GnRH reduced feeding [83]. Treatment with GnRH vaccine suppresses but does not completely block the production of steroid hormones [8]; therefore, the availability of these hormones after treatment had positive implications for the welfare, as lack of steroids could have potentially wide-ranging effects on animal health.

4.2.4.2
Behavioural Changes

Immunocontraception used in free-ranging wildlife should not disrupt species-typical behaviour patterns, like an extension of the breeding season. The presence of treated females could disrupt social interactions in a population. Males coexisting with untreated females spent more time exhibiting aggressive behaviour during rut than males living with PZP-treated females, but males did not differ in time spent in mating behaviour [84]; an extension of breeding season increased movements and ranges were not observed [85]. Even so, social rank of treated wild boars [8] and brushtail possums [86] did not change during treatment with GnRH.

Another potential behavioral change is the risk of prey-switching of predators feeding on immunocontracepted target species. This ecological effect of prey-switching needs to be considered before an immunocontraceptive strategy can be adopted for pest control [58].

4.2.4.3
Population Level Effects of Fertility Control

Immunocontraception which rely on a healthy immune system to achieve contraception may not be effective in animals with compromised immune function. Thus, in wildlife population this could have a negative effect on natural selection for population fitness. Use of immunocontraception could create genetic changes in the target population that would influence disease resistance. Poor scientific description of ecosystem complexity makes it difficult to predict the consequences of immunocontraception on wildlife populations [87].

Also of concern is the changing age structure of population and the potential deleterious effects associated with increasing inbreeding levels in a smaller population. Diminished number of females in the breeding pool increases theoretically the size of a healthy population which is large enough to maintain the lowest levels of inbreeding. In this context, the increasing number of older females, which will not reproduce after prolonged contraception has to be considered. Contracepted animals live significantly longer than noncontracepted [78, 88]. Thus, the improvements in survivorship diminish the effectiveness of contraception in reducing population size [24].

A very useful tool to determine population level effects caused by immunocontraception are mathematical models, which have been developed to guide management decisions for many wildlife species. These models use basic information on a species' life history to predict the effect of various management actions, including contraception [89–91].

4.2.5
Conclusion

Traditional methods to control wildlife, such as culling and poisoning, often turn out to be ineffective, environmentally hazardous, and uneconomic and may have significant welfare costs. Public concerns about lethal control, animal welfare, and restrictions on biocides place increasing constraints on wildlife management options and require the identification of alternative methods. One of these alternatives is population control by immunocontraception. Over the last three decades significant progress has been made in developing immunocontraception for wildlife control, although the wide range of animals for which fertility control is desired makes the development of a single method impossible [92]. Immunocontraception is already used in captive and small population of free-ranging wildlife animals. Further research and concepts are needed to safely apply immunocontraception to overabundant pest or alien species. Contraceptive treatment may alter the health, behavior, and population structure of wildlife animals and therefore must be monitored closely.

References

1. Jewgenow K, Dehnhard M, Hildebrandt TB, Goritz F (2006) Contraception for population control in exotic carnivores. Theriogenology 66:1525–1529
2. Jewgenow K, Göritz F, Hildebrandt TB, Rohleder M, Wegner I, Kolter L (2001) Bestimmung des Antikörpertiters gegen Schweine-Zona-Pellucida bei Zootieren vor und nach Kontrazeption mit porcinen Zona pellucida (pZP) Proteinen. Zool Garten NF 3:1–14
3. Kirkpatrick JF, Calle PP, Kalk P, Kolter L, Zimmermann W, Goodrowe K, Turner JW, Liu IKM, Bernoco M (1992) Immunocontraception of female captive exotic ungulates. Am Assoc Zoo Vet Annu Proc 1992:100–101
4. Kirkpatrick JF, Calle PP, Kalk P, Liu IKM, Turner JW Jr (1996) Immunocontraception of captive exotic species. 2. Formosan sika deer (*Cervus nippon taiouanus*), axis deer (*Cervus axis*), Himalayan tahr (*Hemitragus jemlahicus*), Roosevelt elk (*Cervus elaphus roosevelti*), Reeves' muntjac (*Muntiacus reevesi*), and sambar deer (*Cervus unicolor*). J Zoo Wildl Med 27:482–495
5. Kirkpatrick JF, Liu IKM, Turner JW Jr (1990) Remotely-delivered immunocontraception in feral horses. Wildl Soc Bull 18:326–330
6. Turner JW Jr, Liu IKM, Flanagan DR, Rutberg AT, Kirkpatrick JF (2001) Immunocontraception in feral horses: one inoculation provides one year of infertility. J Wildl Manag 65:235–241
7. Becker SE, Enright WJ, Katz LS (1999) Active immunization against gonadotropin-releasing hormone in female white-tailed deer. Zoo Biol 18:385–396
8. Massei G, Cowan DP, Coats J, Gladwell F, Lane JE, Miller LA (2008) Effect of the GnRH vaccine GonaCon on the fertility, physiology and behaviour of wild boar. Wildl Res 35:540–547
9. Miller LA, Gionfriddo JP, Rhyan JC, Fagerstone KA, Wagner DC, Killian GJ (2008) GnRH immunocontraception of male and female white-tailed deer fawns. Hum Wildl Confl 2:93–101
10. Delsink AK, van Altena JJ, Grobler D, Bertschinger H, Kirkpatrick J, Slotow R (2006) Regulation of a small, discrete African elephant population through immunocontraception in the Makalali Conservancy, Limpopo, South Africa. South Afr J Sci 102:403–405
11. Jacob J, Singleton GR, Hinds LA (2008) Fertility control of rodent pests. Wildl Res 35:487–493

12. Cowan PE, Tyndale-Biscoe CH (1997) Australian and New Zealand mammal species considered to be pests or problems. Reprod Fertil Dev 9:27–36

13. van Leeuwen BH, Kerr PJ (2007) Prospects for fertility control in the European rabbit (*Oryctolagus cuniculus*) using myxoma virus-vectored immunocontraception. Wildl Res 34:511–522

14. Barlow ND (1994) Predicting the effect of a novel vertebrate biocontrol agent: a model for viral-vectored immunocontraception of New Zealand possums. J Appl Ecol 31:454–462

15. Hood GM, Chesson P, Pech RP (2000) Biological control using sterilizing viruses: Host suppression and competition between viruses in non-spatial models. J Appl Ecol 37:914–925

16. Arthur AD, Pech RP, Singleton GR (2005) Predicting the effect of immunocontraceptive recombinant murine cytomegalovirus on population outbreaks of house mice (*Mus musculus domesticus*) in mallee wheatlands. Wildl Res 32:631–637

17. McLeod SR, Saunders G, Twigg LE, Arthur AD, Ramsey D, Hinds LA (2007) Prospects for the future: is there a role for virally vectored immunocontraception in vertebrate pest management? Wildl Res 34:555–566

18. Redwood AJ, Smith LM, Lloyd ML, Hinds LA, Hardy CM, Shellam GR (2007) Prospects for virally vectored immunocontraception in the control of wild house mice (*Mus domesticus*). Wildl Res 34:530–539

19. Rushton SP, Gurnell J, Lurz PWW, Fuller RM (2002) Modeling impacts and costs of gray squirrel control regimes on the viability of red squirrel populations. J Wildl Manag 66:683–697

20. Dolman PM, Waber K (2008) Ecosystem and competition impacts of introduced deer. Wildl Res 35:202–214

21. Bradley MP (1994) Experimental strategies for the development of an immunocontraceptive vaccine for the European red fox, *Vulpes vulpes*. Reprod Fertil Dev 6:307–317

22. Artois M, Delahay R, Guberti V, Cheeseman C (2001) Control of infectious diseases of wildlife in Europe. Vet J 162:141–152

23. Kirkpatrick JF, Turner JW Jr, Liu IK, Fayrer-Hosken R, Rutberg AT (1997) Case studies in wildlife immunocontraception: wild and feral equids and white-tailed deer. Reprod Fertil Dev 9:105–110

24. Rutberg AT, Naugle RE (2008) Population-level effects of immunocontraception in white-tailed deer (*Odocoileus virginianus*). Wildl Res 35:494–501

25. Turner JW, Rutberg AT, Naugle RE, Kaur MA, Flanagan DR, Bertschinger HJ, Liu IKM (2008) Controlled-release components of PZP contraceptive vaccine extend duration of infertility. Wildl Res 35:555–562

26. Deigert FA, Duncan AE, Frank KM, Lyda RO, Kirkpatrick JF (2003) Immunocontraception of captive exotic species. III. Contraception and population management of fallow deer (*Cervus dama*). Zoo Biol 22:261–268

27. Fraker MA, Brown RG, Gaunt GE, Kerr JA, Pohajdak B (2002) Long-lasting, single-dose immunocontraception of feral fallow deer in British Columbia. J Wildl Manag 66:1141–1147

28. Frank KM, Lyda RO, Kirkpatrick JF (2005) Immunocontraception of captive exotic species - IV. Species differences in response to the porcine zona pellucida vaccine, timing of booster inoculations, and procedural failures. Zoo Biol 24:349–358

29. Shideler SE, Stoops MA, Gee NA, Howell JA, Lasley BL (2002) Use of porcine zona pellucida (PZP) vaccine as a contraceptive agent in free-ranging tule elk (*Cervus elaphus nannodes*). In: Kirkpatrick JF, Lasley BL, Allen WR, Doberska C (eds.) Fertility control in wildlife. Cambridge University Press, Cambridge [Reproduction Supplement 60]

30. Kirkpatrick JF, Turner A (2008) Achieving population goals in a long-lived wildlife species (*Equus caballus*) with contraception. Wildl Res 35:513–519

31. Kirkpatrick JF, Turner JW Jr, Liu IK, Fayrer-Hosken R (1996) Applications of pig zona pellucida immunocontraception to wildlife fertility control. J Reprod Fertil Suppl 50:183–189

32. Turner JW Jr, Liu IKM, Kirkpatrick JF (1996) Remotely delivered immunocontraception in free-roaming feral burros (*Equus asinus*). J Reprod Fertil 107:31–35

33. Delsink AK, van Altena JJ, Grobler D, Bertschinger HJ, Kirkpatrick JF, Slotow R (2007) Implementing immunocontraception in free-ranging African elephants at Makalali Conservancy. J South Afr Vet Assoc 78:25–30

34. Fayrer-Hosken RA, Grobler D, Van Altena JJ, Bertschinger HJ, Kirkpatrick JF (2000) Immunocontraception of African elephants. A humane method to control elephant populations without behavioural side effects. Nature 407:149

35. Perdok AA, de Boer WF, Stout TAE (2007) Prospects for managing African elephant population growth by immunocontraception: a review. Pachyderm 42:97–107

36. Lane VM, Liu IKM, Casey K, vanLeeuwen EMG, Flanagan DR, Murata K, Munro C (2007) Inoculation of female American black bears (*Ursus americanus*) with partially purified porcine zona pellucidae limits cub production. Reprod Fertil Dev 19:617–625

37. Miller LA, Bynum K, Zemlicka D (2006) PZP immunocontraception in coyotes: a multi-year study with three vaccine formulations. Proc Vertebr Pest Conf 22:88–95

38. Garrott RA, Cook JG, Bernoco MM, Kirkpatrick JF, Cadwell LL, Cherry S, Tiller B (1998) Antibody response of elk immunized with porcine zona pellucida. J Wildl Dis 34:539–546

39. Fayrer-Hosken RA, Barber MR, Crane M, Collins T, Hodgden R (2002) Differences in immunocontraceptive responses in white-tailed deer (*Odocoileus virginianus*) and goats (*Capra hircus*). In: Kirkpatrick JF, Lasley BL, Allen WR, Doberska C (eds) Fertility control in wildlife. Cambridge University Press, Cambridge [Reproduction Supplement 60]

40. Jewgenow K, Rohleder M, Wegner I (2000) Differences between antigenic determinants of pig and cat zona pellucida proteins. J Reprod Fertil 119:15–23

41. D'Occhio MJ, Fordyce G, Whyte TR, Aspden WJ, Trigg TE (2000) Reproductive response of cattle to GnRH agonists. Anim Reprod Sci 60:433–442

42. Clarke IJ, Fraser HM, McNeilly AS (1979) Active immunization of ewes against luteinizing hormone-releasing hormone neutralisation. Endocrinology 110:1116–1123

43. Esbenshade KL, Britt JH (1985) Active immunization of gilts against gonadotropin-releasing hormone: effects on secretion of gonadotropins, reproductive function, and responses to agonists of gonadotroin-releasing hormone. Biol Reprod 333:569–577

44. Johnson HE, DeAvila DM, Chang CF, Reeves JJ (1988) Active immunization of heifers against luteinizing hormone releasing hormone, human chorionic gonadotropin hormone and bovine luteinizing hormone. J Anim Sci 66:719–726

45. Garza F, Thompson DL, French DD, Wiest JJ, George RLS, Ashley KB, Jones LS, Mitchell PS, McNeill DR (1986) Active immunization of intact mares against gonadotropin-releasing hormone: differential effects on secretion of luteinizing hormone and follicle-stimulating hormone. Biol Reprod 2:347–352

46. Perry KR, Arjo WM, Bynum KS, Miller LA (2006) GnRH single-injection immunocontraception of black-tailed deer. Proc Vertebr Pest Conf 22:72–77

47. Nash PB, James DK, Hui LT, Miller LA (2004) Fertility control of California ground squirrels using GnRH immunocontraception. Proc Vertebr Pest Conf 21:274–278

48. Bradley MP, Geelan A, Leitch V, Goldberg E (1996) Cloning, sequencing, and characterization of LDH-C4 from a fox testis cDNA library. Mol Reprod Dev 44:452–459

49. Strive T, Hardy CM, Reubel GH (2007) Prospects for immunocontraception in the European red fox (*Vulpes vulpes*). Wildl Res 34:523 529

50. Afzalpurkar A, Sacco AG, Yurewicz EC, Gupta SK (1997) Induction of native protein reactive antibodies by immunization with peptides containing linear B-cell epitopes defined by anti-porcine ZP3 beta monoclonal antibodies. J Reprod Immunol 33:113–125

51. Hardy CM, Beaton S, Hinds LA (2008) Immunocontraception in mice using repeated, multiantigen peptides: immunization with purified recombinant antigens. Mol Reprod Dev 75: 126–135

52. Ringleb J, Rohleder M, Jewgenow K (2004) Impact of feline zona pellucida glycoprotein B-derived synthetic peptides on in vitro fertilization of cat oocytes. Reproduction 127:179–186

53. Dubova-Mihailova M, Komori S, Kameda K, Tsuji Y, Koyama K, Isojima S (1994) Identification and characterization of a 27 kDa acrosome protein of human sperm defined by a monoclonal antibody with fertilization-blocking effect. J Reprod Immunol 26:97–110
54. Jackson RJ, Beaton S, Dall DJ (2007) Stoat zona pellucida genes with potential for immuno-contraceptive biocontrol in New Zealand. DOC Res Dev Ser 275:2–21
55. Deakin JE, Belov K, Curach NC, Green P, Cooper DW (2005) High levels of variability in immune response using antigens from two reproductive proteins in brushtail possums. Wildl Res 32:1–6
56. Redwood AJ, Harvey NL, Lloyd M, Lawson MA, Hardy CM, Shellam GR (2007) Viral vec-tored immunocontraception: screening of multiple fertility antigens using murine cytomega-lovirus as a vaccine vector. Vaccine 25:698–708
57. Humphrys S, Lapidge SJ (2008) Delivering and registering species-tailored oral antifertility products: a review. Wildl Res 35:578–585
58. Parkes J, Murphy E (2004) Risk assessment of stoat control methods for New Zealand. Sci Conserv 237:1–38
59. Alexander NJ, Bialy G (1994) Contraceptive vaccine development. Reprod Fertil Dev 6: 273–280
60. Liu IKM, Bernoco M, Feldman M (1989) Contraception in mares heteroimmunized with por-cine zona pellucida. J Reprod Fertil 85:19–29
61. Muller LI, Warren RJ, Evans DL (1997) Theory and practice of immunocontraception in wild mammals. Wildl Soc Bull 25:504–514
62. Killian G, Thain D, Diehl NK, Rhyan J, Miller L (2008) Four-year contraception rates of mares treated with single-injection porcine zona pellucida and GnRH vaccines and intrauter-ine devices. Wildl Res 35:531–539
63. Jewgenow K, Greube A, Naidenko SV, Ringleb J (2004) Immune response of domestic cats (*Felis catus*) to a single injection of feline ZPB derived peptides. Andrologia 36:132–134
64. Ndolo TM, Oguna M, Bambara CS, Dunbar BS, Schwoebel ED (1996) Immunogenicity of zona pellucida vaccines. J Reprod Fertil Suppl 50:151–158
65. Munson L, Moresco A, Calle PP (2005) Adverse effects of contraceptives. In: Asa CS, I.J P (eds.) Wildlife contraception: issue, methods, and application. The John Hopkins University Press, Baltimore
66. Upadhyay SN, Thillai-Koothan P, Bamezai A, Jayaraman S, Talwar GP (1989) Role fo adju-vants in inhibitory influence of immunization with zona pellucida antigen (ZP-3) on ovarian folliculogenesis in bonnet monkeys: a morphological study. Biol Reprod 41:665–673
67. Stohr K, Meslin FX (1997) Zoonoses and fertility control in wildlife–requirements for vac-cines. Reprod Fertil Dev 9:149–155
68. Polkinghorne I, Hamerli D, Cowan P, Duckworth J (2005) Plant-based immunocontraceptive control of wildlife – "potentials, limitations, and possums". Vaccine 23:1847–1850
69. Hardy CM, Hinds LA, Kerr PJ, Lloyd ML, Redwood AJ, Shellam GR, Strive T (2006) Biological control of vertebrate pests using virally vectored immunocontraception. J Reprod Immunol 71:102–111
70. Li H, Piao YS, Zhang ZB, Hardy CM, Hinds LA (2006) Molecular cloning and assessment of the immunocontraceptive potential of the zona pellucida subunit 3 from Brandt's vole (*Microtus brandti*). Reprod Fertil Dev 18:331–338
71. Strive T, Hardy CM, French N, Wright JD, Nagaraja N, Reubel GH (2006) Development of canine herpesvirus based antifertility vaccines for foxes using bacterial artificial chromo-somes. Vaccine 24:980–988
72. Singleton GR, Farroway LN, Chambers LK, Lawson MA, Smith AL, Hinds LA (2002) Ecological basis for fertility control in the house mouse (*Mus domesticus*) using immunocon-traceptive vaccines. Reprod Suppl 60:31–39

73. Strive T, Hardy CM, Wright J, Reubel GH (2007) A virus vector based on Canine Herpesvirus for vaccine applications in canids. Vet Microbiol 119:173–183

74. Arthur AD, Pech RP, Singleton GR (2007) Cross-strain protection reduces effectiveness of virally vectored fertility control: results from individual-based multistrain models. J Appl Ecol 44:1252–1262

75. Hardy CM, Braid AL (2007) Vaccines for immunological control of fertility in animals. Revue Scientifique et Technique Office International des Epizooties 26:461–470

76. Nettles VF (1997) Potential consequences and problems with wildlife contraceptives. Reprod Fertil Dev 9:137–143

77. Hermes R, Hildebrandt TB, Walzer C, Goritz F, Patton ML, Silinski S, Anderson MJ, Reid CE, Wibbelt G, Tomasova K, Schwarzenberger F (2006) The effect of long non-reproductive periods on the genital health in captive female white rhinoceroses (*Ceratotherium simum simum*, C.s. cottoni). Theriogenology 65:1492–1515

78. McShea WJ, Monfort SL, Hakim S, Kirkpatrick J, Liu I, Turner JW Jr, Chassey L, Munson L (1997) The effect of immunocontraception on the behaviour and reproduction of white-tailed deer. J Wildl Manag 61:560–569

79. Kazensky CA, Munson L, Seal US (1998) The effects of melengestrol acetate on the ovaries of captive wild felids. J Zoo Wildl Med 29:1–5

80. Miller LA, Johns BE, Killian GJ (2000) Immunocontraception of white-tailed deer with GnRH vaccine. Am J Reprod Immunol 44:266–274

81. Molenaar GJ, Lugard-Kok C, Meloen RH, Oonk RB, de Koning J, Wensing CJG (1993) Lesions in the hypothalamus after active immunization against GnRH in pigs. J Neuroimmunol 48:1–12

82. Cronin GM, Dunshea FR, Butler KL, McCaughley I, Barnett JL, Hemsworth PH (2003) The effects of immuno- and surgical-castration on the behaviour and consequent growth of group-housed, male finisher pigs. Appl Anim Behav Sci 81:111–126

83. Kiyuma Z, Adams TE, Hess BW, Riley ML, Murdoch WJ, Moss GE (2006) Gonadal function, sexual behaviour, feedlot performance, and arcass traits of ram lambs actively immunized against GnRH. J Anim Sci 78(9):2237–2243

84. Darhower SE, Maher CR (2008) Effects of immunocontraception on behavior in fallow deer (*Dama dama*). Zoo Biol 27:49–61

85. Hernandez S, Locke SL, Cook MW, Harveson LA, Davis DS, Lopez RR, Silvy NJ, Fraker MA (2006) Effects of SpayVac® on urban female white-tailed deer movements. Wildl Soc Bull 34:1430–1434

86. Jolly SE, Scobie S, Cowan PE (1996) Effects of vaccination against gondaotrophin releasing hormone (GnRH) on the social status of brushtailed possum in captivity. New Zealand J Zool 23:325–330

87. Cooper DW, Herbert CA (2001) Genetics, biotechnology and population management of over-abundant mammalian wildlife in Australasia. Reprod Fertil Dev 13:451–458

88. Kirkpatrick JF, Turner A (2007) Immunocontraception and increased longevity in equids. Zoo Biol 26:237–244

89. Ballou JD, Traylor-Holzer K, Turner A, Malo AF, Powell D, Maldonado J, Eggert L (2008) Simulation model for contraceptive management of the Assateague Island feral horse population using individual-based data. Wildl Res 35:502–512

90. Courchamp F, Cornell SJ (2000) Virus-vectored immunocontraception to control feral cats on islands: a mathematical model. J Appl Ecol 37:903–913

91. Saunders G, McIlroy J, Berghout M, Kay B, Gifford E, Perry R, van de Ven R (2002) The effects of induced sterility on the territorial behaviour and survival of foxes. J Appl Ecol 39:56–66

92. Barfield JP, Nieschlag E, Cooper TG (2006) Fertility control in wildlife: humans as a model. Contraception 73:6–22

Experience from Clinical Trials with Fertility Control Vaccines

4.3

G. P. Talwar, Shilpi Purswani, Jagdish Chandra Gupta, and Hemant Kumar Vyas

4.3.1
Introduction and Prologue

Only four vaccines have progressed to the stage of clinical evaluation so far. This stage is reached after successful experimental studies and after conducting preclinical toxicology studies in two species, whereby the safety and reversibility of the vaccine are established. hCG vaccine is intended as a birth control vaccine for use by women, whereas LHRH vaccine is usable in both humans and animals, being given that the structure of this decapeptide is largely conserved in mammals. Furthermore, LHRH is common to both males and females and is thereby a unisex molecule controlling both male and female fertility.

Clinical trials are conducted phase-wise after obtaining the approval of the Drugs Regulatory Authorities and Institutional Ethics Committees. Written, informed consent of the subject opting for clinical trial must also be taken. Phase I trial has the objective of assessing the safety of the vaccine in humans after its safety has been demonstrated in animals during preclinical toxicology studies. The number of subjects enrolled in Phase I trial are between 10 and 20 in one or more centers. The study is intensive and carefully done with not only thorough clinical observations but also with a variety of laboratory investigations. After establishing the safety and reversibility of the procedure, Phase II studies are undertaken to assess the efficacy and extended safety of the candidate vaccine. The number of subjects on which the Phase II trials are conducted varies from 50 to 200. Only one vaccine directed against hCG has so far completed the Phase II efficacy trial in women.

The vaccine(s) against LHRH have been employed not only to control the fertility of animals but also for therapy of hormone-dependent prostatic cancers. LHRH regulates the secretion of FSH and LH from the pituitary which in turn act on gonads to generate sperm and testosterone in males and egg and sex steroid hormones in females. The rationale in employing anti-LHRH vaccine in prostate carcinoma patients is to cut off the androgen support to the prostatic cancer cells. One vaccine against LHRH has undergone Phase I/Phase II trials in prostate carcinoma patients in India and Austria.

G. P. Talwar (✉)
Talwar Research Foundation, E-8 Neb Valley, Neb Sarai, 110068, New Delhi, India
e-mail: gptalwar@gmail.com

W. K. H. Krause and R. K. Naz (eds.), *Immune Infertility*,
DOI: 10.1007/978-3-642-01379-9_4.3, © Springer Verlag Berlin Heidelberg 2009

This chapter reviews the vision of making vaccines against hCG and LHRH and the achievements and limitations of the approaches made.

4.3.2
Counter hCG Vaccine

hCG is made and secreted by early embryo. It is present in the culture medium of the eggs fertilized in vitro [1]. It is critical for implantation; marmoset embryos exposed to antibodies against hCGβ do not implant whereas their incubation with normal immunoglobulins has no such effect [2]. Interception of implantation by circulating anti-hCG antibodies is also deducible in humans. Women carrying antibodies above 50 ng/mL do not become pregnant nor experience lengthening of the leuteal phase [3, 4], whereas anti-hCG antibodies abort early pregnancy with lengthening of the leuteal phase, when these were given postimplantation. The latter action of the anti-hCG antibodies is exercised by block of progesterone synthesized by the corpus luteum and later the cytotrophoblasts under the influence of hCG [5].

It is logical to see that a vaccine against hCG, is an ideal mode of contraception. It does not impair ovulation. Women continue making their normal sex steroids and have no derangement of menstrual regularity and bleeding profiles.

4.3.2.1
Diversity of hCG Vaccines

hCG is a heterodimer, alpha subunit is common to TSH, FSH, and LH, and the beta subunit imparts hormonal identity. hCGβ is a glycosylated peptide of 145 amino acids. It has high homology with hLHβ, but, the carboxy terminal 30–35 amino acids are unique to hCGβ. It is for this reason that Vernon Stevens and WHO Task Force decided to make a vaccine based on the carboxy terminal peptide (CTP) of hCGβ. Our experience with CTPs was not very encouraging. These were very poor immunogens and the antibodies were elicited, only by employing strong adjuvants, which were of low bio-efficacy. Lengthening of the CTP to 45 and 53 terminal amino acids improved immunogenicity [6, 7]. However, the antibodies were still inferior in their affinity and bio-efficacy to those generated by employing the entire hCGβ subunit.

The potential risk of anti-hCG antibodies was the cross-reaction with hLH and may be with other organs expressing hCG determinants. This was not found to be the case. The gonadotrophins and the steroid hormone profiles of women immunized with hCGβ-TT vaccine were similar to their preimmunization profiles as determined by Tapani Luukkainen in Finland, Elsimar Coutinho in Brazil, Elof Johansson in Sweden and Horacio Croxatto in Chile [8]. Even by hyperimmunizing the monkeys with ovine LH (oLH), generating antibodies cross-reactive with the monkey LH had no discernable side effects or immunopathology [9, 10]. A possible explanation is that hLH surge taking place once in a month has enough surplus beyond the amount required to induce ovulation. The antibodies generated by hCGβ and the heterospecies dimer (HSD) consisting of hCGβ associated with alpha subunit of ovine LH, linked to carriers, generate primarily conformation reading antibodies with Ka of 10^{10} M^{-1} or more. Over 80% of antibodies generated by HSD vaccine are directed to an epitope competed by a monoclonal antibody of high specificity with less than 5% cross-reaction with hLH [11]. On the other hand, much to the surprise of all, the antibodies generated by CTP vaccine were cross-reactive with pancreatic cells whereas anti-hCGβ-TT did not have such cross-reaction [12]. The CTP-based vaccine of Stevens promoted by WHO Task Force did undergo Phase I trials in Australia [13]. It was however abandoned in view of the unacceptable side effects it provoked in the first seven women immunized with it in Sweden.

4.3.2.2
Necessity of Employing a Carrier

Although nonpregnant women do not make hCG in measurable amount, the fact that the fetus (male or female) is exposed to high amounts of hCG during pregnancy renders them immunologically tolerant to hCG. Hence, the need of a carrier to mobilize T helper cells. We employed tetanus toxoid (TT) in the very first vaccine conceived for hCG [14]. The reasons were (1) it was an approved low cost vaccine readily available in unlimited quantities and (2) it would prevent in addition, deaths due to tetanus which occurred in large numbers in developing countries following delivery taking place at homes in aseptic conditions. hCGβ-TT vaccine generated both anti-hCG and antitetanus antibodies. The response was reversible. hCG alone did not act as a booster, ruling out the fear of auto-immunization. Repeated immunization with the vaccine containing TT as carrier however led to carrier induced suppression of response to hCGβ. This could be overcome by employing alternate carriers such as diphtheria toxoid (DT) or cholera toxin B subunit (CTB) [15].

4.3.2.3
Phase II Efficacy Trials on HSD-hCG Vaccine

This was the first ever trial conducted with any birth control vaccine [3]. Hundred and eighty women of proven fertility with two living children and one or more medical termination of early pregnancy (MTP) were enrolled in the trial. While all women generated antibodies to hCG, 119 (80%) had titers above 50 ng/mL bioneutralization capacity. But, only 60% women maintained antibody titers above 50 ng/mL threshold for 3 months or longer. All women continued to have regular menstrual cycles and had luteal progesterone indicative of normal ovulation. No pregnancy took place in women at and above 50 ng/mL titers. The antibody titers declined with time but booster injections raised the levels. Eight women completed more than 30 cycles by voluntary intake of boosters without becoming pregnant. Nine completed 24–29 cycles, 12 completed 18–23 cycles, 15 completed 12–17 cycles, and 21 subjects completed 6–11 cycles. Women became readily pregnant in the absence of boosters on antibodies declining to 35 ng/mL or lower levels. The efficacy of the vaccine to prevent pregnancy was very high with only one pregnancy recorded in 1,224 cycles in women having antibody titers above 50 ng/mL [3, 4]. The vaccine was well tolerated. Infact, when we were asked to close the trial for analysis of data, many women wanted to continue and offered to get the booster at their own expense. These women were hyperfertile and had more than one MTP. On interrogation, it was brought home to us that other contraceptives did not suit them. IUD caused extra bleeding and pelvic pain, steroids were unacceptable due to either weight gain or irregularity of menstrual profile and spotting and they were not ready to undergo tubectomy in view of the uncertainty of survival of their children. Thus a contraceptive vaccine against hCG would be their choice, as it did not impair their ovulation nor caused derangement of menstrual regularity and hormonal profiles, while keeping them protected from becoming pregnant in spite of frequent sexual intercourses.

4.3.2.4
What Was the Shortcoming of the HSD Vaccine?

The HSD vaccine was given with alum as adjuvant. The dose and the adjuvant, at which it was given, generated above protective threshold of antibody in 60–80% of recipients. This order of efficacy may be acceptable for vaccines against infectious diseases but as other contraceptives protecting up to 98–99% of recipients are available, this order of efficacy is not sufficient to make it eligible as an option in the family planning basket.

4.3.2.5
Revival of the hCG Vaccine

Two years back research on hCG vaccine was revived under an Indo-US program. While the previous HSD vaccine had hormonal subunits purified from natural sources (hence costly), linked chemically to carrier (DT/TT). The efficiency of conjugation, besides the uncertainties of the numbers and the position at which carrier was conjugated lowered the yield and nonhomogeneity of the product. To overcome these limitations, we decided to make a fully recombinant vaccine. hCGβ was cloned and expressed in Pichia pastoris to obtain a glycosylated hormonal subunit linked in a defined position to LTB. The yield is good and the procedure amenable to Industrial production. This recombinant conjugate has been tested for immunogenicity in Balb/C mice and every mouse immunized so far with this vaccine given on alum with SPLPS (sodium pthylylated derivative of lipopolysaccharide of *Salmonella typhi*) in the first injection has generated above 50 ng/mL antibody titers. We are extending the studies to five inbred strains of mice of different genetic background, encompassing haplotypes $H-2^d$, $H-2^k$, $H-2^b$, $H-2^s$, and $H-2^q$, in order to ascertain the genetic restriction, if any, of antibody response to this vaccine.

An alternate strategy to be adopted along with our US collaborator is to mount the recombinant hCGβ on VLPs of HPV 16. It may be recalled that this laboratory has been responsible in the recent past to generate an anti-HPV vaccine based on VLPs of HPV 16/18 which produce protective antibodies in >99% of women.

4.3.2.6
Additional Benefits of the hCG Vaccine

Immunization against hCG has no doubt applications for preventing pregnancy. A number of recent papers report ectopic expression of hCG or subunits in a variety of cancers: lung [16], bladder [17], colon [18], gastric [19], pancreatic [20], breast [21], cervical [22], oral [23], head and neck [24], vulva/vaginal [25, 26], prostate [27], and renal cancers [28]. It has been further observed that patients with cancers expressing hCGβ ectopically have poor prognosis and adverse survival [17, 28]. It follows that a vaccine against hCG or recombinant antibodies against hCG may have additional applications for therapy of such cancers. We engineered a recombinant chimeric antibody of high affinity and specificity [29, 30]. This antibody, cPiPP, bound to T-lymphoblastic leukemia MOLT-4 cells expressing hCG whereas it had no binding with Peripheral Blood Lymphocytes (PBLs) of normal healthy subjects [31]. Vyas et al. [43] observed that this antibody linked to curcumin, a safe anticancerous compound, killed 100% of MOLT-4 cells as well as histocytic lymphomas U937 cells, both expressing ectopically hCG. On the other hand, the immuno-conjugate had no deleterious effect on PBLs of healthy subjects.

4.3.3
LHRH Vaccine

Besides hCG, the only other vaccine undergoing clinical trial was directed against LHRH. It was a semi-synthetic vaccine in which glycine at position 6 was replaced by D-lysine which created a functional NH_2 group for linking the carrier either TT or DT [32]. The vaccine was highly immunogenic and induced bio-effective response in rodents [33] and in monkeys [34] with alum alone as adjuvant. Immunization caused cessation of spermatogenesis in rodents along with testosterone declining to castration levels [35]. Spermatogenesis and fertility was regained on decline of antibodies. Immunization against LHRH could also block fertility of female rodents in a reversible manner [36].

In male rats and in monkeys, a drastic atrophy of prostate was observed. The vaccine inhibited the growth of Dunning R3327-PAP tumor implanted in rats by suppression of cell division [37]. Preclinical toxicology studies in India and Austria, indicated the safety of semi-synthetic vaccine LHRH vaccine. With permission of the Drugs Regulatory Authority in India and Austria and with the approval of the Institutional Ethics Committees, Phase I/II clinical trials were conducted with this vaccine in 28 patients of carcinoma of prostate, 12 patients each at the All India Institute of Medical Sciences (AIIMS) New Delhi, and Postgraduate Institute of Medical Education and Research (PGIMER) Chandigarh, and four patients at the Urology Department of Salzburg General Hospital. The vaccine was well tolerated in all subjects. No ill effect of immunization was seen. Subjects developing more than 200 pg/mL of antibodies, experienced a decline of testosterone to castration levels with marked reduction of PSA there by reduction of prostatic tissue mass (Fig. 4.3.1). Patients receiving 400 µg LHRH equivalent dose showed better clinical improvement than those receiving 200 µg.

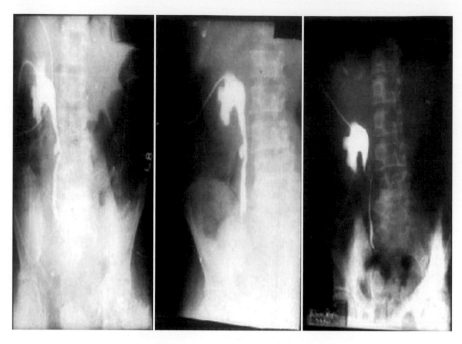

Fig. 4.3.1 Serial Nephrostograms showing the noticeable reduction of prostatic tissue mass at various stages of immunization with anti-LHRH vaccine

Table 4.3.1 Observations of clinical trials conducted with anti-CHRH vaccine

Effect of immunization	Dose level of the vaccine	
	200 µg (n>6)	400 µg (n>6)
Clinically stable/improvement in symptoms	4	5
Reduction in prostatic size/hardness	1	3
Reduction in acid phosphatases	1	4

Table 4.3.1 is a summary of observations on 12 patients of carcinoma of prostate on whom trial was conducted by Prof. S. Wadhwa, at AIIMS.

Delivery of multiple doses of the vaccine at a single contact point was achieved by encapsulating these in biodegradable microspheres, shortening also the lag period for bioeffective response [38].

4.3.3.1
Recombinant LHRH Vaccine

A mutimer recombinant vaccine has been developed against LHRH in which five units of LHRH are interspersed with four different T non-B peptides from *Plasmodium falciparum* circumsporozoite protein, tetanus toxoid, Respiratory Synctial virus, and Measles virus. Knowledge-based computer graph of this multimer shows LHRH moieties are exposed to hydrophilic environment, in which the T non-B peptides are embedded. The gene encoding the multimer vaccine was constructed, and the recombinant protein expressed and purified from *E. coli* [39, 40]. This multimer vaccine caused nonsurgical castration lowering of testosterone and drastic atrophy of the rat prostate [41]. Lowell Miller and coworkers at the National Wildlife Research Center, USA, tested the vaccine in pigs for control of fertility. Given along with Adjuvac, an oily adjuvant approved by USFDA, it sterilized 100% of the pigs tested [42].

Acknowledgment Our current work on the hCG vaccine is supported by Grant from the Dept. of Biotechnology, Govt. of India.

References

1. Fishel SB, Edwards RG, Evans CJ (1984) Human chorionic gonadotropin secreted by preimplantation embryos cultured in vitro. Science 223(4638):816–818
2. Hearn JP, Gidley-Baird AA, Hodges JK (1988) Embryonic signals during the preimplantation period in primates. J Reprod Fertil Suppl 36:49–58
3. Talwar GP, Singh O, Pal R et al (1994) A vaccine that prevents pregnancy in women. Proc Natl Acad Sci U S A 91:8532–8536
4. Talwar GP, Singh O, Gupta SK et al (1997) The HSD-hCG vaccine prevents pregnancy in women, fesability studies of reversibily safe contraception vaccine. Am J Reprod Immunol 37:153–160
5. Dhar R, Karmakar S, Sriraman R et al (2004) Efficacy of a recombinant chimeric anti-hCG antibody to prevent human cytotrophoblasts fusion and block progesterone synthesis. Am J Reprod Immunol 51:358–363
6. Ramakrishnan S, Das C, Dubey SK (1979) Immunogenecity of three C-terminal synthetic peptides of the beta subunit of human chorionic gonadotropin and properties of the antibodies raised against 45-aminoacid C-terminal peptide. J Reprod Immunol 1:249–261
7. Sahal D, Ramakrishnan S, Iyer KSN et al (1982) Immunobiological properties of a carboxy-terminal 53-amino acid peptide of the beta subunit of human chorionic gonadotropin. J Reprod Immunol 4:145–146
8. Nash H, Talwar GP, Segal S et al (1980) Observation on the antigenecity and clinical effects of a candidate antipregnancy vaccine: B-subunit of human chorionic gonadotropin linked to tetanus toxoid. Fertil Steril 34:328–335
9. Thau RB, Witkin SS, Bond MG et al (1983) Effects of long term immunization against the beta-subunit of ovine luteinizing hormone on circulating immune complex formation and on arterial changes in rhesus monkeys. Am J Reprod Immunol 3:83–88
10. Thau RB, Bond MG, Witkins SS (1986) Lack of toxicological effects following seven years of active immunization of rhesus monkeys with the beta subunit of ovine leutinizing hormone. In: Talwar GP (ed) Immunological approaches to contraception and promotion of fertility. Plenum, New York, pp 25–33
11. Deshmukh US, Talwar GP, Gupta SK (1994) Antibody response against three epitopic domains on human chorionic gonadotropins (hCG) in women and rodents immunized with a hCGβ-based immunocontraceptive vaccine. J Clin Immunol 14:162–168

12. Rose NR, Burek CL, Smith JP (1988) Safety evaluation of hCG vaccine in primates: auto-antibodies production. In: Talwar GP (ed) Contraception research for today and nineties. Springer, New York, pp 231–239

13. Jones WR, Bradley J, Judd SJ et al (1988) Phase I clinical trial of a World Health Organization birth control vaccine. Lancet 1:1295–1298

14. Talwar GP, Sharma NC, Dubey SK et al (1976) Isoimmunisation against human chorionic gonadotropin with conjugates of processed beta subunit of the hormone and tetanus toxoid. Proc Natl Acad Sci U S A 73:218–222

15. Gaur A, Arunan K, Singh O, Talwar GP (1990) Bypass by an alternate carrier of acquired unresponsiveness to hCG upon repeated immunization with tetanus conjugated vaccine. Int Immunol 2:151–155

16. Szturmowicz M, Slodkowska J, Zych J et al (1999) Frequency and clinical significance of beta-subunit human chorionic gonadotropin expression in non- small cell lung cancer patients. Tumour Biol 20:99–104

17. Iles RK, Persad R, Trivedi M (1996) Urinary concentration of human chorionic gonadotropin and its fragments as a prognostic marker in bladder cancer. Br J Urol 77:61–69

18. Lundin M, Nordling S, Carpelan-Holmstrom M (2000) A comparison of serum and tissue hCG beta as prognostic markers in colorectal cancer. Anticancer Res 20:4949–4951

19. Rau B, Below C, Liebrich W (1995) Significance of serum hCGβ as a tumor marker for stomach carcinoma. Langenbecks Arch Chir 380:359–364

20. Alfthan H, Haglund C, Roberts P et al (1992) Elevation of free beta subunit of human chorionic gonadotropin and core beta fragment of human chorionic gonadotropin in the serum and urine of patients with malignant pancreatic and biliary diseases. Cancer Res 52:4628–4633

21. Bièche I, Lazar V, Noguès C et al (1998) Prognostic value of chorionic gonadotropin beta gene transcripts in human breast carcinoma. Clin Cancer Res 4:671–676

22. Crawford RA, Iles RK, Carter PG et al (1998) The prognostic significance of beta human chorionic gonadotropin and its metabolites in women with cervical carcinoma. J Clin Pathol 51:685–688

23. Bhalang K, Kafrawy AH, Miles DA (1999) Immunohistochemical study of the expression of human chorionic gonadotropin-beta in oral squamous cell carcinoma. Cancer 85:757–762

24. Scholl PD, Jurco S, Austin JR (1997) Ectopic production of beta-HCG by a maxillary squamous cell carcinoma. Head Neck 19:701–705

25. Carter PG, Iles RK, Neven P et al (1995) Measurement of urinary beta core fragment of human chorionic gonadotropin in women with vulvovaginal malignancy and its prognostic significance. Br J Cancer 71:350–353

26. De Bruijn HW, Ten Hoor KA, Krans M et al (1997) Rising serum values of beta-subunit human chorionic gonadotropin (hCG) in patients with progressive vulvar carcinomas. Br J Cancer 75:1217–1218

27. Sheaff MT, Martin JE, Badenoch DF et al (1996) Beta hCG as a prognostic marker in adeno-carcinoma of the prostate. J Clin Pathol 49:693–694

28. Hotakainen K, Ljungberg B, Paju A (2002) The free beta-subunit of human chorionic gonadotropin as a prognostic factor in renal cell carcinoma. Br J Cancer 86:185–189

29. Kathuria S, Nath R, Pal R et al (2002) Functional recombinant antibodies against hCG expressed in plants. Curr Sci 82:1452–1457

30. Kathuria S, Sriraman R, Nath R et al (2002) Efficacy of plant produced recombinant antibodies against hCG. Hum Reprod 17:2054–2061

31. Kabeer RS, Pal R, Talwar GP (2005) Human acute lymphoblastic leukemia cells make human pregnancy hormone hCG and expose it on the membrane: a case for using recombinant antibody against hCG for selective delivery of drugs and/or radiations. Curr Sci 89:1571–1576

32. Talwar GP, Chaudhuri MK, Jayshankar R (1992) Inventors. Antigenic derivative of GnRH. UK Patent, 2228262

33. Jayashankar R, Chaudhari M, Singh OM (1989) Semisynthetic anti-LHRH vaccine causing atrophy of the prostate. Prostate 14:3–11
34. Giri DK, Jayaraman S, Neelaram GS (1991) Prostatic hypoplasia in Bonnet monkeys following active immunization with semi-synthetic anti-LHRH vaccine. Exp Mol Pathol 54:255–264
35. Rovan E, Fiebiger E, Kalla NR et al (1992) Effect of active immunization to luteinizing-hormone-releasing hormone on the fertility and histoarchitecture of the reproductive organs of male rat. Urol Res 20:323–334
36. Shastri N, Manhar SK, Talwar GP (1981) Important role of the carrier in the induction of antibody response without Freund's complete adjuvant against a "self" peptide hormone LHRH. Am J Reprod Immunol 1:262–265
37. Fuerst J, Fiebiger E, Jungwirth A (1997) Effect of active immunization against luteinizing hormone-releasing hormone on the androgen-sensitive Dunning R3327-PAP and androgen independent Dunning R3327-AT2.1 prostate cancer sublines. Prostate 32:77–84
38. Diwan M, Dawar H, Talwar GP (1998) Induction of early and bioeffective antibody response in rodents with the anti LHRH vaccine given as a single dose in biodegradable microspheres along with alum. Prostate 35:279–284
39. Gupta JC, Raina K, Talwar GP (2004) Engineering, cloning and expression of genes encoding the multimeric luteinising- hormone-releasing-hormone linked to T-cell determinants in *Escherichia coli*. Protein Expr Purif 37:1–7
40. Raina K, Panda AK, Ali MM (2004) Purification, refolding, and characterization of recombinant LHRH-T multimer. Protein Expr Purif 37:8–17
41. Talwar GP, Raina K, Gupta JC et al (2004) A recombinant luteinising-hormone-releasing-hormone immunogen bioeffective in causing prostatic atrophy. Vaccine 22:3713–3721
42. Miller LA, Talwar GP, Killlian GJ (2006) Contraceptive effect of a recombinant GnRH vaccine in adult female pigs. Proc Vertebr Pest Conf 22:106–109
43. Vyas HK, Pal R, Vishwakarma R et al (2009) Selective killing of leukemia and lymphoma cells expressing ectopically hCGβ by a conjugate of curcumin with an antibody against hCGβ subunit. Oncology 76:101–111

Index